Advances in
Drug Therapy
of Gastrointestinal Ulceration

Advances in
Drug Therapy
of Gastrointestinal Ulceration

Edited by

A. Garner
Bioscience Department, ICI Pharmaceuticals, Macclesfield, UK

and

B. J. R. Whittle
Department of Pharmacology, Wellcome Research Laboratories, Beckenham, UK

A Wiley–Interscience Publication

JOHN WILEY & SONS

Chichester · New York · Brisbane · Toronto · Singapore

Distributed in the United States of America, Canada and Japan by Alan R. Liss Inc., 41 East 11th Street, New York, NY 10003, USA.

Library of Congress Cataloging-in-Publication Data

Advances in drug therapy of gastrointestinal ulceration/edited by A. Garner
and B. J. R. Whittle.
    p.   cm.
    Based on proceedings of the 38th Annual Biological Council
Symposium on Drug Action held at the Royal Institution in London on
Apr. 11–12, 1988.
    'A Wiley–Interscience publication.'
    Includes bibliographies and index.
    ISBN 0 471 92051 7
    1. Peptic ulcer—Chemotherapy—Congresses.   2. Antiulcer drugs—
Congresses.   I. Garner, A. (Andrew)   II. Whittle, B. J. R.
(Brendan J. R.)   III. Biological Council Symposium on Drug Action
(38th: 1988: Royal Institution, London)
    [DNLM: 1. Anti-Ulcer—therapeutic use—congresses.   2. Peptic
Ulcer—drug Agents therapy—congresses. WI 350 A2437 1988]
RC821.A36 1989
616.3'43061—dc19
DNLM/DLC
for Library of Congress   89-5370
                                           CIP

British Library Cataloguing in Publication Data

Advances in drug therapy of gastrointestinal ulceration.
   1. Man. Gastrointestinal tract. Peptic
ulcers. Drug therapy
   I. Garner, A. II. Whittle, B. J. R.
   616.3'43061

ISBN 0 471 92051 7

Phototypeset by Dobbie Typesetting Limited, Plymouth, Devon
Printed by The Bath Press, Bath, Avon

The Biological Council and its Coordinating Committee for Symposia on Drug Action are grateful for the financial contributions from the pharmaceutical companies listed below who supported this 1988 Symposium. Without their help it would be impossible to hold these annual meetings.

Abbott Laboratories Ltd
Amersham International PLC
Beecham Pharmaceuticals
Byk Gulden Pharmazeutika
Chugai Pharmaceutical Co. Ltd
Glaxo Group Research Ltd
ICI Pharmaceuticals
Janssen Pharmaceuticals Ltd
Kotobuki Seiyaku Co. Ltd
Eli Lilly & Co. Ltd
Miles Laboratories Ltd
Ortho-Cilag Pharmaceutical Ltd
Pfizer Ltd
Reckitt & Colman
Rorer Pharmaceuticals Ltd
Searle Research
Smith Kline & French Laboratories Ltd
Sumitomo Pharmaceuticals Co. Ltd
The Wellcome Research Laboratories
Wyeth Laboratories

Contents

List of Contributors

*A. ALLEN *Department of Physiological Sciences, Medical School, The University, Newcastle upon Tyne NE2 4HH, UK*

P. BAUERFEIND *Division of Gastroenterology, Department of Internal Medicine, CHUV, 1011 Lausanne, Switzerland*

W. BEIL *Abt. Allgemeine Pharmakologie, Medizinische Hochschule Hannover, D-3000 Hannover 61, FRG*

*A. L. BLUM *Division of Gastroenterology, Department of Internal Medicine, CHUV, 1011 Lausanne, Switzerland*

T. BRZOZOWSKI *Institute of Physiology, Academy of Medicine, 31-531 Krakow, Poland*

A. DEMBINSKI *Institute of Physiology, Academy of Medicine, 31-531 Krakow, Poland*

*G. J. DOCKRAY *MRC Secretory Control Research Group, Department of Physiology, University of Liverpool, Liverpool L69 3BX, UK*

P. DUROUX *Division of Gastroenterology, Department of Internal Medicine, CHUV, 1011 Lausanne, Switzerland*

J. V. ESPLUGUES *Department of Pharmacology, Wellcome Research Laboratories, Beckenham, Kent BR3 3BS, UK*

*G. FLEMSTRÖM *Department of Physiology and Medical Biophysics, Uppsala University, S-751 23 Uppsala, Sweden*

*J. G. FORTE *Department of Physiology–Anatomy, University of California, Berkeley, California 94707, USA*

*A. GARNER *Bioscience Department, ICI Pharmaceuticals, Alderley Park, Macclesfield, Cheshire SK10 4TG, UK*

R. A. GOODLAD *Department of Histopathology, Royal Postgraduate Medical School, Hammersmith Hospital, London W12 0HS, UK*

*Symposium speakers

S.-O. GRANSTAM *Department of Physiology and Medical Biophysics, Uppsala University, S-751 23 Uppsala, Sweden*

*F. HALTER *Gastrointestinal Unit, University Hospital, Inselspital, Bern, Switzerland*

D. K. HANZEL *Department of Physiology–Anatomy, University of California, Berkeley, California 94707, USA*

*C. J. HAWKEY *Department of Therapeutics, University Hospital, Nottingham NG7 2UH, UK*

A. C. HUNTER *Department of Physiological Sciences, Medical School, The University, Newcastle upon Tyne NE2 4HH, UK*

*S. J. KONTUREK *Institute of Physiology, Academy of Medicine, 31-531 Krakow, Poland*

S. K. LAM *Division of Gastroenterology, Department of Medicine, University of Hong Kong, Queen Mary Hospital, Hong Kong*

*M. J. S. LANGMAN *Department of Medicine, Queen Elizabeth Hospital, Birmingham B15 2TH, UK*

A. J. LEONARD *Department of Physiological Sciences, Medical School, The University, Newcastle upon Tyne NE2 4HH, UK*

*R. F. MCCLOY *University Department of Surgery, Manchester Royal Infirmary, Manchester M13 9WL, UK*

*J. J. MISIEWICZ *Department of Gastroenterology and Nutrition, Central Middlesex Hospital, London NW10 7NS, UK*

*M. E. PARSONS *Pharmacology Department, Smith Kline & French Research Ltd, The Frythe, Welwyn, Hertfordshire AL6 9AR, UK*

J. P. PEARSON *Department of Physiological Sciences, Medical School, The University, Newcastle upon Tyne NE2 4HH, UK*

*B. M. PESKAR *Department of Experimental Clinical Medicine, Ruhr-University of Bochum, D-4630 Bochum, FRG*

*R. SCHIESSEL *1st Clinic of Surgery, University Hospital, A-1090 Vienna, Austria*

L. A. SELLERS *Department of Physiological Sciences, Medical School, The University, Newcastle upon Tyne NE2 4HH, UK*

*K.-Fr. SEWING   *Abt. Allgemeine Pharmakologie, Medizinische Hochschule Hannover, D-3000 Hannover 61, FRG*

*W. SILEN   *Department of Surgery, Harvard Medical School, Beth Israel Hospital, Boston, Massachusetts 02215, USA*

*S. SZABO   *Department of Pathology, Brigham & Women's Hospital, Harvard Medical School, Boston, Massachusetts 02115, USA*

T. URUSHIDANI   *Department of Physiology–Anatomy, University of California, Berkeley, California 94707, USA*

Z. WARZECHA   *Institute of Physiology, Academy of Medicine, 31-531 Krakow, Poland*

*B. J. R. WHITTLE   *Department of Pharmacology, Wellcome Research Laboratories, Beckenham, Kent BR3 3BS, UK*

*N. A. WRIGHT   *Department of Histopathology, Royal Postgraduate Medical School, Hammersmith Hospital, London W12 0HS, UK*

J. YAMAZAKI   *Hitachi Chemical Company, Ibraki, Japan*

Series Preface

The Biological Council Symposium on Drug Action is an annual event which is held in London every Spring. International experts are assembled to give presentations centred on a topic chosen by the Coordinating Committee for Symposia on Drug Action. The topic is selected after consideration of a number of criteria, in particular that recent advancement of knowledge has occurred in the field and that it should appeal to clinical and basic biological scientists alike. A major purpose of the Symposium is to provide information for the non-expert as well as the expert. Postgraduate students are encouraged to attend by the waiving of the registration fee. This year witnessed the 38th Symposium, the topic of which covered an extremely important branch of pharmacology. Peptic ulceration is a very common ailment and drugs used in its treatment are currently the most widely prescribed. Nevertheless, there is still room for improvement; hence the title of the meeting. All of the presentations given at the Symposium were of high standard and provided an insight into the future directions of research in this area. I firmly believe that the chapters resulting from these presentations have captured the enthusiasm which was so evident at the Symposium.

Scientific meetings require considerable financial support and the Biological Council Symposia are no different in this respect. Since we endeavour to keep the registration fee as low as possible substantial support is required. The Biological Council is therefore extremely grateful for the support given by the drug industry without which a much larger registration fee would be needed. It is hoped that this wide support attracted by the Symposia may long continue.

Each year the Coordinating Committee chooses not only the topic but also the main organizer. This year we were fortunate to have two organizers, Dr Andrew Garner and Dr Brendan Whittle, who are very much involved in gastrointestinal research and who shared the responsibilities for the symposia. The Biological Council is very grateful to both of them for all their hard work in making the Symposium such a success and for editing this comprehensive volume of the proceedings. Finally, on behalf of the Biological Council, may I thank all of the contributors for their active participation.

Norman G. Bowery

Preface

Treatment of gastric and duodenal ulcer disease has been revolutionized over the last decade following introduction of specific inhibitors of acid secretion. Today, the histamine H_2 antagonists cimetidine and ranitidine provide an effective and convenient means of healing the majority of peptic ulcers with a minimum of side-effects. Recently, more potent antisecretory agents with a longer duration of action have been developed for clinical evaluation. These compounds, which include unsurmountable H_2 blockers and inhibitors of the parietal cell hydrogen pump such as omeprazole, have the ability to induce achlorhydria, which is associated with an increase in the rate of ulcer healing. However, this apparent therapeutic advantage is not without potential risk since the compounds have induced gastric carcinoid tumours during long-term toxicity testing in animals.

Discovery of specific antisecretory agents has provided much of the impetus for studies of parietal cell function. Similarly, drugs which heal ulcers without inhibiting acid secretion have stimulated research on mechanisms of mucosal protection. Although prostaglandins appear to display remarkable anti-ulcer activity in laboratory experiments by a mechanism independent of acid inhibition, clinical performance of current analogues has been disappointing due to a relatively high incidence of side-effects combined with the finding that ulcer healing in patients seems to be a consequence of antisecretory activity alone. Nevertheless, peptic ulcer healing can undoubtedly be achieved without inhibiting acid output as evidenced by the actions of sucralfate and colloidal bismuth preparations, which do not affect acidity, and even antacids, which seem to act by processes in addition to neutralization of luminal acid.

The first half of this volume concentrates primarily on peptic ulcer disease and existing therapy. It provides very up-to-date reviews of the pharmacological properties and clinical performance of current anti-ulcer drugs together with some speculations for future developments based on established mechanisms of action. The second half of the book concentrates on current basic research on gastrointestinal ulceration and protection in order to highlight new targets which may be exploited in the search for alternative anti-ulcer drugs. Considerable progress has been made over recent years in defining the mechanisms which enable the stomach and duodenum to resist autodigestion by luminal acid and pepsin and to recover rapidly from superficial damage induced by exogenous chemical irritants. These processes are reviewed in a series of chapters dealing with acid disposal mechanisms, luminal aggressive factors, endogenous mediators including eicosanoids and related lipids, peptides and growth factors. The potential which each of these topics offers for the discovery of novel drugs to combat gastrointestinal ulceration is also assessed.

Currently available anti-ulcer drugs are clearly very effective in terms of facilitating the healing of symptomatic ulcers. However, none of the agents available at present substantially influences ulcer recurrence unless administered continuously. The challenge for the future is to discover drugs that cure peptic ulcer disease. New drugs may be developed to prevent ulcer formation or enhance the quality of repair. The proposal that colloidal bismuth preparations reduce initial relapse rate via an antibacterial action against the organism *Campylobacter pylori* offers the possibility of designing a treatment which prevents formation of a chronic ulcer. Equally, as knowledge advances of the regulation of mucosal growth and repair, so the possibility emerges of novel drugs which act to improve wound healing throughout the gastrointestinal tract. Indeed, it could be argued that ulcerative conditions of the lower gut provide a more important target in terms of clinical need than does peptic ulceration.

This volume is based on proceedings of the 38th Annual Biological Council Symposium on Drug Action held at the Royal Institution in London on 11–12 April 1988. The conference was addressed by 20 international experts on gastrointestinal ulcer disease ranging from basic scientists to clinical gastroenterologists. Scientific sessions were presided over by four distinguished chairmen (Dr J. H. Baron, Professor R. H. Dowling, Professor W. Silen and Dr K. G. Wormsley) and attended by over 400 delegates from around the world. We thank all these participants. Our particular thanks go to Professor Norman Bowery, Secretary of the Biological Council Symposium Committee, and Yvonne Haseldine, administrative secretary of the Biological Council, who shouldered much of the organizational responsibility, and to all the various sponsors (listed separately) for their generous financial support of the meeting.

Andrew Garner
Brendan J. R. Whittle

Advances in Drug Therapy of Gastrointestinal Ulceration
Edited by A. Garner and B. J. R. Whittle
©1989 John Wiley & Sons Ltd

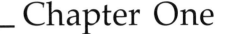

Chapter One

Aetiology of Peptic Ulcer

J. J. Misiewicz
Department of Gastroenterology and Nutrition,
Central Middlesex Hospital, London NW10 7NS, UK

EPIDEMIOLOGY

Gastric ulceration (GU) and duodenal ulceration (DU) are major diseases in many areas of the world. Duodenal ulceration is widely prevalent in the West, and has a varying prevalence in emergent countries. Various factors have combined to make accurate epidemiological studies difficult. Early surveys did not differentiate between GU and DU, as it was not appreciated that these are separate clinical entities with different attributes, outcomes and risks. Peptic ulcers behave differently in young adults than in the elderly and there are also sex-linked differences, so that data have to be corrected for these factors. Most importantly, ulcer disease can only be diagnosed by procedures that are either invasive (fibreoptic endoscopy) or relatively costly (contrast radiology), or both. This makes surveys of larger populations impossible and the technology is often not available in less wealthy countries, which leads to different diagnostic rates. Comparisons between different areas may thus be difficult or impossible.

AUTOPSY SURVEYS

Data from post mortem examinations indicate that more than 20% of males and approximately 10% of females have, or have had, DU or GU (Levi and de la Fuente, 1963; Watkinson, 1960; Table 1.1). Necropsy evidence, however, is flawed on several counts. The frequency at which post mortem examinations are performed varies in different centres and has generally been declining. The sample of population thus surveyed is necessarily selected, and the selection criteria vary with time and with the institution in question. Some ulcers may heal

Table 1.1 Percentage prevalence of gastric and duodenal ulcer at selected ages in Leeds, England and Rotterdam, the Netherlands

Age	Leeds		Rotterdam	
Gastric ulcer				
20–29	2.7	2.0	0.7	0.4
40–49	7.0	3.2	9.8	1.4
60–69	4.1	6.0	9.3	6.4
Duodenal ulcer				
20–29	11.0	3.5	4.9	1.2
40–49	16.8	8.0	10.4	5.7
60–69	12.0	8.0	10.1	4.6

without leaving an easily discernible scar, and others may be missed, depending on the diligence and the interest of the pathologist.

MORTALITY RATES

Mortality rates attributed to GU and DU give information relating to lethal complications of peptic ulcer but these are not a constant fraction of the reservoir of disease. Data obtained in this way are confounded by variations in methods of coding for the cause of death and by variable standards of medical practice. They are strongly related to age (Coggon, Lambert and Longman, 1981) (Figure 1.1) and may reflect prescription of agents, such as non-steroidal anti-inflammatory drugs (NSAIDS), which are associated with complications of ulcer in the elderly (Collier and Pain, 1985; Walt *et al.*, 1986).

CHANGING PATTERNS OF ULCER DISEASE

Environmental factors clearly affect the prevalence of DU and GU, as shown by the changes which occur with time and with geographical location. Identification of environmental influences and the assignment of relative weighting to variables such as race, bodily habits, diet, smoking or consumption of drugs is uncertain, because of difficulties attendant on the collection of reliable data and the impossibility of producing controlled or prospective surveys. Historical surveys are obviously made difficult by changing diagnostic methods; first the introduction of contrast radiology and, more recently, of fibreoptic endoscopy.

TEMPORAL CHANGES

In the second half of the nineteenth century gastric ulcer was the lesion most often described, especially in young women, the diagnosis being established in

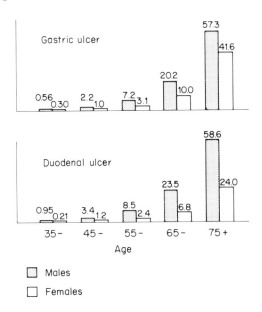

Figure 1.1 Age-specific death rates from peptic ulcer in England and Wales as rates per 100 000/year in 1973–77. (Reproduced from Coggon, Lambert and Langman (1981), by permission of Professor M. J. S. Langman)

those dying from haemorrhage or perforation. Despite the evident inaccuracy of diagnostic techniques at that time, it is remarkable that DU was rarely encountered under these circumstances. A rapid and remarkable increase in the incidence of DU seems to have occurred at the beginning of the present century in Europe and North America. Frequency of GU is gradually declining with time, at least in the West. Since 1960, data relating to trends in incidence of DU are somewhat conflicting. Surveys from Denmark and the USA suggest that the frequency of ulcer has not changed (Bonnevie, 1980; Kurata, Honda and Frankl, 1982). Figures collected in the UK indicate that the ulcer perforation rate has decreased in the younger age groups, but that in the elderly, and especially women, the incidence of perforation is rising (Figure 1.2). One hypothesis advanced to explain this remarkable rise in the frequency of DU at the start of the twentieth century proposes that it was due to influences operating for only a short time which produced a cohort phenomenon (Susser and Stein, 1962). The factors which may be responsible are the deprivation and stress generated by the period of financial recession and unemployment during that period of history. It remains to be seen if the present recession and high unemployment has a similar effect, although the development of the welfare state may have cushioned some of the worst effects.

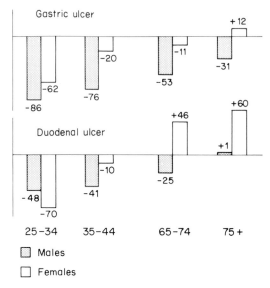

Figure 1.2 Percentage change in admission rates for ulcer perforation in England and Wales as average rates for 1958–62, related to those for 1973–77. (Reproduced from Coggon, Lambert and Langman (1981), by permission of Professor M. J. S. Langman)

GEOGRAPHICAL DIFFERENCES

Comparison of data from different countries is difficult for reasons discussed above. Ulcer complication rates can vary remarkably, even in a small country like the UK. Table 1.2 shows widely differing admission rates for perforated DU between the south and the north in the UK, while perforation rates for GU

Table 1.2 Regional admission rates per 10 000 population with perforated peptic ulcer in the UK

	Duodenal	Gastric
South		
East Anglia	0.07	0.08
Wessex	0.08	0.08
Oxford	0.13	0.04
South-west	0.14	0.02
North		
Leeds	0.22	0.07
Liverpool	0.23	0.03
Manchester	0.23	0.10
Newcastle	0.31	0.10
Scotland	0.45	0.07

do not differ materially between the north and south of England or Scotland (Brown, Langman and Lambert, 1976). The reasons for these observed differences are unknown, but as all those areas have a generally uniform standard of medical care and as virtually everyone with a perforated ulcer is admitted to hospital, where the diagnosis is confirmed at laparotomy, the figures are likely to be reliable.

Prevalence and incidence figures from emergent countries are difficult to interpret. In India, the disease is virtually all DU, predominantly affecting males in the south and in Assam, and associated with a high incidence of pyloric channel obstruction. Duodenal ulceration appears to be common in the Chinese population of Hong Kong (largely Cantonese in origin) and it seems to be the predominant form of peptic ulceration in Africa.

DIET

Diet looms large in the consciousness of patients suffering from peptic ulceration, and avoidance of greasy, fried and spicy foods is almost universal in an attempt to prevent ulcer pain. On the other hand, evidence suggesting that diet has a role in pathogenesis of ulcer disease is difficult to obtain. In a related field, the high incidence of gastric cancer in Japan could be due to dietary influences, but other environmental factors may also operate. For example, a prospective study found gastric cancer in Japanese to be associated not only with a low dietary intake of vegetables, but also with smoking (Hirayama, 1981). Salt intake is high in Japan, where the incidence of gastric ulcer is high, and a significant correlation between salt consumption and mortality from GU (but not from DU) in Western countries has been proposed (Sonnenberg, 1986). The alleged deficiencies in DU frequency between the north and south of India have been linked to the chewable diet in the former, contrasted with the sloppy food eaten in southern parts of the subcontinent. Another hypothesis attributes the decline in incidence and virulence of peptic ulcer disease to an increased availability of dietary fatty acids of the polyunsaturated type, which are precursors of prostaglandins (Hollander and Tarawski, 1986). It is clear that, if diet is important in the causation of peptic ulcer disease, we do not know how this operates.

ATTACK AND DEFENCE

If there is a unifying hypothesis defining the pathogenesis of DU and GU, it is encompassed in the general statement which postulates that ulcers result from an imbalance between influences that damage the integrity of duodenal or gastric mucous membranes (attack factors) and those influences that preserve the mucosal surface intact (defence factors). Attack factors are acid, pepsin, bile and other constituents of duodenal contents, drugs (notably NSAIDs or aspirin), alcohol, smoking and microorganisms (notably *Campylobacter pylori*). Defence factors are less well understood and comprise cellular regeneration and restitution processes, mucosal blood supply, mucus, bicarbonate and prostanoids. 'Cytoprotection' is the term used to describe defence of the gastric mucosa against experimental acute injury; it is possibly mediated by prostanoids and may have a vascular component. It is not at all certain how, or even if, cytoprotection is involved in pathogenesis of chronic peptic ulcer.

How the balance between attack and defence is struck to prevent ulceration and how to assign relative importance to the various factors is at present uncertain. Both GU and DU are likely to be multifactorial disease (Table 1.3).

SECRETION OF ACID

Acid dominates our thinking about ulcer disease. The old dictum 'no acid, no ulcer' remains valid, though it might be rephrased in a more stimulating way as 'if acid, why ulcer?'. Although many patients with DU have high acid outputs, many do not, while patients with GU tend to have normal or even low acid outputs. Despite the multifactorial hypothesis of peptic ulcer aetiology, acid seems to retain a key position in the initiation of the ulcerative process, and in the maintenance of its chronicity or relapse. Evidence for this is circumstantial and is furnished by the remarkable success of histamine H_2-receptor antagonists in accelerating the healing of DU and GU (Walt *et al.*, 1981) and in the significantly lower relapse rate during maintenance therapy with those agents (Gough *et al.*, 1984). There is also a correlation between the degree of inhibition of acid output and the speed and healing rates of DU (McIsaac *et al.*, 1987; Jones *et al.*, 1987). This correlation applies especially to nocturnal acid output, which may therefore be particularly important in maintaining chronicity of ulcers.

Table 1.3 Factors operating in peptic ulcer

Attack	Defence
Acid	Mucus
Pepsin	Bicarbonate
Bile	Cytoprotection
Drugs	Restitution
Smoking	Mucosal blood flow
Campylobacter pylori	
Environment?	
Diet?	
Stress?	
Heredity	

Duodenal ulceration is more strongly linked with acid secretion than GU. As a group, patients with duodenal ulcer secrete more acid, but this abnormality is not present in all patients suffering from DU diathesis. Table 1.4 shows the proportion of subjects with DU exhibiting abnormalities of acid secretion in various studies: the percentage of positive results varied from 0 to 100% depending on the study and the variable examined. Even allowing for errors of experimental technique, the impression remains that abnormal patterns of acid secretion are not present in all patients with DU. Nor has it been possible to integrate the abnormal secretory mechanisms that have been documented in various studies (high basal acid output, high nocturnal acid output, increased sensitivity of the parietal cell mass to gastrin, faulty switch-off mechanism for gastrin release by the antral G cells, increased cephalic phase acid output) into one underlying abnormality. Increased vagal drive remains an attractive hypothesis in many ways, but direct evidence for its existence is lacking. Gastric emptying in patients with DU is said to be faster than normal, thus increasing the acid load delivered to the duodenal cap over unit time, but the data overlap with normal ranges.

On the other hand, it is apparent that the difficulties of showing abnormal acid secretory patterns across the board in patients with DU may be due to difficulties inherent in the techniques used to study this variable. Measurements of acid output are subject to error because of transpyloric losses of acid and duodenogastric reflux of alkaline material. These errors become very appreciable, especially at low rates of acid secretion, when basal and nocturnal acid output are measured. Acquisition of acid output data depends on nasogastric intubation: an invasive method and an unpleasant experience for most subjects and patients. For this reason, virtually all published data on acid output (expressed as mmol acid per unit time) are confined to short (2–3 h) periods of measurement. A notable exception is the recent 24 h study of acid secretion by Feldman and Richardson (1986) showing significantly higher basal, interprandial and nocturnal acid output in DU patients than in controls. These results are extremely interesting, but should be considered in the light of the data

Table 1.4

Variable of acid secretion	Number of studies	Range of subjects with abnormal response (%)
Maximal acid output following histamine or pentagastrin stimulation >normal	17	16–56
Basal acid output >normal	7	10–38
Cephalic acid output >normal	4	7–55
Low D_{50} to pentagastrin	6	0–45
Meal-stimulated acid output >normal	8	10–100

(Modified from Lam, 1984)

in Table 1.4. Many of our ideas concerning the more subtle aspects of faulty acid control mechanisms stem from results based on intensive investigation of small numbers of patients, perhaps studied repeatedly in the same laboratory. It may be unwise to extrapolate such data to all DU patients. For example, the percentage of DU patients with maximal or peak acid output greater than normal following stimulation with histamine or pentagastrin varies from a low of 16–27% in studies done in the USA, to a high of 42–50% recorded in Scottish subjects (Lam *et al.*, 1981).

More recently, many studies have addressed the measurement of intragastric acidity (expressed as mmol/l at the point of measurement) with readings converted from pH recordings (Walt, 1986). The advantage of these studies is that intragastric acidity can be recorded over prolonged periods of time—usually 24 h (Figure 1.3). Aliquots of intragastric contents may be aspirated hourly, although the use of intragastric pH electrodes allows for more comfortable measurement at frequent sampling intervals in ambulant subjects (Merki *et al.*, 1988) (Figure 1.4). The disadvantage is that intragastric acidity does not relate directly to acid output. For example, after meals acid output is high but intragastric acidity remains low due to buffering by food. These techniques show that intragastric acidity is high in DU, especially at night, and that inhibition of nocturnal acid output seems especially important in achieving fast healing of DU. High unbuffered intragastric acidity in DU patients present during the

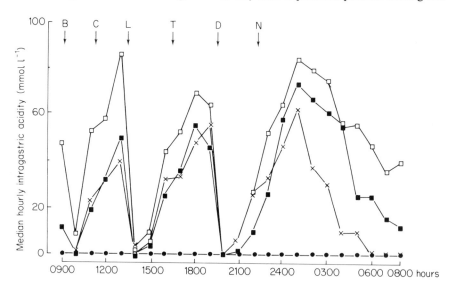

Figure 1.3 Median 24 h intragastric acidity in normals (*n* = 16; ■) and in patients with DU (*n* = 12; □), SU (*n* = 10; ×) or pernicious anaemia (*n* = 8; ●). B = breakfast, C = coffee, L = lunch, T = tea, D = dinner, N = nightcap. (Reproduced from Lanzon-Miller *et al.* (1987), by permission of Blackwell Scientific Publications Ltd)

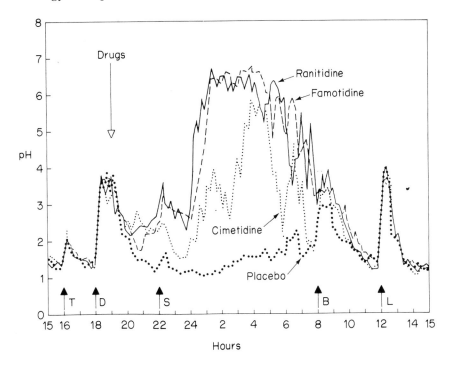

Figure 1.4 Median 5 min values of 24 h intragastric acidity in 30 controls receiving either placebo or a histamine H_2-receptor antagonist (cimetidine 800 mg; ranitidine 300 mg; famotidine 40 mg). T = tea, D = dinner, S = snack, B = breakfast, L = lunch. Horizontal axis = 24 h clock. (Reproduced from Merki *et al.* (1988), by permission of the British Medical Association)

night (low volume/highly concentrated acid) probably explains at least one classical symptom of the disease: the patient is woken by the typical pain in the early hours and the pain is relieved by taking a milky drink or an antacid.

PEPSIN

Secretion of pepsin may also be important, but has not been explored in such detail as acid secretion. In general, secretion of pepsin moves in parallel with the output of hydrochloric acid, but agonists such as secretin can produce a dissociated response. The pharmacology of pepsin secretion is not completely understood. The role of pepsin in the aetiology of peptic ulceration seems to lie in its capacity to disrupt the mucus–bicarbonate barrier, which normally protects the epithelial surface from the injurious effect of luminal acid (Venables, 1986). Precursors of pepsin (pepsinogens) are present in the serum, where they can be measured by radioimmunoassay. Pepsin and pepsinogens exist in more than one molecular form. Serum pepsinogens have been divided into three groups, termed pepsinogen I and II (PgI, PgII) and slow-migrating protease. PgI is itself heterogeneous and has been shown to consist of two immunochemically and electrophoretically distinct components (Taggart and Samloff, 1987). Elevated serum concentrations of PgI are significantly associated with DU and concentrations of PgI above the upper limit of normal are present in about 50% of patients with this disease (Samloff, Liebman and Donitch, 1975). PgI is higher in more severe forms of DU. It has been shown to correlate with the secretory capacity of the stomach, and to be inherited as an autosomal dominant trait; it can be used as a marker for the ulcer diathesis in some families (Rotter et al., 1979). Elevated serum PgI is associated with DU, and raised concentrations of PgII and low PgI/PgII ratios seem to be major risk factors for GU (Samloff et al., 1986). These studies are highly interesting and underline the existence of constitutional factors that predispose certain individuals to the development of ulcer disease: presumably because 'attack' factors in the form of pepsin are more active than normal.

Pepsins secreted in gastric juice have been less intensively studied than serum pepsinogens, probably because it has been difficult to develop reliable techniques for the quantitative estimation of pepsin in the gastric lumen. Pearson et al. (1986) have shown that pure human pepsin I (the enzyme associated with DU) degrades gastric mucus glycoprotein faster and remains active at higher pH than pepsin III, the principal human pepsin. Mucolytic activity of gastric juice from patients with DU resembles that of pepsin I, while the juice from control subjects resembles pepsin III. These observations suggest that the protective coat of mucus is more vulnerable to attack over a broader range of acidity in DU patients than in healthy controls. The implication is that raising the intragastric pH to only 5.0 would still leave pepsin I at least partly active in the ulcer patients. Perhaps this does not matter greatly, as healing of DU appears to occur when the intragastric pH reaches 3.0 or higher. In general, however, these observations define an attack factor on the integrity of the mucus–bicarbonate barrier in patients with DU.

MUCUS AND BICARBONATE

Mucus is secreted by epithelial cells and forms an insoluble gel layer adherent to the mucosal surface. It is the gel layer that is thought to be important in mucosal protection; soluble mucus shed into the gastric lumen and mixed with gastric secretion is probably not important. The gastric mucus glycoprotein is a polymer built up from subunits joined by disulphide bonds. Each subunit has a glycosylated component consisting of a protein core with carbohydrate side chains and a non-glycosylated segment which is susceptible to attack by proteolytic enzymes. Breakdown of mucus by proteolytic enzymes destroys the physico-chemical properties of the gel layer on which its protective properties depend. Normal mucus is not permeable to larger molecules such as pepsins, which are thus prevented from gaining access and damaging the surface epithelium. Pepsins themselves can solubilize mucus by proteolytic action.

Although an intact mucus layer is impermeable to larger molecules, it is permeable to small molecules or solutes, such as H^+ ions. Hollander (1954) and Heatley (1959) have suggested that mucus acts as an unstirred layer, trapping bicarbonate secreted by the mucosa and providing an alkaline protective mantle over the surface epithelium. Direct measurements have confirmed that pH rises sharply as the mucus layer is penetrated by a microelectrode from the lumen inwards towards the mucosa, and reaches near neutrality at the epithelial surface (Allen and Garner, 1980; Rees and Turnberg, 1982).

Isenberg et al. (1986, 1987) have shown that bicarbonate (measured in the lumen) is secreted by the human duodenum. Patients with DU secrete less bicarbonate in their proximal duodenum in response to perfusion with acid than controls. Another source of bicarbonate that may reach the duodenal lumen is pancreatic juice. Studies of luminal bicarbonate secretion document yet another subtle abnormality present in at least some patients with DU without indicating its place in the ranking order of factors responsible for duodenal ulceration. It may be conjectured that the mucus–bicarbonate barrier forming the unstirred layer is likely to be an important mechanism which enables the gastric and duodenal epithelium to survive intact, while ambient luminal hydrogen ion concentrations is at pH of 2.0. Paradoxically, the narrow zone of near neutral pH overlying the mucosal surface also provides an ecosphere for *Campylobacter pylori*: an organism capable of damaging the gastric epithelial cells.

CAMPYLOBACTER PYLORI

The information explosion relating to this spiral, flagellated organism existing in the narrow band between the antral epithelial cells and the surface of mucus layer has been astounding (Rathbone, Wyatt and Heatley, 1986; Bartlett, 1988). The organism was sporadically described by various workers in the past and present century, but Warren and Marshall (1983) rediscovered it for the scientific community by being able to culture it successfully for the first time. There now seems little doubt that the presence of *C. pylori* is strongly associated with chronic active non-specific gastritis affecting the antrum predominantly. It may also be an agent responsible for outbreaks of acute epidemic gastritis associated with hypochlorhydria.

Besides its peculiar habitat, *C. pylori* possesses other interesting features: it is a very powerful producer of urease, and the consequent release of ammonia may provide a microenvironment of raised pH, enabling the organism to survive. Ammonia may be cytotoxic. Electron microscopic studies show damage to the gastric epithelial microvilli in the immediate vicinity of *C. pylori*. Another peculiarity is that the organism will grow only over gastric (mainly antral) epithelium with areas of intestinal metaplasia in the antrum being spared. This has led to an attractive hypothesis to explain the role of *C. pylori* in the pathogenesis of duodenal ulceration: areas of gastric metaplasia arise in the duodenal cap, possibly associated in some way with high gastric acid output (Wyatt *et al.*, 1987). Colonization of these heterotopic islands with *C. pylori* leads to mucosal injury and subsequent ulceration. It can be further imagined that decreased acid perfusion during treatment with H_2-receptor antagonists allows the ulcer to heal, though relapse may follow because the focus of heterotopic mucosa remains. There is some circumstantial evidence to support this view. Relapse rate of DU after treatment with bismuth subcitrate or subsalicylate, which have bactericidal actions, is lower in some, but not all, trials using H_2-blocker treated patients as the comparison group (Coghlan *et al.* 1987; Dobrilla, Vallaperta and Amplatz, 1988). Relapse of DU is associated with recolonization of the antrum with *C. pylori*. However, many of the studies reporting these phenomena are based on small numbers of patients and some have not been published in full. A few studies have reported more normal epithelialization of ulcer craters after bactericidal drugs than after other agents.

On the other hand, the association of *C. pylori* colonization, antral gastritis and the non-ulcer dyspepsia syndrome remains at present conjectural. Those studies that have addressed the problem have reported improvement in histological appearances of gastritis following treatment with bismuth, but it has not been possible to demonstrate a concurrent improvement of symptoms (McNulty *et al.*, 1986). The original source of *C. pylori* and the method of transmission is not as yet clear. No doubt new data will continue to accumulate at a fast rate.

PROSTAGLANDINS

Hawkey and Walt (1986) entitled their review of the therapeutic role of prostaglandins in peptic ulcer 'Prostaglandins—a promise unfulfilled' and this is the view held by many, but not all, workers in this area. The importance of prostaglandins in the aetiology of peptic ulcer is also undecided. Prostaglandins are readily synthesized from fatty acid precursors by an enzyme system present in most mammalian cells, including the gastric and duodenal epithelium. Tissue injury is a powerful stimulus for the synthesis of prostaglandins, which are very powerful pharmacological agents with a variety of actions, depending on their type. Many prostaglandins, such as PGE_2 and synthetic derivatives, are powerful inhibitors of gastric acid secretion, which also affect mucosal blood flow. Animal experiments have demonstrated the ability of prostaglandins to protect the gastric mucosa from injury by acutely administered noxious agents, even when the prostaglandins are given at doses too small to affect gastric acid secretion, or when non-antisecretory prostaglandins are administered. This remarkable property has been termed 'cytoprotection' and debate has continued as to whether deficiency of prostaglandins has an aetiological role in peptic ulcer, and whether exogenous prostaglandins are useful in the treatment of DU or GU.

There are many technical difficulties in making accurate measurements of tissue concentrations, or of synthesis rates of prostaglandins in gastric or duodenal mucosal biopsies, and this may be partly responsible for the discordant results reported by various studies. Some authors find deficiency of at least some prostanoids (Hillier et al., 1985), while others find normal concentrations. It may be difficult to accept intrinsic prostanoid deficiency in subjects eating a diet containing essential fatty acids, and the role of prostaglandins in the pathogenesis of chronic DU and GU remains to be clarified. Different circumstances may obtain during acute mucosal injury secondary to stress, or to ingestion of ethanol or drugs, and a clear distinction has to be made between these two modes of mucosal ulceration. Cytoprotective mechanisms may well be operating to prevent acute mucosal injury and to mediate mucosal restitution processes, but they may not be relevant to chronic, recurrent DU or GU.

ENVIRONMENTAL FACTORS

These are undoubtedly important, but difficult to quantify. Smoking affects ulcer recurrence, since smokers' ulcers relapse sooner and more often. Non-steroidal anti-inflammatory drugs are associated with complications of ulcer disease, such as perforation or haemorrhage. The role of alcohol is more conjectural: excessive consumption of ethanol can cause acute erosive gastritis, but it is doubtful if it plays a role in chronic duodenal or gastric ulcer. Relapses of ulcer and perforations are universally associated in the public mind with stress; whether this is so is uncertain.

SUMMARY

Chronic, recurrent DU and GU are multifactorial diseases (Table 1.3). Gastric acid plays a fundamental role, but a wide variety of other factors (genetic, environmental, dietary, pathophysiological and bacterial) also come into play to finally produce the disease. The relative importance of the various factors in individual patients is difficult to assess.

REFERENCES

Allen, A. and Garner, A. (1980). Gastric mucus and bicarbonate secretion and their possible role in mucosal protection, *Gut*, **21**, 249–62.

Bartlett, J. G. (1988). *Campylobacter pylori*: fact or fantasy, *Gastroenterology*, **92**, 229–38.

Bonnevie, O. (1980). Peptic ulcer in Denmark, *Scand. J. Gastroenterol.* (Suppl. 63) **15**: 163–74.

Brown, R. C., Langman, M. J. S. and Lambert, P. M. (1976). Hospital admissions for peptic ulcer during 1968–72, *Br. Med. J.*, **i**, 35–7.

Collier, D. St. J. and Pain, J. A. (1985). Non-steroidal anti-inflammatory drugs and peptic ulcer perforation, *Gut*, **26**, 359–63.

Coggon, D., Lambert, P. and Langman, M. J. S. (1981). Twenty years of hospital admissions for peptic ulcer in England and Wales, *Lancet*, **i**, 1302–4.

Coghlan, J. G., Gilligan, D., Humphries, H. *et al.* (1987). *Campylobacter pylori* and recurrence of duodenal ulcer—a 12 month follow-up study, *Lancet*, **ii**, 1109–11.

Dobrilla, G., Vallaperta, P. and Amplatz, S. (1988). Influence of ulcer healing agents on ulcer relapse after discontinuation of acute treatment: a pooled estimate of controlled clinical trials, *Gut*, **29**, 181–7.

Feldman, M. and Richardson, C. T. (1986). Total 24-hour gastric acid secretion in patients with duodenal ulcer: comparison with normal subjects and effects of cimetidine and parietal cell vagotomy, *Gastroenterology*, **90**, 540–4.

Gough, K. R., Bardhan, K. D., Crowe, J. P. *et al.* (1984). Ranitidine and cimetidine in prevention of duodenal ulcer relapse, *Lancet*, **ii**, 659–62.

Hawkey, C. J. and Walt, R. P. (1986). Prostaglandins for peptic ulcer: a promise unfulfilled, *Lancet*, **ii**, 1084–6.

Heatley, N. G. (1959). Mucosubstance as a barrier to diffusion, *Gastroenterology*, **37**, 313–23.

Hillier, K., Smith, C. L., Jewell, R., Arthur, M. P. J. and Ross, G. (1985). Duodenal mucosa synthesis of prostaglandins in duodenal ulcer disease, *Gut*, **26**, 237–40.

Hirayama, T. (1981). Methods and results of gastric cancer screening. In J. W. Fielding *et al.* (eds) *Gastric Cancer*, Pergamon Press, Oxford, pp. 77–84.

Hollander, F. (1954). Two two-component mucus barrier, *Arch. Intern. Med.*, **93**, 107–20.

Hollander, D. and Tarawski, A. (1986). Dietary essential fatty acids and the decline in peptic ulcer disease: a hypothesis, *Gut*, **27**, 239–42.

Isenberg, J. I., Hogan, D. L., Koss, M. A. and Selling, J. A. (1986). Human duodenal mucosal bicarbonate secretion: evidence for basal secretion and stimulation by hydrochloric acid and a synthetic prostaglandin E1 analogue, *Gastroenterology*, **91**, 370–9.

Isenberg, J. I., Selling, J. A., Hogan, D. L. and Koss, M. A. (1987). Impaired proximal duodenal mucosal bicarbonate secretion in patients with duodenal ulcer, *New Engl. J. Med.*, **316**, 374–8.

Jones, D. B., Howden, C. W., Burget, D. W. *et al.* (1987). Acid suppression in duodenal ulcer: a meta-analysis to define optimal dosing with antisecretory drugs, *Gut*, **28**, 1120–7.

Kurata, J. H., Honda, G. D. and Frankl, H. (1982). Hospitalization and mortality rates for peptic ulcers: a comparison of large health maintenance organisation and United States data, *Gastroenterology*, **83**, 1008–16.

Lam, S. K., Hasan, M., Sircus, W. *et al.* (1981). Comparison of maximal acid output and gastrin response to meals in Chinese and Scottish normal and duodenal ulcer subjects, *Gut*, **21**, 324–8.

Lam, S. K. (1984). Pathogenesis and pathophysiology of duodenal ulcer, *Clin. Gastroenterol.*, **13**, 447–72.

Lanzon-Miller, S., Pounder, R. E., Hamilton, M. R. *et al.* (1987). 24-hour intragastric acidity and plasma gastrin concentration in healthy subjects and patients with duodenal or gastric ulcer, or pernicious anaemia, *Aliment. Pharmacol. Ther.*, **1**, 228–38.

Levi, I. S. and de la Fuente, A. A. (1963). A post mortem study of gastric and duodenal peptic lesions, *Gut*, **4**, 349–59.

McIsaac, R. L., McCanless, I., Summers, K. and Wood, J. R. (1987). Ranitidine and cimetidine in the healing of duodenal ulcer: meta analysis of comparative clinical trials, *Alimentary Pharmacol. Ther.*, **1**, 369–81.

McNulty, C. A. M., Dear, J. C., Crump, B. *et al.* (1986). *Campylobacter pyloridis* and associated gastritis: investigator-blind placebo-controlled trial of bismuth salicylate and erythromycin succinate, *Brit. Med. J.*, **293**, 645–9.

Merki, H. S., Witzel, L., Walt, R. P. *et al.* (1988). Double blind comparison of the effects of cimetidine, ranitidine, famotidine and placebo on intragastric acidity in 30 normal volunteers, *Gut*, **29**, 81–4.

Pearson, J. P., Ward, R., Allen, A., Roberts, N. B. and Taylor, W. H. (1986). Mucus degradation by pepsin: comparison of mucolytic activity of human pepsin 1 and pepsin 2, *Gut*, **27**, 243–9.

Rathbone, B. J., Wyatt, J. I. and Heatley, R. V. (1986). *Campylobacter pyloridis* — a new factor in peptic ulcer disease?, *Gut*, **27**, 635–41.

Rees, W. D. W. and Turnberg, L. A. (1982). Mechanism of gastric mucosal protection: a role for the 'mucus-bicarbonate' barrier, *Clin. Sci.*, **62**, 343–8.

Rotter, J. L., Sones, J. Q., Samloff, I. M. *et al.* (1979). Duodenal ulcer disease associated with elevated serum pepsinogen 2: an inherited autosomal dominant disorder, *New Engl. J. Med.*, **300**, 63–73.

Samloff, I. M., Liebman, W. L. and Donitch, N. M. (1975). Serum group 1 pepsinogens by radioimmunoassay in control subjects and patients with peptic ulcer, *Gastroenterology*, **69**, 83–90.

Samloff, I. M., Stemmermann, G. N., Hailburn, L. K. *et al.* (1986). Elevated serum pepsinogen I and II levels differ as risk factors for duodenal and gastric ulcer, *Gastroenterology*, **90**, 570–6.

Sonnenberg, A. (1986). Dietary salt and gastric ulcer, *Gut*, **27**, 1138–42.

Susser, S. and Stein, Z. (1962). Civilisation and peptic ulcer, *Lancet*, **i**, 115–18.

Taggart, T. R. and Samloff, I. M. (1987). Immunochemical, electrophoretic and genetic heterogeneity of pepsinogen 1, *Gastroenterology*, **92**, 143–50.

Venables, C. W. (1986). Mucus, pepsin and peptic ulcer, *Gut*, **27**, 233–8.

Walt, R. P., Male, P. J., Rawlings, J. *et al.* (1981). Comparison of the effects of ranitidine, cimetidine and placebo on the 24 hour intragastric acidity and nocturnal acid secretion in patients with duodenal ulcer, *Gut*, **22**, 49–54.

Walt, R. P. (1986). Twenty-four hour intragastric acidity — analysis for the future, *Gut*, **27**, 1–9.

Walt, R., Katschinski, B., Logan, R., Ashley, J. and Langman, M. (1986). Rising frequency of ulcer perforation in elderly patients in the United Kingdom, *Lancet*, **i**, 489–92.

Warren, R. J. and Marshall, B. (1983). Unidentified spiral bacilli on gastric epithelium in active chronic gastritis, *Lancet*, **i**, 1273–5.

Watkinson, G. (1960). The incidence of chronic peptic ulcer found at necropsy, *Gut*, **1**, 14–31.

Wyatt, J. I., Rathbone, B. J., Dixon, M. F. and Heatley, R. V. (1987). *Campylobacter pyloridis* and acid induced gastric metaplasia in the pathogenesis of duodenitis, *J. Clin. Pharmacol.*, **40**, 841–8.

Advances in Drug Therapy of Gastrointestinal Ulceration
Edited by A. Garner and B. J. R. Whittle
©1989 John Wiley & Sons Ltd

Chapter Two

Experimental Studies with Histamine H₂-Receptor Antagonists

M. E. Parsons
*Pharmacology Department, Smith Kline & French Research Ltd,
The Frythe, Welwyn, Hertfordshire AL6 9AR, UK*

INTRODUCTION

Although many of the pharmacological properties of histamine had been described by Dale and co-workers in the first decade of this century, it was not until some ten years later that its potent stimulant effect on gastric acid secretion was identified (Popielski, 1920).

Over the following 40 years, numerous pieces of evidence accumulated to suggest a key role for histamine in the *physiological* control of gastric acid secretion. Histamine was found to be stored in the acid secreting fundic mucosa and McIntosh (1938) demonstrated that stimulation of the vagus nerve (which had long been known to influence acid secretion) led to an increase in gastric acid secretion which was quantitatively paralleled by an increase in the amount of histamine in the gastric juice.

Kahlson *et al.* (1964) showed that food-stimulated acid secretion was accompanied by a decrease in the histamine content of the gastric mucosa of the rat and the concomitant increase in the activity of the histamine-forming enzyme, histidine decarboxylase.

Data of this kind led McIntosh and, in particular, Code (1956, 1965) to propose the common final mediator hypothesis which stated that, whatever the method of stimulation of gastric acid secretion, histamine released from the gastric mucosa was the common and final chemostimulant.

However, as early as 1905, Edkins had proposed that a hormone ('gastrin') was present in the antral gastric mucosa and played an important role in the control of acid secretion. With the discovery of the ability of histamine to stimulate acid secretion and its presence in the gastric mucosa, many investigators concluded that gastrin and histamine were synonymous.

This situation was radically altered in 1961 with the isolation of a peptide from the antral gastric mucosa, identification of its structure and demonstration of its acid secretory stimulant properties (Gregory and Tracy, 1961). Subsequently, histamine was frequently considered not to play a key role in the stomach as exemplified by a special article published in *Gastroenterology* (Johnson, 1971) which in essence relegated histamine to a purely *pharmacological* role unrelated to the normal *physiological* control of gastric acid secretion.

DEVELOPMENT OF THE
HISTAMINE H₂-RECEPTOR ANTAGONISTS

One of the problems hindering our understanding of the interrelationships between the three chemical messengers for acid secretion (i.e. histamine, gastrin and acetylcholine) was the lack of adequate pharmacological tools and, in particular, specific receptor antagonists.

Anticholinergic drugs such as atropine had been available for many years and had been shown to inhibit acid secretion stimulated by the parasympathetic vagus nerve and exogenously administered cholinergic agents and indeed synthetic analogues such as probanthene had been used in the treatment of acid-related diseases such as duodenal ulcer. However, no such specific antagonist existed (and still does not exist) for gastrin and up until 1972 did not exist for histamine. The latter situation was somewhat surprising since the first antihistamine drugs were developed in the 1920s and were rapidly followed by more potent and specific antagonists such as Benadryl and mepyramine.

However, without exception, these compounds failed to inhibit histamine-stimulated gastric acid secretion. Other actions of histamine were also found to be refractory to inhibition by the classical antihistamine drugs, for example the chronotropic effect of histamine on the heart and the ability of histamine to inhibit evoked contractions of the rat uterus. These data prompted speculation that two populations of histamine receptor may exist as had been found with α and β receptors in the adrenergic system.

In 1964 research commenced at Smith Kline & French to address this question of possible histamine receptor heterogeneity. It became clear that relatively minor modifications of the structure of the histamine molecule lead to compounds showing relative agonist selectivity depending on the tissue studied. For example, 4-methylhistamine had only 0.2% of the agonist activity of histamine on the guinea-pig ileum (a tissue containing H_1-histamine receptors), but retained 40% of the activity of histamine on the heart or as a stimulant of gastric acid secretion.

Further structural modification led to a series of partial agonists and weak antagonists at the hypothetical second histamine receptor and culminated in 1972 with the publication of a paper in *Nature* (Black *et al.*, 1972) defining a second class of histamine receptor (designated the H_2-receptor) and describing the properties of a relatively specific and competitive antagonist of this receptor, burimamide.

Although burimamide was studied in human pharmacological experiments, its relatively low oral potency precluded its clinical development. However, Smith Kline & French developed two further potent H$_2$-receptor antagonists, metiamide and cimetidine (Figure 2.1). Metiamide was taken into clinical studies but its development was halted by the occurrence of granulocytopenia in a small number of patients. This was associated with the chemical structure of metiamide and not its pharmacological activity as an H$_2$-antagonist. Subsequently, cimetidine was shown not to have this side-effect and has proved a major success in the therapy of acid-related diseases.

All three compounds have been demonstrated to be selective and competitive antagonists at the H$_2$-receptor on non-gastric tissues and to inhibit histamine-stimulated gastric acid secretion in a wide variety of species, including man, indicating the involvement of H$_2$-receptors in this response.

The development of H$_2$-receptor antagonists provided basic scientists and clinical gastroenterologists with powerful tools to dissect out the interrelationships between the triad of chemical secretagogues and, in turn, their relationship to the normal physiological control of gastric acid secretion. With the establishment of a central role for histamine in the process (see below), clinicians were also provided with important new therapeutic agents in the field of acid-related diseases.

Histamine

Burimamide

Metiamide

Cimetidine

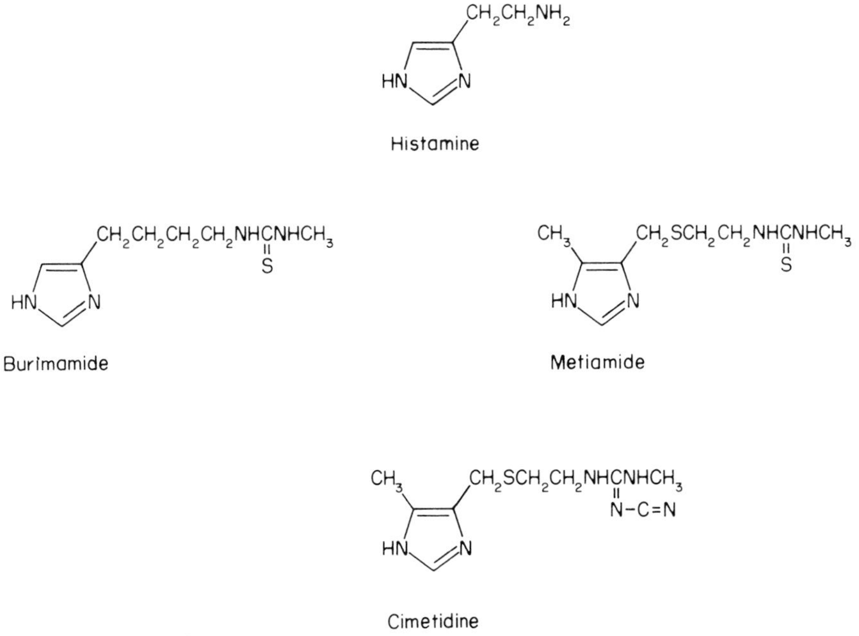

Figure 2.1 Structures of burimamide, metiamide and cimetidine

HISTAMINE AND THE PHYSIOLOGICAL
CONTROL OF GASTRIC ACID SECRETION

It was demonstrated at an early stage (Black *et al.*, 1972) that H_2 antagonists were effective inhibitors of gastrin (or pentagastrin) stimulated gastric acid secretion both in experimental animals and in man (Aadland and Bersted, 1978) with potencies similar to those obtained against histamine (Figure 2.2). The markedly different chemical structures of the two secretagogues, together with cimetidine's established selectivity at H_2-receptors on non-gastric tissues, render it unlikely that they are both acting directly on H_2-receptors in the gastric mucosa and hence the data could be seen to support Code's hypothesis that gastrin acts via a mobilization of endogenous mucosal histamine.

Subsequently, numerous studies have demonstrated that histamine H_2-receptor antagonists can inhibit the effects of virtually all acid secretory stimulants in both experimental animals and man. However, under certain experimental conditions, cholinergically stimulated secretion does tend to be more resistant to H_2 antagonist inhibition than secretion evoked by other secretagogues, while the inhibition of gastrin-stimulated secretion appears to be non-competitive or unsurmountable in nature.

Gastric acid secretion resulting from activation of the vagus nerve by 2-deoxyglucose, insulin (Carter *et al.*, 1976) or sham feeding (Schoon and Olbe,

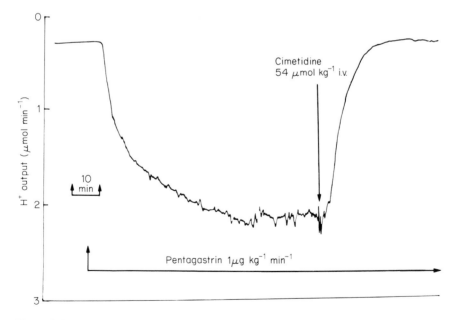

Figure 2.2 Inhibition of pentagastrin-stimulated gastric acid secretion by intravenous cimetidine in the stomach lumen perfused anaesthetized rat preparation

1978) is also inhibited by H$_2$-antagonists. Acid secretion in response to the more physiological stimulus of food administration is also inhibited and in a manner quantitatively similar to that obtained against pentagastrin (Figure 2.3). Basal acid secretion (both daytime and nocturnal) can be inhibited by H$_2$-antagonists in both rodents and man (Longstreth, Go and Malagelada, 1976).

From these data it is clear that histamine plays a central role in the physiological control of acid secretion, although the precise nature of this role is still not entirely clear.

RECEPTORS ON THE PARIETAL CELL

Various observations, for example, the relatively greater resistance of cholinergic-stimulated secretion to H$_2$-receptor blockade, suggested that a hypothesis requiring an obligatory histamine step in secretagogue-induced acid secretion might be oversimplistic.

Clearly *in vivo* studies on the control of acid secretion are complex and involve not only direct parietal cell receptor activation but also modulating influences such as vagal and local cholinergic tone, blood flow and local hormone release. To gain a clearer view of the receptors involved in the control of acid secretion necessitates moving to *in vitro* studies. Thus, a wide range of experimental

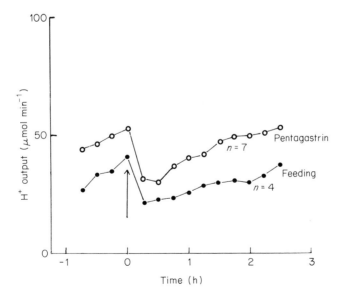

Figure 2.3 A comparison of the inhibition by intravenous metiamide (arrow) of pentagastrin and food stimulated gastric acid secretion in the conscious Heidenhain pouch dog

preparations have been used ranging from isolated whole stomachs and sections of isolated fundic mucosa through to isolated whole gastric glands and purified parietal cell preparations.

In all the preparations studied, H_2-receptor antagonists inhibited histamine-stimulated acid secretion over a concentration range similar to that effective at H_2-receptors on *in vitro* non-gastric tissues (Bunce and Parsons, 1976).

The situation regarding gastrin is more complex. In an isolated whole rat stomach preparation, metiamide was found to inhibit gastrin-stimulated acid secretion over the concentration range effective against histamine although, as *in vivo*, the inhibition was only partially surmountable (Bunce and Parsons, 1976). Inhibition of gastrin-stimulated acid secretion *in vitro* has been confirmed in other species, e.g. the kitten isolated mucosa, the isolated mouse stomach and the isolated primate mucosa. However, further studies using both whole stomach and isolated fundic mucosal preparations have indicated that a small residual response can be obtained to gastrin even in the presence of extremely high concentrations $(10^{-3} M)$ of an H_2-antagonist, suggesting the possible existence of a separate gastrin receptor on the mucosa.

Further refinement of the experimental model from whole muscosa to isolated cell adds a further complication. For example, Berglindh and Öbrink (1979), using an isolated gastric gland preparation from the rabbit, found that the tissue responded to histamine and carbachol but not to pentagastrin.

It is unlikely that these data indicate the lack of specific receptors for gastrin since the secretagogue could stimulate acid secretion in the presence of isobutylmethylxanthine, a phosphodiesterase inhibitor.

Using isolated parietal cells Soll (1978a) found that gastrin could stimulate parietal cell activity, although the magnitude of the response was very small relative to that found with histamine and acetylcholine. The gastrin response was not blocked by an H_2-antagonist or atropine. Stimulation of parietal cell function has been confirmed by other workers using parietal cells isolated from rat (Cheret, Girodet and Lewin, 1977; Jennewein, Herbst and Waldeck, 1979) and guinea-pig (Albinus, 1979).

What is clearly established is that *in vitro* gastric preparations will respond to cholinergic stimulation (Figure 2.4) and that the responses are totally refractory to inhibition by H_2-antagonists, suggesting the existence of specific cholinergic receptors (e.g. Bunce, Parsons and Rollings, 1976).

The existence of specific receptors for gastrin on canine parietal cells has been confirmed by binding studies using ([^{125}I] Leu^{15})gastrin (Soll *et al.*, 1984) and also demonstrated in the rat gastric mucosa (Speir, Takeuchi and Johnson, 1979). In addition the existence of specific muscarinic receptors has been confirmed using tritiated QNB binding (Rosenfeld *et al.*, 1978; Hammer *et al.*, 1980).

If there are three separate receptors for histamine, gastrin and acetylcholine, how can the apparent non-specific inhibitory effects of H_2-antagonists *in vivo* be explained? One suggestion, which is supported by experimental data, is that

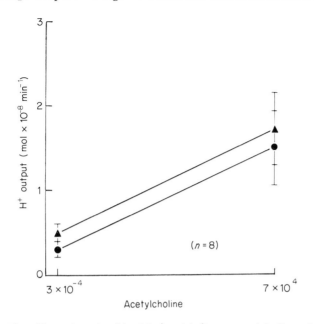

Figure 2.4 The effect of metiamide (10^{-4} mol l^{-1}) on acetylcholine-stimulated acid secretion in the isolated lumen-perfused whole stomach of the rat. ○ Control, ● Metiamide 10^{-4} mol l^{-1}. (Reproduced from Bunce, Parsons and Rollings (1976) by kind permission of Macmillan Press Ltd)

there are potentiating interactions between the agonists in their ability to stimulate acid secretion. Using canine parietal cells, Soll (1978a,b,c) found that, for example, the response to gastrin plus histamine is much greater than additive. Since all of the potentiating interactions involved histamine, blockade of the H$_2$-receptor to remove the potentiating effect of histamine might account, at least in part, for the apparent lack of selectivity of H$_2$-antagonists. For the hypothesis to be tenable requires that the parietal cell is subject to a 'tonic' level of histamine under circumstances when gastrin and acetylcholine are the primary stimulants.

The basis of these potentiating interactions is unclear, although Grossman and Konturek (1974) proposed that they occurred at the receptor level with blockade of one receptor changing the properties of one or both of the other receptors. Experimental evidence to support this hypothesis was not provided, however.

POST-RECEPTOR EVENTS

An alternative point at which amplifying interactions could occur might be at the post-receptor stage. Our understanding of the second messengers involved in signal transduction within the parietal cells has increased significantly in the past 20 years. It is now clear that activation of the parietal cell by histamine depends on the stimulation of adenylate cyclase and a concomitant increase in mucosal cyclic AMP levels. Scholes *et al.* (1976), using isolated gastric mucosal cells from canine mucosa, showed that histamine caused a dose-dependent increase in cyclic AMP levels and this effect was competitively antagonized by the histamine H_2-receptor antagonist metiamide.

Dibutyryl cyclic AMP will stimulate gastric acid secretion *in vitro*, an effect predictably refractory to H_2-receptor antagonists since the agent is acting beyond the receptor stage (Bunce, Parsons and Rollings, 1976). Elevation of endogenous cyclic AMP levels by the use of phosphodiesterase inhibitors such as isobutylmethylxanthine has also been shown to stimulate gastric acid secretion (Figure 2.5) and to potentiate the secretory response to histamine (Bunce and Parsons, unpublished observations). This result is interesting in the light of the fact that gastrin will stimulate acid secretion in the isolated rabbit gland preparation only in the presence of a phosphodiesterase inhibitor (Berglindh and Öbrink, 1979).

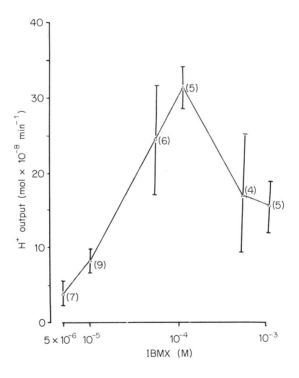

Figure 2.5 The stimulant effect of isobutylmethylxanthine on acid secretion in the isolated lumen-perfused whole stomach of the rat

Activation of the muscarinic receptor on the parietal cell appears, in contrast, to be calcium dependent and linked to an increase in cytosolic calcium (Muallem and Sachs, 1984). The source of calcium appears to be extracellular, since acetylcholine-stimulated acid secretion is abolished by removal of calcium from the extracellular bathing fluid (Bunce, Honey and Parsons, 1979) (Figure 2.6). Also, lanthanum, which blocks calcium fluxes across plasma membranes, caused marked inhibition of cholinergic stimulation (Soll, 1981). Finally, carbachol-stimulated aminopyrine accumulation into isolated parietal cells is associated with enhanced $^{45}Ca^{2+}$ influx (Soll, 1981).

The transduction mechanism for gastrin has not been clearly established although it has recently been suggested that gastrin stimulation does lead to a transient increase in cell calcium which is not blocked by calcium channel blockers and may involve an increase in inositol triphosphate (Sachs, 1986).

However, although the potential for amplifying interactions exists within the parietal cell, there is no direct experimental evidence to support the hypothesis that this is the basis for the ability of H₂-antagonists to inhibit gastrin and cholinergically evoked secretion *in vivo*.

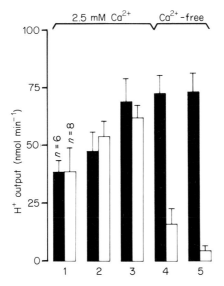

Figure 2.6   The effect of the removal of extracellular Ca^{2+} on the acid-secretory response to acetylcholine in the isolated lumen-perfused whole stomach of the rat: □ , control; ■ , test. (Reproduced from Bunce, Honey and Parsons (1979) by kind permission of Macmillan Press Ltd)

HISTAMINE STORAGE IN THE GASTRIC MUCOSA

By far the most attractive hypothesis to account for the ability of H_2-antagonists to inhibit gastrin and cholinergically evoked secretion still resides in the ability of these agonists to release endogenous histamine as an obligatory step in their action on the parietal cell.

To this end, a considerable body of research has been directed towards identifying storage sites for histamine in the gastric mucosa and its release by secretagogues.

High concentrations of histamine are found in the acid-secreting portion of the stomach in all species studied, although the absolute amount varies. This may, however, reflect differences in the assay techniques employed. In the rat, rabbit and frog, histamine appears to be stored in the so-called enterochromaffin-like cells located in the fundic mucosa. These cells also contain the histamine-forming enzyme, histidine decarboxylase. In contrast, in dog, man and pig, histamine appears to be stored in a type of mast cell.

As mentioned earlier, histamine release by vagal stimulation and by feeding was established at an early date and provided one of the cornerstones of Code's final common mediator hypothesis. Subsequently, release of histamine induced by either gastrin or acetylcholine has been reported from the isolated rat stomach (Main and Pearce, 1977), from the amphibian mucosa *in vitro* (Rangachari, 1975) and in isolated rabbit gastric glands (Bergqvist *et al.*, 1980). However, these data have been derived from studies containing a variety of cell types. Soll (1982, 1986) performed studies using mast cells obtained from the canine fundic mucosa and, although these cells released histamine in response to the cross-linking of IgE receptors and treatment with the calcium ionophore A 23187, they were totally refractory to the effects of gastrin and acetylcholine. Thus, although further experimental work is required, it is clear that the site of histamine storage and its susceptibility to release by gastric secretagogues is markedly species dependent. This in turn makes it difficult to provide a unifying hypothesis for the central role of histamine in the control of gastric acid secretion.

DEVELOPMENTS SINCE CIMETIDINE

Although its exact nature is not entirely understood, the central role of histamine in the control of acid secretion and the effectiveness of H_2-antagonists in inhibiting all forms of basal and stimulated acid secretion has led to a revolution in the treatment of acid-related diseases and in particular duodenal ulcer. This in turn has led to a rapid proliferation in the number of histamine H_2-receptor antagonists both on the market and in development, although some have failed because of toxicological problems.

Ranitidine was the second histamine H$_2$-receptor antagonist to reach the market. In animal experimental studies this compound was found to have a similar acid-secretory inhibitory profile to that of cimetidine (Figure 2.7). Depending on the experimental design, the secretagogue used and the species being studied, ranitidine had a potency three to ten times greater than that of cimetidine. However, the duration of action of the two compounds was very similar after both parenteral and oral administration.

In the development of new H$_2$-antagonists, the issue of duration of action became of considerable importance. The dosing regimens for the therapeutic use of H$_2$-antagonists in acid-related diseases was initially three or four times per day since both cimetidine and ranitidine were relatively short acting and 24 h control of gastric acid secretion was considered desirable. Thus, the search for a long-acting H$_2$-antagonist made sense, particularly from the point of view of patient compliance.

Smith Kline & French synthesized a potent and long-acting histamine H$_2$-receptor antagonist, SK&F 93479 (lupitidine). The compound was more potent than either cimetidine or ranitidine in animal experimental studies (Figure 2.8). However, in the 2 year rat carcinogenicity study, animals receiving the top dose of 1000 mg kg^{-1} p.o. daily showed a significant incidence of carcinoid tumours in the fundic mucosa (Betton and Salmon, 1985). On histological examination, these tumours were found to be associated with the

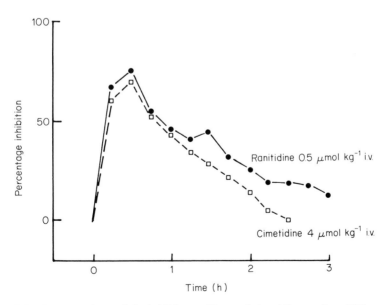

Figure 2.7 A comparison of the inhibitory effects of cimetidine and ranitidine, given as bolus intravenous injection, on a maximal plateau secretory response to an intravenous infusion of histamine in the dog

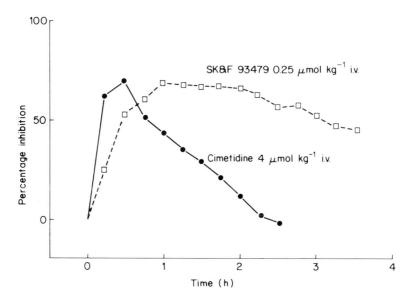

Figure 2.8 A comparison of the inhibitory effects of cimetidine and SK&F 93479 (lupitidine), given as bolus intravenous injection, on a maximal plateau secretory response to an intravenous infusion of histamine in the dog

histamine-containing enterochromaffin-like cells. A similar problem was found with loxtidine, a very long acting H_2-antagonist synthesized by Glaxo (Poynter *et al.*, 1985), and both compounds were withdrawn from development.

The Glaxo group suggested that the phenomenon was associated with 'unsurmountable' antagonism, but the primary cause appears to be the sustained duration of action. At the high toxicological doses used, virtually complete inhibition of acidity will be produced over a 24 h period. This effect has led to the elaboration of the so-called gastrin hypothesis.

The release of gastrin from the pyloric antrum is controlled in part at least by the pH of the fluid bathing the antral mucosa. At pH values below approximately 3.5, gastrin release is inhibited, whereas elevation above this level, as would occur with high doses of H_2-antagonists, results in elevated plasma gastrin levels. With long-acting H_2-antagonists, this hypergastrinaemia would be sustained over long periods. In addition to its ability to stimulate gastric acid secretion, gastrin is a trophic hormone stimulating growth of the gastric mucosa. It is assumed that this trophic effect acts on the enterochromaffin-like cells leading to hyperplasia and eventually carcinoid formation.

It is interesting to note that a similar toxicological problem has been found with omeprazole, an H^+/K^+-ATPase inhibitor acting on the final step of acid production, which also has a very long duration of action, and the 'gastrin hypothesis' has been used to explain the effects of this compound. Clinical studies with omeprazole are continuing, but to date no truly long-acting histamine H$_2$-receptor antagonist has entered the market place although several are under development.

While the search for long-acting H$_2$-antagonists went on, the pattern of dosing of the short-acting H$_2$-antagonists such as cimetidine and ranitidine in clinical practice was changing. Frequency of dosing was reduced and clinical trials showed that, at least in duodenal ulcer disease, single night-time doses produced healing rates similar to those obtained with divided doses. Two new H$_2$-antagonists, famotidine and nizatidine, have been recently introduced on to the market with a recommended dosage of a single tablet at night.

Whether or not new potent long-acting H$_2$-antagonists will reach the marketplace remains to be seen. If so, it will be of interest to see if they can match the rapidity and high incidence of healing achieved with omeprazole.

CONCLUSIONS

The identification of a second type of histamine receptor and the discovery of specific antagonists for this receptor led to a great increase in our understanding of the physiological control of gastric acid secretion. The ability of histamine H$_2$-receptor antagonists to inhibit virtually all forms of acid secretion established a central role for histamine, although the precise nature of this role has yet to be completely elucidated.

This antisecretory activity of H$_2$-antagonists has led to a revolution in the therapy of acid-related diseases. Further development of our understanding of the role of histamine in gastric physiology and pathophysiology, together with the discovery of new histamine H$_2$-receptor antagonists, will be awaited with interest.

REFERENCES

Aadland, E. and Berstad, A. (1978). Effect of cimetidine on pentagastrin-stimulated gastric acid and pepsin secretion before and after 6 weeks of cimetidine treatment, *Scand. J. Gastroenterol.*, **13**, 193–7.

Albinus, M. (1979). Action of gastric secretagogues on the oxygen consumption in isolated gastric mucosal cells of the guinea-pig, *N.S. Arch. Pharmacol.*, **307** (Suppl. R52).

Berglindh, T. and Öbrink, K. J. (1979). Histamine as a physiological stimulant of gastric parietal cells. In T. O. Yellin (ed.) *Histamine Receptors*, SP Medical and Scientific Books, New York, pp. 35–56.

Bergqvist, E., Waller, M., Hammer, L. and Öbrink, K. J. (1980). Histamine as the secretory mediator in isolated gastric glands. In I. Schulz, G. Sachs, J. G. Forte and K. J. Ulrich (eds) *Hydrogen Ion Transport in Epithelia*, Elsevier/North-Holland Biomedical Press, Amsterdam, pp. 429–37.

Betton, G. R. and Salmon, G. K. (1985). Neuroendocrine carcinoid tumours of the glandular stomach of the rat following treatment with the H$_2$-receptor antagonist SK&F 93479, *26th Congress of European Society of Toxicology*, Kupio, Abstract P32.

Black, J. W., Duncan, W. A. M., Durant, G. J., Ganellin, C. R. and Parsons, M. E. (1972). Definition and antagonism of histamine H$_2$-receptors, *Nature*, **236**, 385–90.

Bunce, K. T. and Parsons, M. E. (1976). A quantitative study of metiamide, a histamine H$_2$-receptor antagonist, on the isolated whole rat stomach, *J. Physiol. (Lond.)*, **258**, 453–65.

Bunce, K. T., Parsons, M. E. and Rollings, N. A. (1976). The effect of metiamide on acid secretion stimulated by gastrin, acetylcholine, and dibutyryl cyclic adenosine 3′,5′-monophosphate in the isolated whole stomach of the rat, *Br. J. Pharmacol.*, **58**, 149–56.

Bunce, K. T., Honey, A. C. and Parsons, M. E. (1979). Investigation of the role of extracellular calcium in the control of acid secretion in the isolated whole stomach of the rat, *Br. J. Pharmacol.*, **67**, 123–31.

Carter, D. C., Forrest, J. A. H., Logan, R. A. *et al.* (1976). Effect of the histamine H$_2$-receptor antagonist, cimetidine, on gastric secretion and serum gastrin during insulin infusion in man, *Scand. J. Gastroenterol.*, **11**, 565–70.

Cheret, A. M., Girodet, J. and Lewin, M. (1977). Stimulation of isolated rat parietal cell by gastrin. In S. Bonfils, P. Fromageot and G. Rosselin (eds) *Hormonal Receptors in Digestive Tract Physiology*, Elsevier/North-Holland, Amsterdam, p. 405.

Code, C. F. (1956). Histamine and gastric secretion. In G. E. W. Wolstenholme and C. M. O'Connor (eds) *Histamine*, Churchill, London, pp. 189–219.

Code, C. F. (1965). Histamine and gastric secretion: a later look, 1955–1965, *Fed. Proc.*, **24**, 1311–33.

Edkins, J. S. (1905). On the chemical mechanism of gastric secretion, *Proc. R. Soc. (Lond.) Ser. B. Biol. Sci.*, **76**, 376.

Gregory, R. A. and Tracy, H. J. (1961). The preparation and properties of gastrin, *J. Physiol.*, **156**, 523–43.

Grossman, M. I. and Konturek, S. J. (1974). Inhibition of acid secretion in dog by metiamide, a histamine antagonist acting on H$_2$-receptors, *Gastroenterology*, **66**, 517–21.

Hammer, R., Berrie, C. P., Birdsall, N. J. M., Burgen, A. S. V. and Hulme, E. C. (1980). Pirenzepine distinguishes between different subclasses of muscarinic receptors, *Nature*, **283**, 90–92.

Jennewein, H. M., Herbst, M. and Waldeck, F. (1979). Functional oxygen consumption of isolated rat gastric mucosal cells in comparison to the *in vivo* function of the rat gastric mucosa, *N.S. Arch. Pharmacol.*, **307** (Suppl. R52).

Johnson, L. R. (1971). Control of gastric secretion: no room for histamine?, *Gastroenterology*, **61**, 106–18.

Kahlson, G., Rosengren, E., Svahn, D. and Thunberg, R. (1964). Mobilization and formation of histamine in the gastric mucosa as related to acid secretion, *J. Physiol.*, **174**, 400–16.

Longstreth, G. F., Go, V. L. W. and Malagelada, J. R. (1976). Cimetidine suppression of nocturnal acid secretion in active duodenal ulcer, *New Engl. J. Med.*, **294**, 801–4.

McIntosh, F. C. (1938). Histamine is a normal stimulant of gastric secretion, *Q. J. Exp. Physiol.*, **28**, 87–98.

Main, I. H. M. and Pearce, J. B. (1977). Histamine output from the rat isolated gastric mucosa during acid secretion stimulated by pentagastrin, methacholine and dibutyryl-cyclic adenosine 3′,5′-monophosphate, *Br. J. Pharmacol.*, **61**, 461.

Muallem, S. and Sachs, G. (1984). Changes in cytosolic free Ca^{2+} in isolated parietal cells: differential effects of secretagogues, *Biochim. Biophys. Acta*, **805**, 181–6.

Popielski, L. (1920). β-Imidazolylathylamine und de Organextrakte: β-Imidazolylathylamin als Machtiger Erreger der Magendruson, *Pflug. Arch. Eur. J. Physiol.*, **178**, 214–26.

Poynter, D., Pick, C. R., Harcourt, R. A. *et al.* (1985). Association of long lasting unsurmountable histamine H$_2$-blockade and gastric carcinoid tumours in the rat, *Gut*, **26**, 1284–95.

Rangachari, P. K. (1975). Histamine release by gastric stimulants, *Nature*, **253**, 53–5.

Rosenfeld, G. C., Ecknauer, R., Johnson, L. R. and Thompson, W. J. (1978). Purified gastric mucosal parietal cells: demonstration of [^{3}H] QNB binding to cholinergic receptors, *7th International Congress of Pharmacology*, Paris, Abstract 319.

Sachs, G. (1986). The parietal cell as a therapeutic target, *Scand. J. Gastroenterol.*, **21** (Suppl. 118), 1–10.

Scholes, P., Cooper, A., Jones, D., Major, J., Walters, M. and Wilde, C. (1976). Characterization of an adenylate cyclase system sensitive to histamine H$_2$-receptor excitation in cells from dog gastric mucosa, *Agents Actions*, **6**, 677–82.

Schoon, I. M. and Olbe, L. (1978). Inhibitory effect of cimetidine on gastric acid secretion vagally activated by physiological means in duodenal ulcer patients, *Gut*, **19**, 27–31.

Soll, A. H. (1978a). The action of secretagogues on oxygen uptake by isolated mammalian parietal cells, *J. Clin. Invest.*, **61**, 370–80.

Soll, A. H. (1978b). The interaction of histamine with gastrin and carbamylcholine on oxygen uptake by isolated mammalian parietal cells, *J. Clin. Invest.*, **61**, 381–9.

Soll, A. H. (1978c). Three-way interactions between histamine, carbachol and gastrin on aminopyrine uptake by isolated canine parietal cells, *Gastroenterology*, **74**, 1146.

Soll, A. H. (1981). Extracellular calcium and cholinergic stimulation of isolated parietal cells, *J. Clin. Invest.*, **68**, 270–8.

Soll, A. H. (1982). Histamine and gastric acid secretion: studies with isolated canine fundic mucosal cells. In B. Uvnas and K. Tasaka (eds) *Advances in Histamine Research*, Pergamon Press, Oxford, pp. 189–201.

Soll, A. H. (1986). Mechanisms of action of antisecretory drugs, *Scand. J. Gastroenterol.*, **21** (Suppl. 125), 1–6.

Soll, A. H., Amerian, D. A., Thomas, L. P., Reedy, T. J. and Elashoff, J. D. (1984). Gastrin receptors on isolated canine parietal cells, *J. Clin. Invest.*, **73**, 1434–47.

Speir, G. R., Takeuchi, K. and Johnson, L. R. (1979). Binding characteristics and assay standardization of the gastrin receptor on rat gastric mucosa, *Gastroenterology*, **76**, 1253.

Advances in Drug Therapy of Gastrointestinal Ulceration
Edited by A. Garner and B. J. R. Whittle
© 1989 John Wiley & Sons Ltd

Chapter Three

Mechanisms of Parietal Cell Function

John G. Forte, David K. Hanzel and Tetsuro Urushidani
Department of Physiology–Anatomy, University of California, Berkeley, California 94707, USA

INTRODUCTION

The gastric parietal cell is responsible for the secretion of a voluminous juice which is isotonic hydrochloric acid. Because of its unusual secretory function, the parietal cell has evolved a number of structures and activities that might at first appear as very highly specialized, but on closer inspection they can be viewed as exaggerations of more typical cellular processes. The formation of a highly acidic secretory juice requires an enormous energetic commitment, and parietal cells have high oxidative metabolic capacity to meet the demand. The gastric proton pump is closely related to other, widespread cation pumps, but the gastric enzyme has specifically evolved to meet the power requirements of transport against high gradient and flow. The very acts of turning hydrochloric acid secretion on and off, in collaboration with digestive activities, employ intracellular messengers common to many cells, but the effector pathways are exaggerated in parietal cells, involving massive cytological rearrangements of the cell membranes containing the ion transport pathways. For every mole of acid secreted into the gastric lumen, an equivalent amount of base is produced and released into the blood stream. Thus, parietal cells must have efficient ways to deal with intracellular base. Finally, the parietal cell must have specialized means for protecting itself from its own acidic secretions. This review focuses on the structural and functional changes in parietal cells related to physiological secretory states. In particular, it examines processes of membrane recycling, ion pumps and transport pathways, and possible paths of regulation through protein phosphorylation.

MORPHOLOGICAL CHANGES
ASSOCIATED WITH SECRETION

Parietal cells are located within the tubular glands, interspersed among other epithelial cells, in the mucosa of the fundus and body of the stomach.

They are readily distinguished (1) as being larger than their neighbours, (2) by their position towards the wall of the gland, and (3) by their unique system of secretory canaliculi that invaginate from the apical surface and ramify throughout the cell (Helander, 1981; Ito, 1987). Numerous large mitochondria, to power the energetic demands of hydrochloric acid secretion, are another characteristic feature of parietal cells. Nearly 100 years ago, Camillo Golgi (1893) used the light microscope to identify the network of parietal cell canaliculi and to document that the secretory canaliculi become enlarged in cells of the 'digesting stomach', as compared to the fasting animal.

The electron microscope has provided a more detailed view of the elaborate ultrastructural changes that accompany parietal secretory activity. In resting, or non-secreting, cells the apical plasma membrane bordering the canaliculi is characterized by short stubby microvilli, and the sub-adjacent cytoplasmic space is literally packed with tubular and vesicular membrane structures, called tubulovesicles (Figure 3.1). Actin microfilaments support the apical microvilli, anchoring at the microvillar tip, running their length, and often extending up to $1 \mu m$ into the cytoplasm (Black, Forte and Forte, 1982). In maximally stimulated parietal cells the tubulovesicles have all but disappeared; on the other hand, the apical microvilli have become greatly elongated (Figure 3.2). Helander and Hirschowitz (1972) applied morphometric analysis to parietal cells of dog stomach to show that the five- to ten-fold increase in apical plasma membrane area of stimulated cells could be accounted for by the decrease in equivalent membrane surface area of tubulovesicles. When the stimulus is withdrawn, or appropriate inhibitors are added, secretory canaliculi collapse and the parietal cell is ultimately transformed to the resting morphology by sequestration of apical plasma membrane back into intracellular tubulovesicles (Forte, Machen and Forte, 1977; Helander and Hirschowitz, 1972). These ultrastructural changes form the basis for the membrane recycling hypothesis of hydrochloric acid secretion (Forte *et al.*, 1981). When the parietal cell is stimulated, tubulovesicles fuse with apical canalicular membranes, bringing the transport machinery into operation; withdrawal of the stimulus leads to conservative uptake of the membrane back into the resting form (Figure 3.3).

H^+,K^+-ATPase: THE PRIMARY GASTRIC PROTON PUMP

The concentration of primary oxyntic juice is about $0.16 \, mol \, l^{-1}$ hydrochloric acid, and this is ultimately derived from blood where the H^+ concentration is $10^{-7.4} \, mol \, l^{-1}$, i.e. pH 7.4. Thus, the gastric epithelium, and parietal cells in particular, can produce and sustain a gradient of H^+ concentration greater than a million fold. The ionic pump that produces the primary transport event is a K^+-stimulated ATP-hydrolysing membrane-bound enzyme called the H^+,K^+-ATPase. Fundic gastric mucosa is rich in H^+,K^+-ATPase activity and

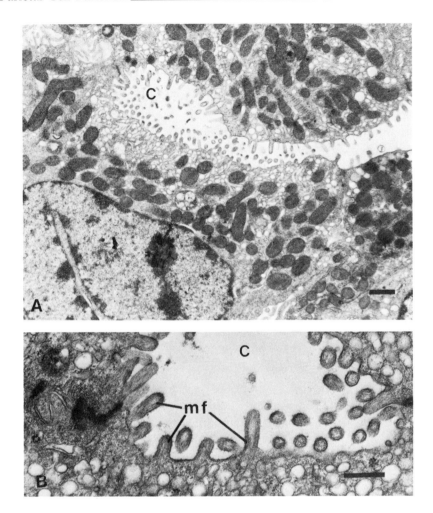

Figure 3.1 Electron micrographs of non-secreting (resting) parietal cells in piglet gastric mucosa. A: Short microvilli line the lumen of a secretory canaliculus (C). Numerous tubular and vesicular membrane profiles (called tubulovesicles) are found in the apical region of the cell. Many mitochondria are also evident. Bar marker, 1 μm. B: Apical surface of resting parietal cell at higher power showing microfilaments (mf) within the short microvilli. Subadjacent tubulovesicles are also readily apparent. Bar marker, 0.5 μm.
(Reproduced from Forte *et al.* (1983) by permission of Raven Press)

the enzyme appears to be unique to parietal cells (Forte *et al.*, 1975; Smolka *et al.*, 1983), although reports have suggested that it might also be represented at low levels in several other tissues. The enzyme was first isolated as a K^+-stimulated ATPase activity, and an associated *p*-nitrophenyl phosphatase (pNPPase) activity, in a purified microsomal fraction from amphibian gastric

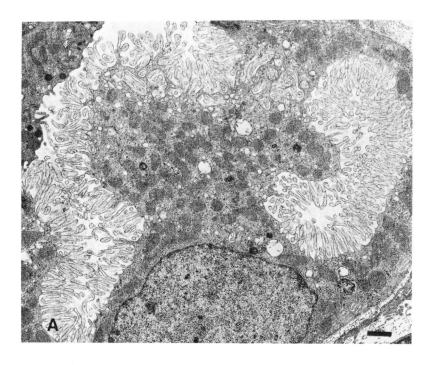

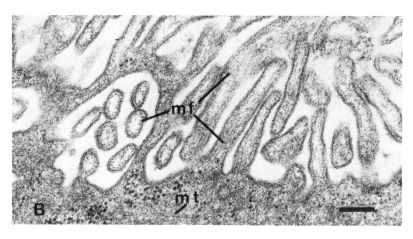

Figure 3.2 Electron micrographs of histamine-stimulated parietal cells. A: Apical microvilli are extensive and greatly elongated, whereas cytoplasmic tubulovesicles are drastically reduced compared to resting (cf. Figure 3.1). Bar marker, 1 μm. B: Apical microvilli shown at higher magnification to demonstrate microfilaments (mf). A microtubule (mt) can also be seen near the cell surface. Bar marker, 0.2 μm. (Reproduced from Forte *et al.* (1983) by permission of Raven Press)

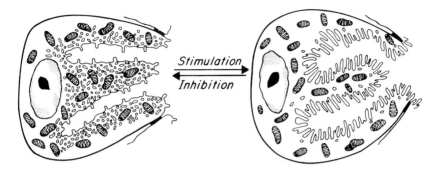

Figure 3.3 Schematic representation of parietal cells at rest and after stimulation. The membrane transformations between cytoplasmic tubulovesicles and apical plasma membrane bordering the secretory canaliculi form the basis of the membrane recycling hypothesis of hydrochloric acid secretion

mucosa (Ganser and Forte, 1973). The general occurrence of the enzyme in the oxyntic mucosa of many species was subsequently established (Forte *et al.*, 1975; Forte, Ganser and Ray, 1976). The highly purified gastric microsomal fraction that is rich in H^+,K^+-ATPase has now been shown to be derived from tubulovesicles from parietal cells. A crude microsomal fraction is obtained from fundic mucosal homogenates as the membrane fraction that sediments between $14\,000\,g \times 10\,\text{min}$ and $100\,000\,g \times 1\,\text{h}$, and contains 70–90% of the total H^+,K^+-ATPase from non-secreting stomach (see discussion below). The microsomes are purified of contaminants, such as submitochondrial particles, rough endoplasmic reticulum and basolateral membranes, by density gradient centrifugation, yielding a homogeneous, low-density (1.08–1.11), vesicular fraction (Forte *et al.*, 1975; Saccomani *et al.*, 1977).

Purified gastric microsomal vesicles have been used to study the characteristics of proton transport *in vitro* (e.g. Lee, Simpson and Scholes, 1974; Sachs *et al.*, 1976; Lee and Forte, 1978). When supplemented with ATP, Mg^{2+} and K^+ the microsomal vesicles transport H^+ into the vesicles and K^+ out of the vesicles. Sachs *et al.* (1976) demonstrated that the microsomal proton pump was non-electrogenic, that is, ATP hydrolysis drives the one-for-one exchange of H^+ for K^+. The non-electrogenic nature of the gastric proton pump, as well as its sensitivity to inhibitors and subunit structure, has been used to differentiate it from F_0-F_1 proton pumps that operate in mitochondria, chloroplasts and microorganisms (Sachs *et al.*, 1976).

The H^+,K^+-ATPase utilizes ATP to catalyse the transmembrane exchange of H^+ from cell to lumen and K^+ from lumen to cell. Biochemical studies on the enzyme and its partial reactions have yielded a considerable amount of detail (Ray and Forte, 1976; Wallmark *et al.*, 1980; Sachs, 1987). The gastric

H^+K^+-ATPase belongs to the class of enzymes known as E_1–E_2 ATPases, all of which have two distinct sequential forms of phosphorylated intermediate and have molecular weights of about 100 000. Although the catalytic cycle of the H^+,K^+-ATPase is not completely established, a reasonable sequence of reaction can be described as follows:

(1) $\quad H_C^+ + ATP + E_1 \rightleftharpoons H \cdot E_1 \cdot ATP \rightleftharpoons H \cdot E_1 - P + ADP$

(2) $\quad H \cdot E_1 - P + K_L^+ \rightleftharpoons H_L^+ + K \cdot E_2 - P$

(3) $\quad K \cdot E_2 - P \rightleftharpoons K \cdot E_2 \cdot P \rightleftharpoons E_1 + P_i + K_C^+$

$$H_C^+ + ATP + K_L^+ \rightleftharpoons H_L^+ + ADP + P_i + K_C^+$$

where E_1 and E_2 represent two different conformational forms of the enzyme; the 'dash' forms (e.g. E_1–P) represent covalent association as a phosphoenzyme; the 'dot' forms (e.g. $K \cdot E_2 \cdot P$) represent ionic associations; and the subscripts C and L represent cytoplasmic and luminal locations, respectively, for the transported ions. The overall cycle is described here as three sets of partial reactions:

(1) kinase activity involving formation of a phosphoenzyme intermediate,
(2) transition between an H^+ binding form and a K^+ binding form (possibly the major ion translocation step),
(3) phosphatase activity.

In many regards the catalytic cycle of the H^+,K^+-ATPase is similar to that of two other cation-transporting E_1–E_2 ATPases, the ubiquitous Na^+,K^+-ATPase and the Ca^{2+}-ATPase of sarcoplasmic reticulum. In fact, the primary amino acid sequences of these three ATPases show remarkable homologies (Shull and Lingrel, 1986), suggesting a common ancestry and the structural importance of certain sequential groupings in conveying membrane transport function. Although the similarities are informative, there are differences as well. It has been suggested that the greatest structural divergence among the three ATPases occurs in the domains that confer ion specificity, while the regions involved in nucleotide binding, phosphorylation and energy transduction are highly conserved (Shull and Lingrel, 1986). The H^+,K^+-ATPase operates against the most stringent transmembrane gradient (i.e. greater than 10^6-fold). The enormous proton gradient sets an energy requirement that must be met by that available from ATP hydrolysis. Because of this thermodynamic constraint, the H^+,K^+-ATPase has a 'unitary' stoichiometry for its turnover under physiological conditions, that is $1H^+ : 1K^+ : 1ATP$ (Reenstra, Lee and Forte, 1980), in comparison to higher orders for the other enzymes.

The general features of ion transport in gastric microsomal vesicles are shown schematically in Figure 3.4. The model depicts the electroneutral H^+/K^+ pump as well as the pathways for passive flux of the principal ionic species K^+, Cl^- and H^+. In the presence of an ample supply of Mg^{2+}-ATP, turnover of the pump is limited by the availability of K^+ at intravesicular sites; thus vesicular permeability to K^+ is critical for pump operation. Moreover, if the vesicles are to produce a net transport of H^+ as HCl, the rate of Cl^- entry, as the anion that must accompany K^+, could also be limiting. These particular limitations of K^+ and Cl^- permeability in gastric microsomes are demonstrated in the proton uptake data of Figure 3.5 (Lee *et al.*, 1979). The addition of ATP to microsomes causes very little proton uptake until a K^+ ionophore, valinomycin, is added. Under these latter conditions, when K^+ permeability is high, the rate of proton uptake can be seen to be limited by the concentration of permeant anion (in this case Cl^-). Anions that are more permeable than Cl^- have been shown to promote an even faster rate of microsomal proton accumulation (Lee *et al.*, 1979). The membrane permeability to H^+ also represents a limitation, especially in the maximum gradient that is formed, since it represents a pathway for proton backflux, or leakage. We can conclude that the

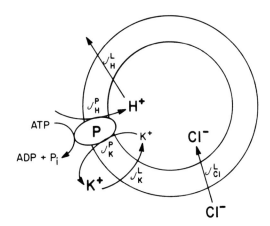

Figure 3.4 Model of H^+ pumping and ion transport in gastric membrane vesicles. The pump (P) is an H^+,K^+-ATPase that uses ATP to pump H^+ into vesicles and K^+ out of vesicles. Pathways are also shown for the passive flux (J^L) of K^+, Cl^- and H^+. When [ATP] is not limiting, the turnover of the pump is limited by [K^+] at an intravesicular site, which in turn is limited by the rate of K^+ entry and, to satisfy electroneutrality, the rate of anion (Cl^-) entry. For gastric microsomes derived from tubulovesicles the intrinsic permeabilities to K^+ and Cl^- are low, thus the use of valinomycin and high [Cl^-] and [K^+] are required for rapid vesicular uptake of HCl. Isolated apical plasma membrane vesicles from stimulated parietal cells (s.a. vesicles) have intrinsic conductance pathways for rapid flux of K^+ and Cl^-, uptake of HCl can process at rapid rates determined by the turnover number of the pump. (Reproduced from Lee *et al.* (1979) by permission of Elsevier Science Publishers BV)

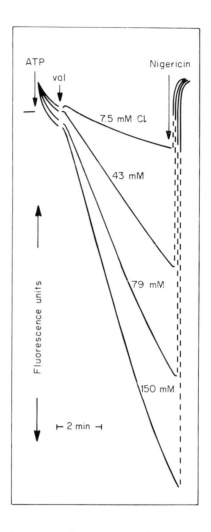

Figure 3.5 H^+ uptake in gastric microsomal vesicles is dependent on Cl^- concentration and K^+ ionophores. H^+ uptake was monitored by the acridine orange method, and is proportional to the rate of fluorescence quenching. Addition of ATP to a suspension of microsomal vesicles resulted in a small uptake of H^+ that was accelerated by the subsequent addition of the K^+ ionophore valinomycin (val). K^+ concentration was constant at $150\,\mathrm{mmol\,l^{-1}}$ in all cases. Cl^- concentration was varied as shown, with isethionate being used as the balance anion. The rate of H^+ uptake was greatly enhanced by increasing the concentration of the permeant anion, Cl^-. All H^+ gradients were abolished by the H^+–K^+ exchange ionophore nigericin. (Reproduced from Lee and Forte (1978) by permission of Elsevier Science Publishers BV)

most effective HCl transport based on the H^+/K^+ pump would take place in vesicles with high permeability to K^+ and Cl^- and low permeability to H^+. This is not the state of gastric microsomes (tubulovesicles) since they have relatively low K^+ and Cl^- permeability.

CELLULAR LOCALIZATION AND SECRETORY DYNAMICS OF H^+,K^+-ATPase

The measured distribution of H^+,K^+-ATPase among cell fractions derived from gastric homogenates by differential centrifugation provides important information on functional dynamics of the enzyme during the secretory cycle (Wolosin and Forte, 1981). For resting gastric mucosa the enzyme was found predominantly (~80%) in the microsomal fraction, that is the smallest membrane particles represented as P3 in Table 3.1. These gastric microsomes

Table 3.1 H^+,K^+-ATPase is redistributed among subcellular fractions during stimulation or inhibition of acid secretion

	H^+ secretory rate		Percentage of total H^+,K^+-ATPase activity in cell fraction				Redistribution ratio
	n	μeq min^{-1}	P1	P2	P3	S3	P1/P3
Resting stomach	5	4.8 ± 2.3	12.0	8.1	78.1	1.8	0.15
Histamine-stimulated	5	78.9 ± 9.0	60.4	19.0	20.7	1.2	2.92
Time after H_2 blocker							
10 min	4	37.3 ± 7.6	38.8	14.6	42.4	4.1	0.92
15 min	4	26.6 ± 6.6	35.0	21.8	39.4	3.8	0.89
20 min	3	17.5 ± 6.6	28.7	12.5	59.5	0	0.48
45 min	3	4.8 ± 2.2	22.2	14.2	61.5	2.1	0.36

Rabbits were fasted overnight, anaesthetized and a plastic cannula secured into the stomach for collecting gastric juice; the juice was subsequently titrated to determine H^+ secretory rates. The experimental design was to compare stomachs from animals under various functional states of rest (i.e. non-secreting), maximal histamine-stimulation, and after H^+ secretion was inhibited by a powerful H_2-receptor antagonist (i.e. 12.5 μmol SKF 93479 i.v., Blakemore *et al.*, 1981). Under conditions and/or times as indicated, stomachs were removed, and the fundic mucosa was scraped, homogenized and separated by centrifugation into cell fractions (Hirst and Forte, 1985). After removing a very low speed fraction of tissue debris ($40 \times g \times 5$ min), the following fractions were separated: P1, $4000 \times g \times 10$ min; P2, $14\,000 \times g \times 10$ min; P3, $49\,000 \times g \times 90$ min; and S3, supernatant. K^+-stimulated *p*-nitrophenylphosphatase was measured as a marker of H^+,K^+-ATPase activity, and values are shown for percentage of total enzyme activity in each fraction. The redistribution ratio, P1/P3, demonstrates the large redistribution of H^+,K^+-ATPase activity among particulate fractions associated with histamine stimulation and recovery after H_2-receptor blockade can be further purified by density gradient centrifugation, providing a homogeneous population of vesicles, highly enriched in H^+,K^+-ATPase, which is derived from cytoplasmic tubulovesicles.

When gastric mucosa from maximally stimulated stomach was subjected to the same homogenization/centrifugation described above there was a surprise in store; H^+,K^+-ATPase activity was greatly reduced in microsomes and was distributed to larger membrane particles, e.g. P1 in Table 3.1 (Wolosin and Forte, 1981). Further purification of H^+,K^+-ATPase from this latter fraction produced a preparation of large, dense, often structurally complex, membrane vesicles derived from the apical canalicular membrane of the stimulated parietal cells. Hence they are called stimulation-associated (s.a.) vesicles. Furthermore, going from rest to maximal histamine-stimulated hydrochloric acid secretion and back to conditions of no secretion produced a defined and apparently cyclic redistribution of H^+,K^+-ATPase activity, as shown by the data of Table 3.1. These secretion-dependent changes in distribution of H^+,K^+-ATPase are consistent with the transformations and recycling of membranes seen through electron microscopy.

Important structural and functional differences exist between the H^+,K^+-ATPase-rich membranes from resting and stimulated parietal cells. The purified microsomes are homogeneous, primarily unilamellar, vesicles oriented with their ATP-hydrolysing sites (i.e. cytoplasmic surface) facing outside. Analysis of microsomal composition shows that the 94 000 molecular weight H^+,K^+-ATPase is the dominant protein (Figure 3.6); a broad band of glycoprotein (mol. wt 60 000–80 000) is also characteristically present. H^+,K^+-ATPase-rich vesicles from stimulated parietal cells are structurally complex, as would be expected from the fragmentation of the elaborate apical canalicular surfaces. Membrane orientation appears more random than for the microsomes; about 25–40% of the ATP-hydrolysing sites are exposed to the exterior, and the rest of the H^+,K^+-ATPase activity is 'cryptic', being contained as vesicles within vesicles and/or in vesicles oriented with their cytoplasmic surface inside (Hirst and Forte, 1985). Compositional analysis reveals that these stimulation-associated membranes contain an abundance of H^+,K^+-ATPase (mol. wt 94 000) and also shows additional major bands (Figure 3.6), such as actin (mol. wt 40 000) and an 80 000 mol. wt protein (Forte *et al.*, 1983). The significance of these two latter proteins will be discussed below.

The most interesting functional differences between microsomal vesicles and s.a. vesicles concern their transport and permeability characteristics. Proton transport activity proceeds at high rates in s.a. vesicles without the requirement for any exogenous ionophore (Figure 3.7), which is in contrast to the situation observed for gastric microsomes (Figures 3.5 and 3.7). To date, we have observed no differences in the basic catalytic activity of the H^+,K^+-ATPase, that is, no activation of the enzyme *per se*. The reason for the functional differences in proton transport by the two types of gastric membrane vesicles concerns their

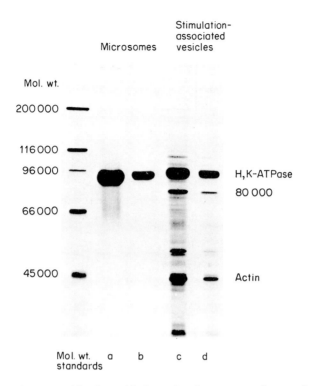

Figure 3.6 Protein composition in purified gastric microsomes and s.a. vesicles revealed by SDS-PAGE. Molecular weight of standards are indicated. Lanes a and c have 50 μg total protein; lanes b and d have 25 μg protein. The single most prominent band in microsomes is the H^+,K^+-ATPase at mol. wt 94 000. There is also a very broad band of glycoprotein in the region of 60 000–80 000 mol. wt that does not stain well with Coomassie blue. In addition to H^+,K^+-ATPase the s.a. vesicles have prominent bands at 40 000 (actin) and 80 000 mol. wt (see text)

permeability to potassium chloride. In addition to H^+,K^+-ATPase, s.a. vesicles have pathways for the rapid flux of K^+ and Cl^-, actually high conductance pathways, whereas microsomes are relatively impermeable to K^+ and Cl^- (Wolosin and Forte, 1984, 1985). The general model presented in Figure 3.4 must be expanded for s.a. vesicles to include specific channels whereby permeabilities to K^+ and to Cl^- greatly exceed the permeability to H^+.

These observations on H^+,K^+-ATPase redistribution and changes in transport properties of the H^+,K^+-ATPase-rich membranes suggest a means by which gastric hydrochloric acid secretion is regulated, as shown in Figure 3.8. In resting cells the H^+,K^+-ATPase is localized to tubulovesicles. The low permeabilities to K^+ and Cl^- limit the turnover of the H^+/K^+ pump, and there is no accessibility to the lumen. Fusion of tubulovesicles with the apical canalicular membrane provides a luminal access for the pump. In addition, the

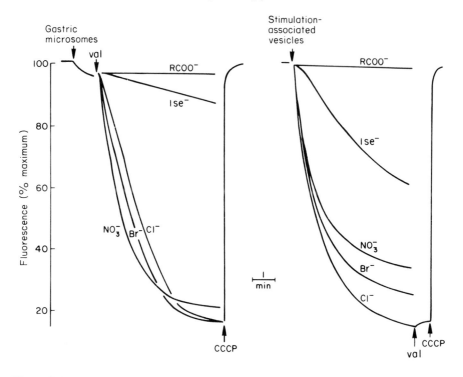

Figure 3.7 Patterns of H^+ uptake by gastric microsomes compared with s.a. vesicles. All tests were performed in 150 mmol l^{-1} K^+ solution with the balance anion being as indicated (Ise$^-$ is isethionate and RCOO$^-$ is either acetate or gluconate). The medium also contained buffer, pH 7.05, 0.5 μmol l^{-1} Mg^{2+}, 0.5 μmol l^{-1} ATP and 4 μmol l^{-1} acridine orange. The rate of H^+ uptake was measured by the rate of acridine orange fluorescence quenching. The most significant difference between microsomes and s.a. vesicles is the dependence upon valinomycin: microsomes require the K^+ ionophore to effect rapid H^+ uptake; s.a. vesicles do not. Carboxylate ions are impermeable, therefore H^+ uptake is nil with acetate or gluconate. Microsomes demonstrate an anionic preference to support H^+ uptake, suggestive of simple passive membrane permeability: $NO_3^- > Br^- > Cl^- > Ise^-$. The dependence of initial H^+ uptake rate on anions in s.a. vesicles shows a different order: $Cl^- > Br^- > NO_3^- > Ise^-$; with sulphonates, such as Ise$^-$ or methylsuphonate, promoting measurable uptake rates. For all cases where H^+ permeability was greatly increased by adding CCCP (carbonylcyanide-*m*-chlorophenyl hydrazone), the proton gradient dissipated. (Adapted from Wolosin and Forte (1983) by permission of Springer-Verlag NY Inc.)

luminal membrane is highly permeable to K^+ and Cl^-. The flow of potassium chloride from cell to lumen provides K^+ for which the pump exchanges H^+, and Cl^- which will be the co-ion for net hydrochloric acid secretion. At the present time, it is uncertain as to how K^+ and Cl^- channels get into the apical membrane. For example, they might be permanent residents of the apical membrane or they might be part of another vesicle type that fuses under the

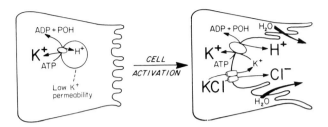

Figure 3.8 Schematic representation of parietal cell activation as the cell is transformed from rest to active hydrochloric acid secretion. In the resting cell, tubulovesicles contain H^+,K^+-ATPase, but because of low membrane permeability to K^+ (and Cl^-) there is very little H^+ accumulation and virtually no ATP turnover. Cell activation brings about a fusion of tubulovesicles with the apical plasma membrane, transferring the H^+,K^+-ATPase to that surface. In addition the participation of conductive pathways (possibly activated?) for K^+ and Cl^- movement provides the means for KCl movement into the secretory canaliculi. The H^+/K^+ exchange pump recycles K^+ back into the cytoplasm with the net effect of HCl transfer and ATP turnover. Water flux into the canaliculus is osmotically driven by net solute flux

influence of stimulation (e.g. Im, Blakeman and Davis, 1985). Moreover, it is not known whether the channels are always active or whether they undergo a change in state with stimulation. These are questions of critical importance for future study.

CHANGES IN PHOSPHORYLATION ASSOCIATED WITH STIMULATION

The question of secretagogue–receptor relationships in parietal cells is beyond the scope of this review, and is addressed by other authors in this volume. However, we have recently examined some of the intracellular changes that occur when parietal cells are stimulated to secrete hydrochloric acid. Stimulus–secretion coupling in many systems is regulated by activation of intracellular kinases and the subsequent phosphorylation of substrate effector proteins. It was of interest for us to search for those proteins that serve as substrates for phosphorylation in the activation of parietal cell secretion. To do this we needed an *in vitro* system that was physiologically responsive to activation. The isolated gastric gland preparation (Berglindh, Helander and Obrink, 1976) was used, and tested for those secretagogues that were competent to bring about the functional changes in membrane distribution and properties that were associated with hydrochloric acid secretion (Urushidani and Forte, 1987). In our hands the histamine/cyclic AMP pathway was the most effective in the isolated gland preparation. That is, the addition of cyclic AMP analogues, or agents that cause an elevation of intracellular cyclic AMP (e.g. histamine, histamine plus isobutylmethylxanthine or forskolin), produced functional changes in rabbit gastric glands that were most similar to intact stomach. For the phosphorylation studies, glands were preincubated in $^{32}P_i$ for 40 min, washed with unlabelled buffer, and divided into aliquots to receive secretagogues, or not. After an appropriate experimental period the glands were homogenized, separated into cell fractions, and the fractions examined for enzyme activity, protein and ^{32}P incorporation (Urushidani, Hanzel and Forte, 1987).

In order to measure protein phosphorylation and turnover of ^{32}P, we subjected the cell fractions to sodium dodecyl sulphate–polyacrylamide gel electrophoresis (SDS-PAGE) so that protein bands could be visualized by Coomassie Blue staining and ^{32}P by autoradiography. It was clear that many protein bands in the various cell fractions were phosphorylated, but the most consistent changes, between resting and stimulated glands, occurred in the fraction of s.a. vesicles. An example of experimental results is shown in Figure 3.9. There it can be seen that histamine plus isobutylmethylxanthine caused an increase in the relative amount of H^+,K^+-ATPase in the fraction that was harvested as s.a. vesicles, and an increase in the incorporation of ^{32}P into 80 000 and 120 000 mol. wt proteins of those same s.a. vesicles.

In the case of the 120 000 mol. wt protein, we now have evidence to suggest that the increased ^{32}P activity in the s.a. vesicle fraction is correlated with a redistribution of the protein from the cytosol to the apical plasma membrane at the time of stimulation (Urushidani, Hanzel and Forte, 1988). We have identified the same protein in the cytosolic, supernatant fraction from parietal cell-rich homogenates. As indicated by the data shown in Figure 3.9, the ^{32}P activity of 120 000 mol. wt protein in the supernatant fraction was virtually unchanged with stimulation, while there was an increase in both ^{32}P and quantity of the protein in the s.a. vesicles from histamine-stimulated glands. The 120 000 mol. wt protein of the s.a. vesicles was relatively tightly associated with the membranes, in that it could not be easily removed by sonication or treatment with high salt concentration. These data are consistent with a hypothesis whereby the 120 000 mol. wt protein migrates from the cytosol to the apical plasma membrane at the time of stimulation. However, as yet there is no clue that would specify the function of the protein.

Unlike the 120 000 mol. wt protein, the 80 000 mol. wt phosphoprotein can be considered a membrane protein in that it co-purifies with, and is restricted to, the fraction harvested as s.a. vesicles. In fact, the fraction isolated as s.a. vesicles, whether from resting or stimulated glands, is always rich in the 80 000 mol. wt protein, even though the amount of ^{32}P incorporation into this protein and the amount of H^+,K^+-ATPase associated with s.a. vesicles are both correlated with stimulation. On the other hand, microsomes, the other gastric membrane fraction rich in H^+,K^+-ATPase, are virtually devoid of the 80 000 mol. wt phosphoprotein. This suggests to us that the 80 000 mol. wt protein is a permanent resident of the apical plasma membrane, and that it is excluded

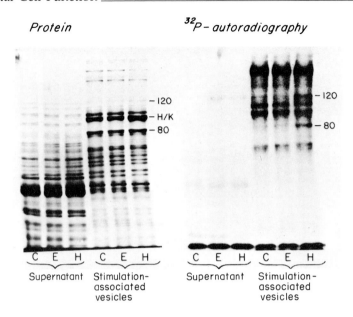

Figure 3.9 Analysis of proteins and ^{32}P-labelled phosphoproteins in cell fractions from resting and stimulated gastric glands. Rabbit glands were prelabelled with ^{32}P and divided into aliquots for treatment to produce control, non-secreting glands (C, 10^{-4} mol l^{-1} cimetidine) or glands maximally stimulated by the histamine/cyclic AMP pathway (H, 10^{-4} mol l^{-1} histamine + 10^{-5} mol l^{-1} isobutylmethylxanthine (IBMX)). In the experiment shown here an aliquot of glands was also treated 10^{-7} M epidermal growth factor (E). After treatment for 40 min, the glands were homogenized and separated into cell fractions; here we show the s.a. vesicle fraction, rich in apical membranes, and the cytosolic (supernatant) fraction. Invariably, the s.a. vesicle fraction from glands stimulated via the histamine/cyclic pathway showed increased ^{32}P-labelling of an 80 000 mol. wt protein and a 120 000 mol. wt protein. The 120 000 mol. wt protein can also be identified in the supernatant fraction, but stimulation did not effect changes in labelling in the supernatant fraction

from the endocytic recycling of H^+,K^+-ATPase into the tubulovesicles when the stimulated cells return to the resting state.

When s.a. vesicles are subjected to two-dimensional electrophoresis, as shown in Figure 3.10, the 80 000 mol. wt protein is focused in a relatively neutral region (about pH 6.7), with a series of spots streaking from the main spot toward the anode. Invariably the ^{32}P radioactivity is seen to focus over the minor more acidic spots (Figure 3.10). We have succeeded in separating the 80 000 mol. wt protein into a series of six distinct isoforms whose isoelectric points vary by 0.03–0.04 pH units. We have confirmed that these are indeed isomers of the same protein by peptide mapping. In our ^{32}P incorporation experiments, measuring the incorporation of ^{32}P in the 80 000 mol. wt protein, we have found that radioactivity is always associated with the three most acidic isoforms,

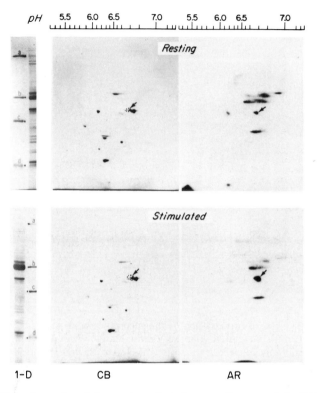

Figure 3.10 Two-dimensional electrophoresis and autoradiogram of the D18 fractions obtained from resting (upper pair) and stimulated (lower pair) gastric glands. Samples of 75 μg protein were first subjected to isoelectric focusing (horizontal dimension) and then the SDS-PAGE using 7.5% acrylamide (vertical direction). The column on the left of each gel (1-D) shows the corresponding sample separated simultaneously only in the second dimension. The pH scale of the isoelectric focusing gel is shown on the top. The regions surrounded by dotted lines on the Coomassie Blue stained gel (CB, left panel) indicate the regions corresponding to radioactive regions on the autoradiogram (AR, right panel). Note that the radioactivity is located on the more acidic end of the series of spots. The molecular weight standards shown are: (a) 200 000, (b) 96 000, (c) 66 000, and (d) 45 000

and for these species we have been able to ascertain that the site of phosphorylation is a serine residue. We are still in the process of working out the interplay among the 80 000 mol. wt isoforms and the enhanced phosphorylation associated with stimulation of hydrochloric acid secretion.

Recently, we have developed monoclonal antibodies against the purified 80 000 mol. wt protein. When fixed gastric glands were probed with these antibodies, visualized with a fluorescent-labelled second antibody, an intense staining of parietal cells was observed (Hanzel, Urushidani and Forte, 1988). The antibody was localized to a network of interconnecting structures emanating from the apical pole and continuing throughout the parietal cell, exclusive of the nucleus (Figure 3.11A). This pattern of staining is morphologically most consistent with a localization within the canalicular network that runs throughout parietal cells.

A characteristic pattern of staining for F-actin has also been identified in gastric glands (Wolosin *et al.*, 1983). This is of particular interest because of the possible involvement of the cytoskeleton, especially the actin microfilaments, in the membrane transformations associated with stimulation of the parietal cell. As demonstrated in Figure 3.11B, F-actin is localized as a fine layer, outlining the entire gastric lumen, including the most luminal aspects of parietal, chief and neck cells. In addition, parietal cells have a more extensive pattern of F-actin staining in the form of a fibrillar network, distributed similarly to the 80 000 mol. wt protein (compare Figures 3.11A and B). These localizations

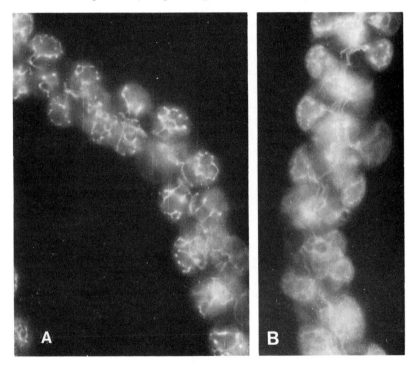

Figure 3.11 Immunohistological localization of 80 000 mol. wt protein and F-actin in resting gastric glands. Gastric glands from rabbit were fixed in formaldehyde, permeabilized with Triton X-100, and probed with either (A) antibodies to the 80 000 mol. wt protein, visualized with FITC-goat-antimouse or (B) NBD-phallicidin which recognizes F-actin. The 80 000 mol. wt protein is present in the parietal cells only, localized to a network which extends from the apical pole to fill the cell. In addition to similar networks throughout the parietal cell, F-actin is localized along the entire length of the gland lumen, including the most luminal aspects of parietal, chief and neck cells

of F-actin are consistent with the known distribution of microfilaments, within microvilli of parietal cells extending throughout the canalicular network, as well as the short microvilli of chief cells and neck cells that line the gland lumen.

It was pointed out above that actin and the 80 000 mol. wt phosphoprotein are major components of the parietal cell apical membranes isolated as s.a. vesicles (see Figure 3.6). This along with their co-localization in parietal cells suggests that there may be some interaction between the 80 000 mol. wt protein and actin microfilaments. Recent experiments have demonstrated that the protein retains a co-localization with actin networks in detergent-resistant cytoskeletons from gastric glands. This actin-binding property is the first hint of a function for the 80 000 mol. wt protein; the effect of phosphorylation on the actin-binding properties remains to be uncovered.

Important characteristics of the 80 000 mol. wt protein include: restriction to the apical membrane of parietal cells; co-localization with actin networks; and specific phosphorylation with the stimulation of gastric acid secretion and translocation of H^+,K^+-ATPase into the apical membrane. These features suggest that the protein may function to facilitate the incorporation of H^+,K^+-ATPase into the apical membrane and that this process may be regulated by phosphorylation of the protein.

Preliminary experiments have demonstrated that immunoreactive 80 000 mol. wt protein is present in several transporting epithelia in addition to stomach, including ileum, duodenum and kidney (Hanzel, Urushidani and Forte, 1988). Appreciation of the role of membrane recycling in the control and modulation of epithelial transport processes has recently widened to include students of intestinal and renal function. Perhaps the exaggerated nature of functional responses in the parietal cell will again lead to an insight of general physiological consequence.

REFERENCES

Berglindh, T., Helander, H. F. and Obrink, K. J. (1976). Effects of secretagogues on oxygen consumption, aminopyrine accumulation and morphology in isolated gastric glands, *Acta Physiol. Scand.*, **97**, 401–14.

Black, J. A., Forte, T. M. and Forte, J. G. (1982). The effects of microfilament disrupting agents on HCl secretion and ultrastructure of piglet oxyntic cells, *Gastroenterology*, **83**, 595–604.

Blakemore, R. C., Brown, T. H., Durant, G. J. *et al.* (1981). Smith Kline and French-93479, A potent and long-acting histamine H_2-receptor antagonist, *Br. J. Pharmacol.*, **74**, 200.

Forte, J. G., Ganser, A. L. and Ray, T. K. (1976). The K^+-stimulated ATPase from oxyntic glands of gastric mucosa. In D, Kasbekar, G. Sachs and W. Rehm (eds) *Gastric Hydrogen Ion Secretion*, Marcel Dekker, New York, pp. 302–30.

Forte, T. M., Machen, T. E. and Forte, J. G. (1977). Ultrastructural changes in oxyntic cells associated with secretory function: a membrane recycling hypothesis, *Gastroenterology*, **73**, 941–55.

Forte, J. G., Ganser, A. L., Beesley, R. C. and Forte, T. M. (1975). Unique enzymes of purified microsomes from pig fundic muscosa, *Gastroenterology*, **69**, 175–89.

Forte, J. G., Black, J. A., Forte, T. M., Machen, T. E. and Wolosin, J. M. (1981). Ultrastructural changes related to functional activity in gastric oxyntic cells, *Am. J. Physiol.*, **241**, G349–58.

Forte, J. G., Forte, T. M., Black, J. A., Okamoto, C. and Wolosin, J. M. (1983). Correlation of parietal cell structure and function, *J. Clin. Gastroenterol.*, **5** (Suppl. 1), 17–27.

Ganser, A. L. and Forte, J. G. (1973). K^+-stimulated ATPase in purified microsomes of bullfrog oxyntic cells, *Biochim. Biophys. Acta*, **307**, 169–80.

Golgi, C. (1893). Sur la fine organisation des glandes peptiques des mammifères, *Arch. Ital. Biol.*, **19**, 448–53.

Hanzel, D. K., Urushidani, T. and Forte, J. G. (1988). Localization and characterization of an 80kDa phosphoprotein associated with gastric acid secretion using antibodies, *FASEB J.*, **2**, A732 (Abstract 2501).

Helander, H. F. (1981). The cells of the gastric mucosa, *Int. Rev. Cytol.*, **70**, 217–89.

Helander, H. F. and Hirschowitz, B. I. (1972). Quantitative ultrastructural studies of microvilli and changes in the tubulovesicular compartment of mouse parietal cells in relation to gastric acid secretion, *J. Cell Biol.*, **63**, 951–61.

Hirst, B. H. and Forte, J. G. (1985). Redistribution and characterization of $(H^+ + K^+)$-ATPase membranes from resting and stimulated gastric parietal cells, *Biochem. J.*, **231**, 641–68.

Im, W. B., Blakeman, D. P. and Davis, J. P. (1985). Studies on K^+ permeability of rat gastric microsomes, *J. Biol. Chem.*, **260**, 9452–60.

Ito, S. (1987). Functional gastric morphology. In L. R. Johnson (ed.) *Physiology of the Gastrointestinal Tract*, Vol. 1, Raven Press, New York, pp. 817–25.

Lee, H. C. and Forte, J. G. (1978). A study of H^+ transport in gastric microsomal vesicles using fluorescent probes, *Biochim. Biophys. Acta*, **508**, 339–56.

Lee, J., Simpson, G. and Scholes, P. (1974). An ATPase from dog gastric mucosa: changes of outer pH in suspensions of membrane vesicles accompanying ATP hydrolysis, *Biochim. Biophys. Acta*, **60**, 825–32.

Lee, H. C., Brietbart, H., Berman, M. and Forte, J. G. (1979). Potassium-stimulated ATPase activity and H^+ transport in gastric microsomal vesicles, *Biochim. Biophys. Acta*, **553**, 107–31.

Ray, T. K. and Forte, J. G. (1976). Studies on the phosphorylated intermediate of a K^+-stimulated ATPase from rabbit gastric mucosa, *Biochim. Biophys. Acta*, **443**, 451–67.

Reenstra, W., Lee, J. C. and Forte, J. G. (1980). Functional studies on the gastric K^+-stimulated ATPase. In I. Schulz, G. Sachs, J. G. Forte and K. J. Uldrich (eds) *Hydrogen Ion Transport in Epithelia*, Elsevier, Amsterdam, pp. 155–64.

Saccomani, G., Stewart, H. B., Shaw, D., Lewin, M. and Sachs, G. (1977). Characterization of gastric mucosal membranes: fractionation by zonal centrifugation and free flow electrophoresis, *Biochim. Biophys. Acta*, **465**, 311–30.

Sachs, G. (1987). The gastric proton pump: the H^+,K^+-ATPase. In L. R. Johnson (ed.) *Physiology of the Gastrointestinal Tract*, Raven Press, New York, pp. 865–82.

Sachs, G., Chang, H. H., Rabon, E., Schackmann, R., Lewin, M. and Saccomani, G. (1976). A non-electrogenic H^+ pump in plasma membranes of hog stomach, *J. Biol. Chem.*, **251**, 7690–8.

Shull, G. E. and Lingrel, J. B. (1986). Molecular cloning of the rat stomach $(H^+ + K^+)$-ATPase, *J. Biol. Chem.*, **261**, 16788–91.

Smolka, A., Helander, H. F. and Sachs, G. (1983). Monoclonal antibodies against H$^+$ + K$^+$-ATPase. *Am. J. Physiol.*, **245**, G589-96.

Urushidani, T. and Forte, J. G. (1987). Stimulation-associated redistribution of H$^+$,K$^+$-ATPase activity in isolated gastric glands, *Am. J. Physiol.*, **252** (*Gastrointest. Liner Physiol.* 15), G458-65.

Urushidani, T., Hanzel, D. K. and Forte, J. F. (1987). Protein phosphorylation associated with stimulation of rabbit gastric glands, *Biochim. Biophys. Acta*, **930**, 209-19.

Urushidani, T., Hanzel, D. K. and Forte, J. G. (1988). A 120kDa phosphoprotein associated with the apical membrane of stimulated parietal cells, *Biophys. J.*, **53**, 524a.

Wallmark, B., Stewart, H. B., Rabon, E., Saccomani, G. and Sachs, G. (1980). The catalytic cycle of gastric (H$^+$ + K$^+$)-ATPase, *J. Biol. Chem.*, **255**, 5313-19.

Wolosin, J. M. and Forte, J. G. (1981). Changes in the membrane environment of the (K$^+$ + H$^+$)-ATPase following stimulation of the gastric oxyntic cell, *J. Biol. Chem.*, **256**, 3149-52.

Wolosin, J. M. and Forte, J. G. (1983). Kinetic properties of the KCl transport at the secreting apical membrane of the oxyntic cell, *J. Membr. Biol.*, **71**, 195-207.

Wolosin, J. M. and Forte, J. G. (1984). Stimulation of oxyntic cell triggers K$^+$ and Cl$^-$ conductances in apical (H$^+$ + K$^+$)-ATPase membrane, *Am. J. Physiol.*, **246**, C537-45.

Wolosin, J. M. and Forte, J. G. (1985). K$^+$ and Cl$^-$ conductances in the apical membrane from secreting oxyntic cells are concurrently inhibited by divalent cations, *J. Membr. Biol.*, **83**, 261-72.

Wolosin, J. M., Okamoto, C., Forte, T. M. and Forte, J. G. (1983). Actin and associated proteins in gastric epithelial cells, *Biochim. Biophys. Acta*, **761**, 171-82.

Advances in Drug Therapy of Gastrointestinal Ulceration
Edited by A. Garner and B. J. R. Whittle
©1989 John Wiley & Sons Ltd

Chapter Four

Experimental Studies with Proton Pump Inhibitors

K.-Fr. Sewing and W. Beil
*Abt. Allgemeine Pharmakologie, Medizinische Hochschule
Hannover, D-3000 Hannover 61, FRG*

INTRODUCTION

Peptic ulcer disease is a disturbance in integrity of the upper gastrointestinal mucosa in which the presence of gastric acid plays an important permissive role. Therefore scientists have made great efforts to eliminate gastric hydrochloric acid. There are several ways of achieving this, e.g. neutralization of acid already secreted (by antacids) or blockade of parietal cell receptors (most successfully achieved by histamine H_2-receptor antagonists and less effectively by antimuscarinic agents). Compounds acting by any one of these mechanisms have

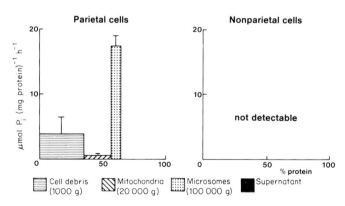

Figure 4.1 Subcellular distribution of K^+-stimulated ATPase activity in isolated and enriched parietal cells (left) and non-parietal cells (right) from the guinea-pig gastric mucosa. (Reproduced from Beil and Sewing, 1984)

53

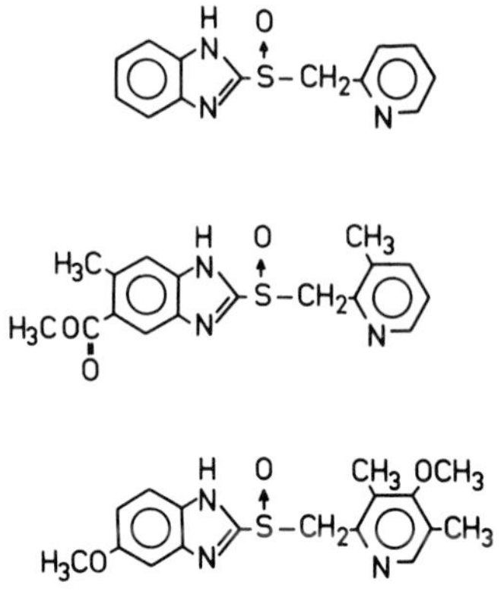

Timoprazole

Picoprazole

Omeprazole

Figure 4.2 Structures of the substituted benzimidazoles timoprazole, picoprazole and omeprazole

proved to be effective anti-ulcer agents. Much attention has been paid to the mechanisms of acid stimulation or inhibition. However, it was not until 1973 that an enzyme from the oxyntic gland area was discovered and characterized which is regarded as the final secretory mechanism for H^+ transport (for review see De Pont and Bonting, 1981). This enzyme is localized in the parietal cell membranes separating the cytosol from the tubulovesicles. Upon parietal cell stimulation the tubulovesicles open up and merge into a canalicular system, providing communication with the oxyntic gland lumen to give hydrochloric acid eventual access into the gastric lumen. There is some controversy with regard to the intracellular mechanisms involved in parietal cell stimulus–secretion coupling, but there is no doubt that a steep pH gradient exists between the cytosol

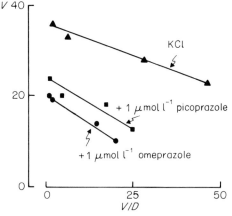

Figure 4.3 Eadie–Hofstee plots demonstrating non-competitive inhibition of the guinea-pig parietal cell K^+-stimulated ATPase by picoprazole and omeprazole ($1\,\mu\mathrm{mol}\,l^{-1}$). (Reproduced from Beil and Sewing, 1984)

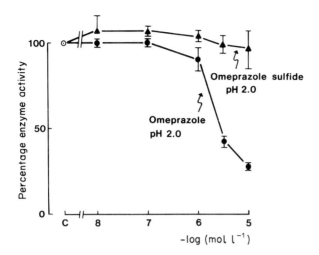

Figure 4.4 Effect of omeprazole and omeprazole sulfide (both dissolved at pH 2.0) on K⁺,H⁺-ATPase of guinea-pig parietal cells

and the intracellular canalicular system from an intracellular pH of 7.4 to a pH of 1–2 in the canaliculi. Such a gradient could not be achieved without utilizing an active transport system pumping protons against a concentration gradient. The enzyme system along the canalicular membrane plays a pivotal role in proton pumping. This has been characterized as an ATPase which

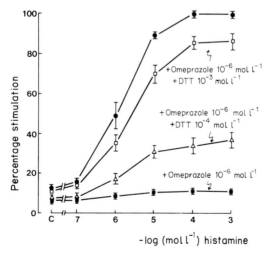

Figure 4.5 Effect of dithiothreitol (DTT) on the inhibitory effect of omeprazole $(10^{-6} \text{ mol l}^{-1})$ on histamine stimulated $[^{14}C]$ aminopyrine accumulation in isolated and enriched guinea-pig parietal cells. (Reproduced from Sewing *et al.*, 1986)

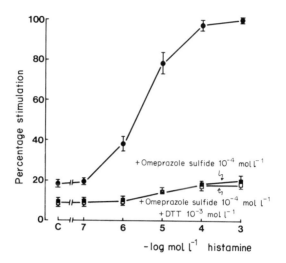

Figure 4.6 Effect of dithiothreitol (DTT) on the inhibitory effect of omeprazole sulfide (10^{-4} mol l^{-1}) on histamine-stimulated [^{14}C]aminopyrine accumulation in isolated and enriched guinea-pig parietal cells

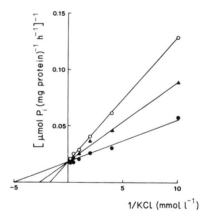

Figure 4.7 Lineweaver–Burk plot of the K^+-stimulated ATP hydrolysis rate by K^+,H^+-ATPase versus concentrations of KCl (0.1–5 mmol l^{-1}) in the absence (●) or presence of 30 (▲) and 50 (○) μmol l^{-1} omeprazole sulfide. Values are the mean from three different enzyme preparations. (Reproduced from Beil *et al.*, 1985)

transports protons in exchange for K^+ on a 1:1 stoichiometric basis. There are several synonyms for the enzyme (e.g. proton pump and K^+,H^+-ATPase), but an international code number does not yet exist. The enzyme can be isolated and partially purified from the microsomal fraction (Beil and Sewing, 1984) as shown in Figure 4.1.

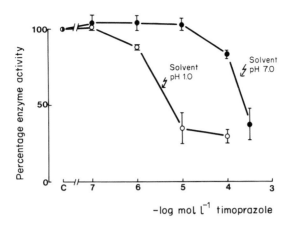

Figure 4.8 Effect of timoprazole (dissolved at pH 1 or pH 7) on guinea-pig parietal cell K^+,H^+-ATPase

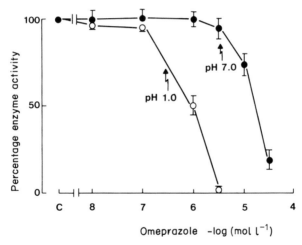

Figure 4.9 Effect of omeprazole (dissolved at pH 1 or pH 7) on guinea-pig parietal cell K^+,H^+-ATPase

INHIBITORS OF THE PROTON PUMP

In the 1970s a group of scientists from Hässle, Mölndal, Sweden, described a series of compounds, generally referred to as 'substituted benzimidazoles' capable of selectively blocking this enzyme and thereby acting as powerful inhibitors of gastric acid secretion. The compounds timoprazole, picoprazole and omeprazole (Figure 4.2) can be regarded as prototypes of this class and were followed by numerous derivatives which are now in the pipeline of different pharmaceutical companies. Since they block proton transport from the parietal

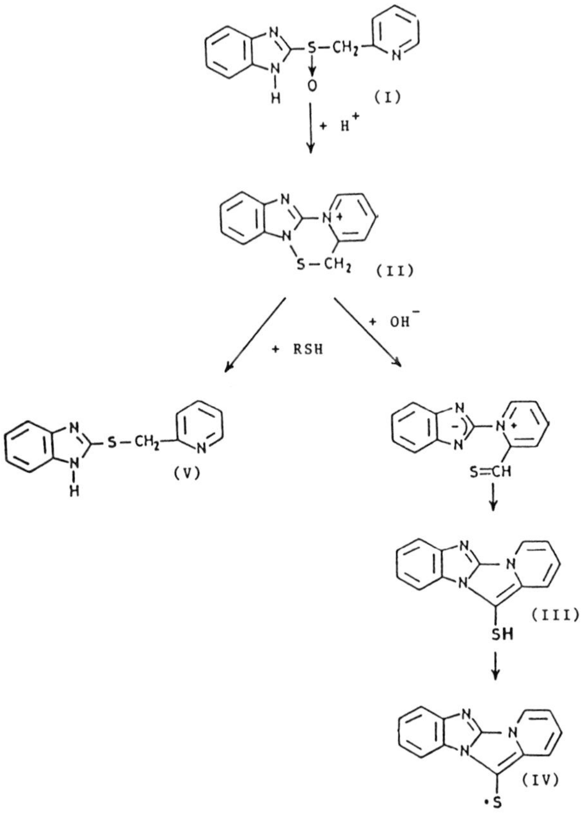

Figure 4.10 Metabolic pathway of timoprazole after acidification (adapted from Rackur *et al.*, 1985 and Figala *et al.* 1986)

cell cytosol into the gastric lumen they are known in more general and functional terms as 'proton pump inhibitors'. This is not the place to review every single compound in detail. It is more interesting to describe the possible mechanisms of interaction of various types of proton pump inhibitor.

MECHANISM OF ACTION OF BENZIMIDAZOLES

Proton pump inhibitors of the timoprazole type block the enzyme in a non-competitive fashion (Beil and Sewing, 1984) as shown in Figure 4.3. Studies of structure–activity relationships revealed that the sulphoxide moiety of the molecule is an essential requirement for proton pump inhibition since the sulphide form of omeprazole and of other sulphoxidized substituted benzimidazoles do not inhibit the enzyme in the same way (Figure 4.4).

Nevertheless, all substituted benzimidazole-derived sulphides inhibit acid secretion in isolated parietal cells, suggesting a different type of interaction with the pump. Such a difference can be demonstrated in protection studies with mercaptanes.

In isolated and enriched guinea-pig parietal cells the inhibitory effect of omeprazole on acid formation, as measured by [^{14}C] aminopyrine uptake, can be prevented by dithiothreitol (DTT) in a concentration-dependent manner (Sewing *et al.*, 1986) as shown in Figure 4.5. Inhibition of [^{14}C] aminopyrine accumulation by the omeprazole sulfide cannot be surmounted by DTT in concentrations which fully counteract the effect of omeprazole (Sewing *et al.*, 1986), as shown in Figure 4.6. The failure of DTT to prevent the

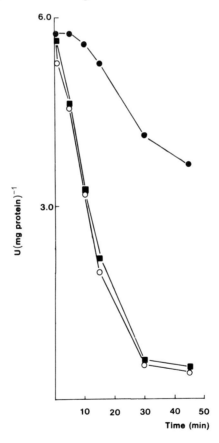

Figure 4.11 Time course for inactivation of glutaminase from *E. coli* by 50 μmol l^{-1} omeprazole and omeprazole cyclic sulphenamide. Glutaminase (80 μg protein ml^{-1}) was incubated at pH 2.5 in the absence (●) or presence of 50 μmol l^{-1} omeprazole (○) and omeprazole cyclic sulphenamide (■). Each time point is the mean of three different determinations (s.e.m. < 10%). (Reproduced from Beil, Staar and Sewing, 1988)

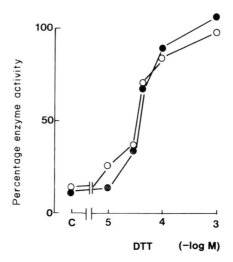

Figure 4.12 Effect of dithiothreitol (DTT) on the inhibitory action of omeprazole and omeprazole sulphenamide on glutaminase from *E. coli*. Glutaminase (20 μg protein) was incubated with increasing concentrations of DTT at pH 2.5 with $100 \, \mu \text{mol} \, l^{-1}$ omeprazole (●) and omeprazole cyclic sulphenamide (○) for 15 min. Each point is the mean of three different determinations (s.e.m. < 10%). (Reproduced from Beil, Staar and Sewing, 1988)

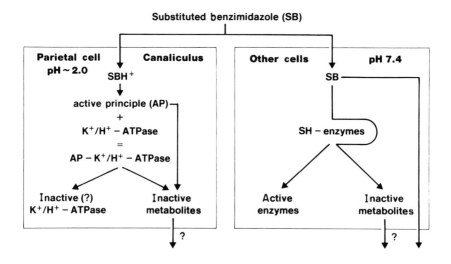

Figure 4.13 Schematic summary of the mechanism of action and specificity of substituted benzimidazoles

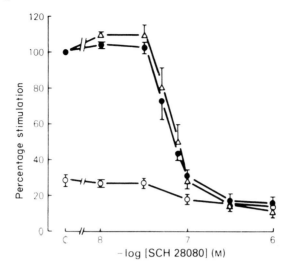

Figure 4.14 Effect of SCH 28080 on basal (○), histamine- (●) and K⁺- (△) stimulated uptake and accumulation of [¹⁴C]aminopyrine in guinea-pig parietal cells. Values are the mean ± s.e.m. from six different cell preparations. (Reproduced from Beil *et al.* 1986)

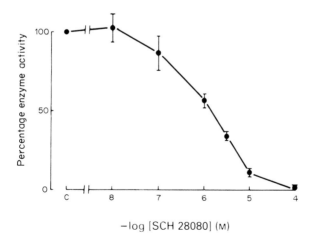

Figure 4.15 Inhibition of guinea-pig parietal cell K^+,H^+-ATPase by SCH 28080. SCH 28080 was preincubated with 5–10 μg enzyme protein at pH 7.5 for 30 min at 22 °C. Enzyme activity was then determined after incubation for 15 min at 37 °C in the presence of 5 μmol/l⁻¹ KCl. Values are the mean ± s.e.m. from three different enzyme preparations. (Reproduced from Beil *et al.*, 1986)

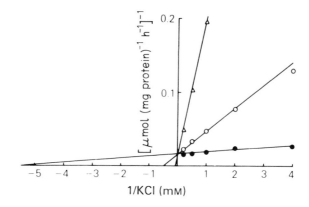

Figure 4.16 Lineweaver–Burk plots of the rate of K^+-stimulated ATP hydrolysis versus concentration of KCl (0.25–5 mmol l^{-1}) in the absence (●) or presence of 0.5 (○) and 3 (△) μmol l^{-1} SCH 28080. (Reproduced from Beil *et al.*, 1986)

inhibitory effect of the omeprazole sulfide may be caused by interaction of the omeprazole sulfide with the potassium site of the enzyme (Beil *et al.*, 1985), as shown in Figure 4.7.

The omeprazole–DTT interaction strongly suggests that substituted benzimidazoles interact with SH-groups in the active centre of the molecule for which we now have evidence. If that is the case one would have to ask why substituted benzimidazoles do not block other SH-enzyme systems. The answer comes from the following investigations, which suggest that an active metabolite is generated only at low pH.

An acidified omeprazole solution left on the bench for a while changes from a colourless into a yellowish coloured solution. Furthermore, Wallmark *et al.*

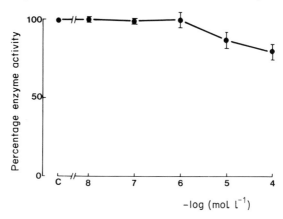

Figure 4.17 Effect of SCH 28080 on dog kidney Na^+,K^+-ATPase. (Reproduced from Beil, Staar and Sewing, 1987)

(1983) noted that the inhibitory effect of omeprazole is enhanced in an acidic environment. Timoprazole and omeprazole are more potent inhibitors of the guinea-pig K^+,H^+-ATPase when dissolved at a low pH than at pH 7 (Figures 4.8 and 4.9). The data suggest some kind of structural change. Three groups independently described the metabolic pathway of substituted benzimidazoles when exposed to a highly acidic environment (Im et al., 1985; Figala et al., 1986; Rackur et al., 1985). As a result of these studies it was discovered that a cyclic sulphenamide (Figure 4.10) formed from substituted benzimidazoles in the presence of a high proton concentration is the active principle which reacts with the enzyme. Under in vitro conditions, the K^+,H^+-ATPase loses activity at low pH. Therefore we used the glutaminase (EC 3.5.1.2) from Escherichia coli as a model enzyme to study interaction of the omeprazole-derived cyclic sulphenamide with an SH-enzyme at low pH (Beil, Staar and Sewing, 1988). The time course of inhibition of this enzyme at pH 2.5 was identical for omeprazole and the omeprazole-derived cyclic sulphenamide (Figure 4.11). Furthermore, the inhibitory effect of both compounds on glutaminase was prevented by DTT (Figure 4.12). A summary of the mechanism of action and specificity of substituted benzimidazoles is depicted in Figure 4.13.

OTHER INHIBITORS

SCH 28080 (2-methyl-8-(phenylmethoxy)imidazole[1,2-a]pyridine-3-acetonitrile) is a powerful antisecretory agent (Long et al. 1983) which was shown in vitro to act distal to cyclic AMP (Chiu et al. 1983). In isolated and enriched guinea-pig parietal cells and gastric membranes purified and enriched with K^+,H^+-ATPase we have been able to show that SCH 28080 is a potent

Table 4.1 IC_{50} values (mean $\pm$ s.e.m.) for H^+ secretion as measured by [^{14}C]aminopyrine uptake in isolated and enriched parietal cells stimulated by 1 mmol l^{-1} histamine or 1 mmol l^{-1} dibutyryl cAMP (n = 4 different cell preparations)

	Histamine (μmol l^{-1})	Dibutyryl (μmol l^{-1})
Chlorpromazine	0.19 ± 0.03	0.22 ± 0.02
Triflupromazine	0.14 ± 0.02	0.15 ± 0.02
Trifluoperazine	0.54 ± 0.10	0.52 ± 0.05
Trimipramine	0.22 ± 0.05	0.24 ± 0.04
Nortriptyline	0.36 ± 0.04	0.38 ± 0.05
Doxepin	0.56 ± 0.07	0.65 ± 0.08
Haloperidol	0.43 ± 0.10	0.46 ± 0.11
Fluspirilene	0.17 ± 0.03	0.12 ± 0.02
Pirenzepine	inactive	inactive

Table 4.2 IC_{50} values (mean $\pm$ s.e.m.) for guinea-pig parietal cell K^+, H^+-ATPase and its partial reactions ($n = 4$ different enzyme preparations)

	K^+,H^+-ATPase reaction	Phosphoenzyme formation	p-NPPase reaction
Chlorpromazine	31.3 ± 2.1	NT	43.6 ± 4.2
Triflupromazine	22.6 ± 4.3	23.0 ± 10.7	42.3 ± 10.7
Trifluoperazine	13.3 ± 0.9	NT	26.0 ± 6.4
Trimipramine	77.3 ± 16.3	NT	153 ± 17.6
Nortriptyline	70.6 ± 4.7	42.8 ± 18.6	116 ± 11.8
Doxepin	283 ± 31	NT	> 300
Haloperidol	190 ± 11.6	> 300	255 ± 14.0
Fluspirilene	5.2 ± 0.2	16.4 ± 1.4	12.5 ± 0.3

NT = not tested

K^+,H^+-ATPase inhibitor interacting competitively and selectively with the K^+ site of the enzyme (Figures 4.14, 4.15 and 4.16). This selectivity can be shown in comparison with the dog kidney Na^+,K^+-ATPase, another SH-enzyme, which is almost resistant to inhibition by SCH 28080 (Figure 4.17). These findings indicate that the proton pump can be specifically attacked by different mechanisms.

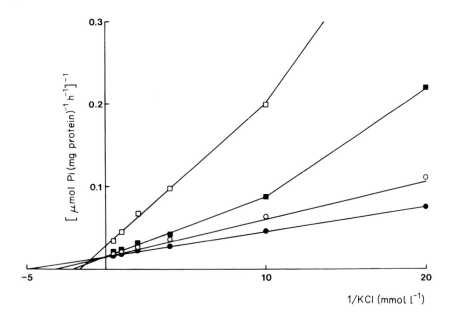

Figure 4.18 Lineweaver–Burk plots of the hydrolysis rate of ATP by K^+,H^+-ATPase versus concentrations of KCl (0.05–2 mmol l^{-1}) in the absence ($\bullet$) or presence of 5 ($\bigcirc$), 10 ($\blacksquare$) and 30 ($\square$) μmol l^{-1} chlorpromazine. Values represent the mean from three different enzyme preparations. (Reproduced from Beil *et al.*, 1987)

Recently Batzri (1985) reported that the antidepressants amitriptyline and nortriptyline inhibit histamine and dibutyryl-cAMP-induced H^+ secretion in rabbit isolated gastric glands, suggesting that they have a site of action distal to the membrane receptor. A series of antidepressants and neuroleptics were tested for their inhibitory activity in isolated and enriched guinea-pig parietal cells and gastric membranes purified and enriched with K^+,H^+-ATPase (Beil et al. 1987). All the compounds tested inhibited [^{14}C]aminopyrine accumulation in response to $1\,mmol\,l^{-1}$ histamine or dibutyryl cAMP with rather similar IC_{50} values (Table 4.1). The same compounds were somewhat less potent inhibitors of K^+,H^+-ATPase (Table 4.2). Enzyme kinetics for chlorpromazine revealed competitive inhibition of the enzyme at low concentrations and non-competitive inhibition at higher concentrations (Figure 4.18). Summarizing these findings we concluded that neuroleptics and antidepressants, because of their basic properties, accumulate in the secretory canaliculi. Dependent on their lipophilicity, the drugs react with hydrophilic areas within the apical plasma membrane and induce conformational changes which interfere with K^+ activation of the K^+,H^+-ATPase.

CONCLUSIONS

The parietal cell proton pump, because of its unique localization and properties, represents a complex system which can be attacked by different mechanisms, both specific and non-specific. It is a challenge for scientists to discover and characterize drugs which effectively inhibit the system and leave other mechanisms of the organism intact.

REFERENCES

Batzri, S. (1985). Tricyclic antidepressants and acid antisecretory response of rabbit gastric cells, Am. J. Physiol., 248, G360-8.

Beil, W. and Sewing, K.-Fr. (1984). Inhibition of partially purified K^+/H^+-ATPase from guinea pig isolated and enriched parietal cells by substituted benzimidazoles, Br. J. Pharmacol., 82, 651-7.

Beil, W., Hackberth, I. and Sewing, K.-Fr. (1986). Mechanism of the gastric antisecretory effect of SCH 28080. Br. J. Pharmacol., 88, 19-23.

Beil, W., Staar, U. and Sewing, K.-Fr. (1987). SCH 28080 is a more selective inhibitor than SCH 32651 at the K^+ site of gastric K^+/H^+-ATPase, Eur. J. Pharmacol., 139, 349-52.

Beil, W., Staar, U. and Sewing, K.-Fr. (1988). Studies on the mechanisms of action of the omeprazole-derived cyclic sulphenamide, Biochem. Pharmacol., 37, 843-8.

Beil, W., Mädge, S., Hannemann, H., Zimmer, K. O. and Sewing, K.-Fr. (1985). Characteristics of K^+/H^+-ATPase inhibition by omeprazole and omeprazole-sulfide, Hepato-Gastroenterology, 32, 47.

Beil, W., Stünkel, P., Pieper, A. and Sewing, K.-Fr. (1987). The gastric proton pump, a target for neuroleptics and antidepressant drugs, Aliment. Pharmacol. Ther., 1, 141-51.

Chiu, P. J. S., Casciano, C., Tetzloff, G., Long, J. F. and Barett, A. (1983). Studies on the mechanisms of the antisecretory and cytoprotective actions of SCH 28080, *J. Pharmacol. Exp. Ther.*, **226**, 121–5.

De Pont, J. J. H. H. M. and Bonting, S. L. (1981). $(K^+ + H^+)$-ATPase. In S. L. Bonting and J. J. H. H. M. De Pont (eds) *New Comprehensive Biochemistry*, Vol. 2, *Membrane Transport*, Elsevier, Amsterdam, pp. 222–34.

Figala, V., Klemm, K., Kohl, B. *et al.* (1986). Acid activation of $(H^+ - K^+)$-ATPase inhibiting 2-(2-pyridylmethylsulphinyl)benzimidazoles: isolation and characterisation of the thiophilic 'active principle' and its reactions, *J. Chem. Soc., Chem. Commun.*, **20**, 125–7.

Im, W. B., Sih, J. C., Blakeman, D. P. and McGrath, J. P. (1985). Omeprazole, a specific inhibitor of gastric $(H^+ - K^+)$-ATPase, is a H^+-activated oxidizing agent of sulfhydryl groups, *J. Biol. Chem.*, **260**, 4591–7.

Long, J. F., Chiu, P. J. S., Derelanko, M. J. and Steinberg, M. (1983). Gastric antisecretory and cytoprotective activities of SCH 28080, *J. Pharmacol. Exp. Ther.*, **226**, 114–20.

Rackur, G., Bickel, M., Fehlhaber, H.-W. *et al.* (1985). 2-((2-pyridylmethyl)sulfinyl)-benzimidazoles: acid sensitive suicide inhibitors of the proton transport system in the parietal cell, *Biochem. Biophys. Res. Commun.*, **128**, 477–84.

Sewing, K.-Fr., Beil, W., Hackbarth, I. and Hannemann, H. (1986). Effect of substituted benzimidazoles on K^+/H^+-ATPase of isolated guinea pig parietal cells, *Scand. J. Gastroenterol.*, **21** (Suppl. 118), 52–3.

Wallmark, B., Jaresten, B.-M., Larsson, H. *et al.* (1983). Differentiation among inhibitory actions of omeprazole, cimetidine, and SCN^- on gastric acid secretion, *Am. J. Physiol.*, **245**, G964–71.

Advances in Drug Therapy of Gastrointestinal Ulceration
Edited by A. Garner and B. J. R. Whittle
©1989 John Wiley & Sons Ltd

Chapter Five

Antisecretory Treatment and Predisposition to Cancer

M. J. S. Langman
*Department of Medicine, Queen Elizabeth Hospital, Birmingham
B15 2TH*

In considering the risk of gastric cancer occurring as a consequence of antisecretory therapy the following important possibilities must be borne in mind. Firstly, drugs themselves, or their metabolic products, may be directly mutagenic or carcinogenic. Secondly, carcinomatous changes may be more likely to occur in circumstances where gastric hypoacidity is induced, possibly as a consequence of intragastric bacterial metabolism of drugs, drug products or substances ingested in the diet. Thirdly, individuals who receive antisecretory treatment may be inherently more liable to develop gastric or other cancers than the rest of the population. Fourthly, treatment may be given inappropriately to patients who already have established, but as yet undetected, cancers.

PRECLINICAL STUDIES

These may be useful in preventing the introduction of drugs which cause carcinomatous change in experimental animals and in eliminating from consideration drugs which are obviously mutagenic. However, it has to be accepted that mutagenicity in early toxicological studies does not necessarily indicate carcinogenicity, and, by the same token, freedom from mutagenicity, does not of itself imply freedom from carcinogenic potential.

In seeking greater safety, it is usual to overdose animals grossly for a lifetime, but there is no good reason for believing that such studies do indeed indicate safety. Paradoxically, these experiments may eliminate drugs which were, in fact, safe and useful.

Examination of individual tissue responses may help, to some extent, in deciding if observed changes indicate general properties of a class of agent or individual idiosyncratic behaviour. Thus Table 5.1 shows recorded abnormalities in animal studies associated with the use of three antisecretory drugs in high doses in experimental animals. The data suggest at least two sets of responses. Firstly, enterochromaffin hyperplasia followed the use of four agents, three of which were histamine H_2-antagonists; SKF 93479, tiotidine and loxtidine. The fourth agent, omeprazole, is a proton pump inhibitor with strong affinity for gastric mucosal tissue. Secondly, both squamous and adenocarcinomatous change were induced, but by different agents, one also causing enterochromaffin hyperplasia.

Taken together, this evidence suggests that there may be a general propensity of antisecretory agents to cause enterochromaffin hyperplasia and that certain specific drugs may be carcinogenic. However, the distinction may not be clear cut because hyperplasia or carcinoid tumour nodules may occasionally develop following use of, in particular, loxitidine and omeprazole. We therefore have to ask whether carcinoid nodules simply express the intensity and duration of antisecretory response to drugs, or whether they occur because the drugs which cause hyperplasia also have separate and distinct carcinogenic properties. Any explanatory hypothesis also has to take account of the lack of carcinoid formation with the classical antisecretory agents cimetidine and ranitidine, although the latter has been found to induce enterochromaffin cell hyperplasia only.

Experimental studies on rats which had, and had not, been subjected to antrectomy have indicated that enterochromaffin hyperplasia does not occur when the antrum has been excised, and that hyperplasia occurs in association with raised serum gastrin levels. At least two mechanisms could explain such results. Firstly, the stimulus to hyperplasia might be gastrin itself, and secondly, another unknown, antral factor might be responsible. The more economical

Table 5.1 Gastric abnormalities observed during animal testing of selected antisecretory agents

	Drug action	Abnormalities observed
Loxitidine	H_2-antagonist	Enterochromaffin hyperplasia and carcinoid nodules
Omeprazole	Proton pump inhibitor	Enterochromaffin hyperplasia and carcinoid nodules
SKF 93479	H_2-antagonist	Squamous tumours and enterochromaffin hyperplasia
Tiotidine	H_2-antagonist	Dysplasia + adenocarcinoma

(Reproduced from Langman, 1985)

theory is the first, and this is compatible with clinical evidence that the gross hypergastrinaemia of the Zollinger–Ellison syndrome and of pernicious anaemia are occasionally associated with carcinoid tumour formation (Larsson *et al.*, 1986; Lanzon Miller *et al.*, 1987).

An unexpected light has been thrown upon this problem by the finding that the fibrates, such as ciprofibrate, ordinarily considered to be hypolipidaemic drugs, can in experimental animals cause enterochromaffin hyperplasia in the stomach. These results were obtained with three different agents, all of which proved to be weak gastric antisecretories. Use of large doses of the most potent and long lasting of these agents caused carcinoid nodules to form (Spencer *et al.*, 1988).

Taken overall, therefore, the evidence would seem to suggest that intensity and/or duration of antisecretory effect may matter above all. Stronger evidence to support this view would be the demonstration that the individual animals developing carcinoids were those with the highest gastrin levels.

STUDIES IN MAN

Experimental studies

Experimental investigations have limited value in aiding attempts to detect carcinogenic agents. Thus, the complexities of nitrosamine measurement, the difficulties inherent in deciding which compounds matter, and whether the experimental method in use will detect them, and whether any detectable level is likely to be significant, make interpretation well nigh impossible. Acid secretory suppression leads inevitably to rises in serum gastrin concentrations, but the levels reached are far lower than those obtained using very high doses of antisecretory drugs in experimental animals (Lanzon Miller *et al.*, 1987). It seems unlikely that these modest changes in gastrin levels are important, given that in patients with pernicious anaemia, who have very high levels, carcinoid changes are only rarely described.

Clinical models of hyposecretory states

Gastric secretory capacity is consistently reduced in three situations—after gastric resection or vagotomy, in pernicious anaemia and in the Zollinger–Ellison syndrome—where continued potent suppressant treatment is essential.

Gastric surgery

The long-term consequences described have been of four general types:

(1) *No change in cancer frequency:* North American studies, conducted where gastric cancer is comparatively rare, have failed to detect an increased risk of gastric malignancy (Sandler, Johnson and Holland, 1984). Whether such results are generally transposable to the situation existing in all geographical areas, including those where cancer is common, must be doubtful. Thus countries with low disease rates have generally been those where the intestinalized type of cancer has become less prevalent and the diffuse type persists. This argues that underlying predisposing factors to gastric malignancy are of at least two types. It should be noted, however, that some non-US data sets have also shown no increase in rates of gastric malignancy (Kalina and Kivilaasko, 1983).

(2) *Increased gastric cancer risk:* A variety of data sets indicated a modest, perhaps two-fold, increase in the risk of gastric cancer many years after gastric resection, and perhaps after vagotomy (Lundegardh *et al.*, 1988).

(3) *Increased lung cancer risk:* Data from Edinburgh suggest that the risk of lung cancer death, in particular, is increased after gastric surgery (Ross *et al.*, 1982). The assumption is made, without supportive evidence though it is plausible, that this reflects the influence of tobacco consumption in predisposing to both lung cancer and peptic ulcer.

(4) *General increase in cancer frequency:* One follow-up study has suggested that, by comparison with community expectation, the frequency of several varieties of cancer is increased, comparatively uniformly, after gastric surgery (Caygill *et al.*, 1987). Whether this unexpected result indicates a real difference, or whether it could have arisen through an underestimation of ordinary population disease frequency is unclear. Trends in the same direction have, however, been observed (Watt, Patterson and Kennedy, 1984).

Pernicious anaemia. Gastric cancer is about twice as frequent in pernicious anaemia sufferers as in the rest of the population. In addition, carcinoid tumours of the stomach have occasionally been described and are probably more frequent than in the ordinary population, where they rarely arise. Whether this disease provides any clues to mechanism in the general population must be doubtful, since not only is there complete anacidity but the mucosa is generally abnormal, and probably inherently unstable.

Zollinger–Ellison syndrome. Carcinoid tumours of the stomach are well described (Bardram, Thompson and Stadil, 1986), but it is unclear why these arise. Possibilities include a stimulant effect of gastrin (Larsson *et al.*, 1988) and a general predisposition to endocrine tumours of any type.

DEMOGRAPHIC TRENDS

The widespread use of antisecretory drugs since their introduction 10 years ago suggests that it might be prudent to examine cancer incidence trends to try and detect any following change in disease frequency. Whether such studies can yield useful information is doubtful. Firstly, gastric cancer mortality and incidence taken overall have been decreasing steeply in the last 20 years. Where disease incidence is changing, it becomes correspondingly harder to detect the superimposed influence of a second factor unless it is very strong indeed. Secondly, although antisecretory treatment has been widely used, the intermittent pattern and long latency make a cohort increase or period effect difficult to detect.

SURVEILLANCE OF DRUG TAKERS

Follow-up studies of takers of drugs have an obvious logic if there are concerns about risks of drug-induced disease. Before undertaking these, it is sensible to be aware of the weaknesses of the data. Firstly, most diseases in which we are likely to be interested will occur at a frequency of 1 in 1000 or less. It therefore follows that study cohorts must be very large if they are to give useful data. Secondly, controlled comparisons may be difficult, or impossible, to make. Cohorts of takers and non-takers cannot be collected by random allocation techniques and so basic similarity at the starting point cannot be assumed even if a comparator group is obtainable.

Experience in conducting surveillance studies of cimetidine takers confirms that the difficulties are real (Colin Jones et al., 1983, 1985, 1987). Comparisons were made initially between a cohort of 10 000 individuals all prescribed cimetidine in 1977–79 in four centres in the UK. Data obtained were matched with information about 10 000 age and sex matched individuals with recent attendances with their general practitioners. Recent attendance was specified for two reasons. Firstly, it made it likely that individuals selected were in fact still truly members of the general practitioners' lists. Secondly, it helped to provide a group with an equivalent amount of recent illness. Dyspeptic controls could not be selected because of the likelihood that during the course of the study cimetidine would be prescribed for them.

Examination of mortality rates in control individuals showed that these conformed to community expectation, giving some confidence that any deviations in the drug recipient group from these observed values could represent true differences from ordinary expectation, and hence would require explanation. However, it transpired that increases both in morbidity, as measured by hospital outpatient and inpatient statistics, and in mortality occurred, and these were general increases for all disease categories.

In such circumstances, it was difficult or well nigh impossible to detect drug-induced disease, which could not be differentiated from disease occurring spontaneously. The reasons for the increases are likely to have been complex. Firstly, drug recipients were likely to have included more smokers and heavy drinkers than the controls (although a subsample survey failed to detect an increased proportion of smokers among the drug takers). Secondly, it seemed possible that, despite efforts to match controls for recent practitioner attendance, there was, nevertheless, a greater proportion of patients with coincident disease in the takers than in the controls. Thirdly, the scrutiny associated with drug prescription was likely to have brought other disease to light in the takers.

Having taken all these points into account, it seemed that drug-induced disease was only likely to be detected, and then by the alert, when there was a close relationship between treatment exposure and disease occurrence, and when the disease itself possessed features to differentiate it from spontaneously occurring disease.

Where cancer might be induced, the problems plainly become more severe. The latent interval between drug exposure and disease occurrence would be unknown, but would be very long, perhaps 10 years or more, and the likelihood would exist that the disease would mimic spontaneously occurring cancer. If that cancer were of a rare type, it might be possible to link its appearance to drug exposure. However, if it were of a common type, establishing a link could be very difficult. A further problem might arise in considering a common variety of cancer, even if a particular treatment increased the risk. Thus, if exposure to treatment was very frequent, a very modest increase in risk would result in a large number of cases which, nevertheless, would be difficult or impossible to link with treatment. The obvious example would be breast cancer. So far no coherent body of data exists to suggest an increased risk associated with oral contraceptive use, and generally data indicate an absence of risk. However, a very modest increase in risk could result in thousands of extra cases. Data examining the long-term outcome of antisecretory treatment have to be viewed in this perplexing context.

Following the initial study year, mortality rates fell and after four years have, taken overall, approached those of general population expectation. Scrutiny of individual causes shows no discordant patterns except a tendency for death rates from lung cancer to remain high. This change has been attributed to an excess of smokers in the study group, although a subsample survey of individuals included had failed to show any notable increase in smoking habits.

Succeeding years may present problems in data interpretation and thus any increase in individual cancer frequency has to be assessed for the possibility that it represents random variation. Furthermore, any finding of an increased frequency of small tumours, particularly gastric, could simply represent early diagnosis of naturally occurring disease in a population under frequent scrutiny.

CONCLUSION

Available clinical and epidemiological data do not support the contention that current antisecretory treatment may be predisposing to gastric or other varieties of cancer. Considerable interpretational difficulties exist which do, however, engender caution in coming to conclusions.

REFERENCES

Bardram, L., Thomson, P. and Stadil, F. (1986). Gastric endocrine cells in omeprazole treated and untreated patients with the Zollinger–Ellison syndrome, *Digestion*, **35** (Suppl.), 116–22.

Caygill, C. P. J., Hill, M. J., Hall, C. N., Kirkham, J. S. and Northfield, T. C. (1987). Increased risk of cancer at multiple sites after gastric surgery for peptic ulcer, *Gut*, **28**, 924–8.

Colin Jones, D. G., Langman, M. J. S., Lawson, D. H. and Vessey, M. P. (1983). Postmarketing surveillance of the safety of cimetidine: 12 month mortality report, *Br. Med. J.*, **286**, 1713–16.

Colin Jones, D. G., Langman, M. J. S., Lawson, D. H. and Vessey, M. P. (1985). Postmarketing surveillance of the safety of cimetidine: 12 month morbidity report, *Q. J. Med.*, **54**, 253–68.

Colin Jones, D. G., Langman, M. J. S., Lawson, D. H. and Vessey, M. P. (1987). Review: postmarketing surveillance of the safety of cimetidine — the problems of data interpretation, *Aliment. Pharmacol. Ther.*, **1**, 167–78.

Kalina, T. V. and Kivilaasko, E. (1983). Is the risk of stump cancer increased after partial gastrectomy?, *Scand. J. Gastroenterol.*, **18** (Suppl. 86), 35–6.

Langman, M. J. S. (1985). Antisecretory drugs and gastric cancer, *Br. Med. J.*, **290**, 1850–3.

Lanzon Miller, S., Pounder, R. E. and Hamilton, M. R. *et al.* (1987). Twenty-four-hour intragastric acidity and plasma gastrin concentration in healthy subjects and patients with duodenal or gastric ulcer, or pernicious anaemia, *Aliment. Pharmacol. Ther.*, **1**, 225–37.

Larsson, H., Carlsson, E., Mattson, H. *et al.* (1986). Plasma gastrin and gastric enterochromaffin-like cell activation and proliferation: studies with omeprazole and ranitidine in intact and antrectomized rats, *Gastroenterology*, **90**, 391–9.

Lundegardh, G., Adami, H., Helnick, C., Zack, H. and Meirik, O. (1988). Stomach cancer after partial gastrectomy for benign ulcer disease. *New Engl. J. Med.*, **319**, 195–200.

Ross, A. H. M., Smith, M. A., Anderson, J. R. and Small, W. P. (1982). Late mortality after surgery for peptic ulcer, *New Engl. J. Med.*, **307**, 519–22.

Sandler, R. S., Johnson, M. C. and Holland, K. L. (1984). Risk of stomach cancer after gastric surgery for benign conditions: a case-control study, *Dig. Dis. Sci.*, **29**, 703–8.

Spencer, A. J., Eason, C. T., Henry, D. C. and Bonner, F. W. (1988). Gastric morphological changes leading to carcinoid tumours in rats given phenoxyisobutyrate derivatives, *Human Toxicol.* Abstr. (in press).

Watt, P. C. H., Patterson, C. C. and Kennedy, T. L. (1984). Late mortality after vagotomy and drainage for duodenal ulcer, *Br. Med. J.*, **288**, 1335–8.

Advances in Drug Therapy of Gastrointestinal Ulceration
Edited by A. Garner and B. J. R. Whittle
©1989 John Wiley & Sons Ltd

Chapter Six

Clinical Evaluation of Antisecretory Agents

André L. Blum, Philippe Duroux and Peter Bauerfeind
Division of Gastroenterology, Department of Internal Medicine, CHUV, 1011 Lausanne, Switzerland

Clinical studies with antisecretory agents have increased enormously over the last ten years due to introduction of histamine H_2-antagonists and consequent expansion of the worldwide anti-ulcer market. On the basis of a recent survey, the sales for histamine H_2-antagonists amounted to $1.862 million in 1987 and a further rise of sales was predicted for 1988 (R. F. Randall Medac, 1987, unpublished observation). The Lugano Conference on controlled clinical trials (Blum *et al.*, 1986, 1987) came to the conclusion that 'controlled clinical trials are a must because they represent the best way to advance diagnosis and therapy in medicine', but 'controlled clinical trials are in a crisis because they are corrupted by too many purely commercial trials' and 'the number of controlled clinical trials is increasing because so many me-too drugs are being developed'. This is particularly true for the field of antisecretory agents.

In the following sections this development and some of its consequences will be analysed.

ROUTINE PREREGISTRATION TRIALS OF ULCER HEALING

In the routine preregistration trial of duodenal ulcer healing with antisecretory agents, a new drug is compared with a standard drug or placebo and endoscopy is performed before treatment and at fixed time intervals thereafter, e.g. 2 and 4 weeks later. The following questions are asked:

(1) Is the new drug more effective than placebo; or, more usually, is the new drug as effective or possibly more effective than a standard drug?

(2) In some of the trials, is the response to treatment with a new drug, standard drug or placebo affected by 'risk factors' such as smoking?

The use of placebo in duodenal ulcer trials is often justified by the argument that the registration of a drug with regulatory bodies such as the Food and Drug Administration (FDA) is facilitated when placebo-controlled trials are available. However, it is common knowledge that active, safe and efficacious therapy of duodenal ulcer exists. The Lugano Conference came to the conclusion that 'withholding active, safe and efficacious therapy in controlled clinical trials is acceptable provided that the omission causes minimal and short-term discomfort and an ethics committee and the informed patient agree'. The risk of harming the patient by giving placebo in duodenal and gastric ulcer has recently been assessed (Tables 6.1 and 6.2). It is obvious that the omission of active therapy in ulcer attacks is not innocuous. We consider this widely used technique as unethical, particularly when the motivation for giving placebo is purely commercial. During the Lugano Conference, 91% of the academic participants came to the conclusion that 'it is difficult to justify controlled clinical trials which are not performed with the motivation to improve the practice of medicine, but simply to facilitate the registration of new drugs'.

Table 6.1   Risk of adverse events during placebo treatment of duodenal ulcer in controlled clinical trials

	Active drug	Placebo
Patients at risk	1911	1560
Bleeding (%)	0.1 (1)	0.1 (2)
Perforation	0	0
Obstruction (%)	0.2 (3)	0.1 (1)
Severe pain (%)	0.3 (6)	2.1 (33)

(Data from Schiller and Fordtran, 1986)
The number of patients is given in brackets.

Table 6.2   Risk of adverse events during placebo treatment of gastric ulcer in controlled clinical trials

	Active drug	Placebo
Patients at risk	781	665
Bleeding (%)	0	0.8 (5)
Perforation (%)	0	0.4 (3)
Severe pain (%)	0.6 (5)	3.2 (21)

(Data from Coenen and Brösch, 1987)
The number of patients is given in brackets.

The sharp increase in the number of routine preregistration trials with antisecretory drugs appears undesirable to many observers (Blum *et al.*, 1986). Not only does it make the development of new drugs unduly expensive, but it also neutralizes the energy of many investigators which otherwise could be used in more meaningful trials. An argument which might speak in favour of conducting multiple clinical trials is the fact that one single trial is often too small to answer certain questions. For example, 20 comparative trials have been conducted with cimetidine and ranitidine and in most of these trials a statistically significant difference between the two drugs could not be detected. When McIsaac *et al.* (1987) conducted a meta-analysis of the 20 trials (Table 6.3), ranitidine was shown to be superior to cimetidine. It could be argued that a difference which requires such a large patient population in order to become statistically significant is clinically not relevant.

Routine preregistration trials might arouse more interest when the effect of so-called risk factors on the outcome is examined. In 22 controlled clinical trials the effect of smoking was examined (Table 6.4). There is in fact an interaction between the effect of histamine antagonists and smoking (Bauerfeind *et al.*, 1988), but the difference between the healing rate in smokers and non-smokers is small. However, analyses which are not based on prospectively formulated hypotheses should be regarded with caution. The Lugano Conference came to the conclusion that 'results from subgroup analysis are of use in the designing of new trials but are not very useful in determining how to treat patients'. In order to exclude bias from factors such as heterogenicity and geographical variation, we are presently conducting a large-scale epidemiological study in

Table 6.3 Effectiveness of ranitidine and cimetidine in the healing of duodenal ulcer

| | 4-week healing rate (%) | | Difference (R − C) | |
| | Ranitidine (R) | | | |
Number of patients	(2 × 150)	Cimetidine	χ^2	P
2213	76	70*	8.6	<0.01
540	81	70†	12.9	<0.01

(Data from McIsaac *et al.*, 1987)
*1000 mg day^{-1} in 15 trials
†800 mg day^{-1} in 5 trials

Table 6.4 Four-week healing rate of duodenal ulcer with histamine antagonists: effect of smoking

	22 controlled clinical trials	RUDER study
Smokers	455/646 (71%)	352/509 (69%)
Non-smokers	312/384 (82%)*	359/463 (78%)*

(Data from Bauerfeind, Siewert and Blum, 1987, and unpublished observations)
*P<0.01.

Germany, the RUDER (Ranitidin beim Ulcus Duodeni, Epidemiologie und Rezidivverhütung, A. L. Blum, 1988, unpublished data) where all duodenal ulcer patients receive standard treatment with ranitidine and the effect of smoking is assessed. This study has confirmed the impression obtained in controlled clinical trials (Table 6.4).

Routine preregistration trials usually fail to give answers to questions which are crucial in the treatment with antisecretory agents.

Mode of administration and supportive treatment

Do the mode of administration and supportive treatment modify the effectiveness of antisecretory agents? A typical example is the modification of the effect of histamine antagonists by a meal. There is a prolongation of the antisecretory effect when the drug is taken with dinner, compared with intake before or after dinner (Figure 6.1). This improvement is offset when a snack is taken later in the evening. Merki et al. (1988) reported a median nocturnal pH of 5.9 when 300 mg ranitidine was taken with dinner and a median nocturnal pH of 3.1 when a late snack was taken after dinner.

In a controlled clinical trial in patients with duodenal ulcer, Merki et al. (1988) observed a two-week healing rate of 74% when ranitidine was taken with dinner and a 50% healing rate when it was taken at bedtime. In this study no late snacks were allowed. Other studies with an apparently similar protocol failed to show a difference between ranitidine taken with dinner and ranitidine taken at bedtime; however, in these studies, late snacks were allowed which are known to reduce the effectiveness of histamine antagonists (Kempf, 1988; Kogut, 1988).

Johnston and Wormsley (1988) have recently shown that histamine antagonists are most effective when the patients fast. This study is the most striking evidence for a reduction in efficacy of histamine antagonists by food.

The competitive interaction between inhibition of acid secretion by histamine antagonists and its stimulation by a meal illustrates that apparently minor modifications of the study protocol may lead to differing results and that the particularly good or bad effect of a drug in a given trial may depend on concomitant treatment as much as true geographical variations of the disease or the population at risk.

Combination of drugs

Is a combination of drugs more effective in healing ulcers than either drug alone? In most routine preregistration trials, combinations of drugs are never examined. The question of combining drugs with different mechanisms of action has become particularly pertinent since the discovery of the role of *Campylobacter pylori* in antral gastritis and the presence of *C. pylori* in almost all patients with duodenal ulcer. Bismuth compounds and amoxicillin but not cimetidine

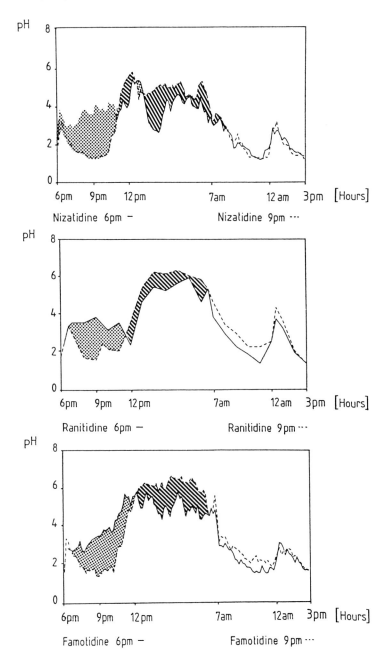

Figure 6.1 Circadian rhythm of intragastric pH with histamine antagonists given either at dinner or 3 h after dinner. (Bauerfeind *et al.*, 1987*a*, and Ph. Duroux *et al.*, unpublished data)

and sucralfate eradicate *C. pylori* (Rauws *et al.*, 1988; Humphreys *et al.*, 1988). *C. pylori* is more effectively eradicated by a combination of colloidal bismuth subcitrate plus amoxycillin than by either drug alone. Histamine antagonists accelerate duodenal ulcer healing independently of whether *C. pylori* is present or not, but bismuth preparations are more effective in the presence than in the absence of infection with *C. pylori*. Finally, one group observed in preliminary studies more rapid healing of duodenal ulcer, healing of resistant ulcers (Bayerdörfer *et al.*, 1987a,b, 1988) and fewer recurrences (Bayerdörfer *et al.*, 1988, personal communication) when an antisecretory agent was combined with an antibacterial agent than when the antisecretory agent was given alone. However, extensive reports of these studies are not yet available and no studies confirming these observations have appeared. Furthermore, the combination of cimetidine plus a bismuth compound has been reported to be no more effective than either drug alone in the treatment of duodenal ulcers (Salmon, 1987). It is uncertain, therefore, whether ulcer patients who harbour *C. pylori* should be treated with a combination of antisecretory agents and antibacterial agents in order to obtain an optimal therapeutic effect. Many more studies will be needed to clarify this question.

Frequency of recurrence

Are recurrences after treatment with a new drug less frequent than after treatment with a standard drug or with placebo? In most routine preregistration trials, no follow-up examinations are performed. Dobrilla, Vallaperta and Amplatz (1987) re-examined previously published trials with adequate follow-up examinations and came to the conclusion that the administration of bismuth compounds during acute attacks reduced the subsequent recurrence of duodenal ulcer. No other drug had this effect; the claim that antibiotics reduce the recurrence rate is discussed above. In Figure 6.2, three trials are depicted in which the treatment with bismuth compounds led to a reduction of the recurrence rate of duodenal ulcer provided, at the end of the treatment, *C. pylori* had been eradicated. Observations of this kind are important since the reduction of the recurrence rate might be more relevant than further acceleration of the healing rate.

In gastric ulcer, the recurrence rate does not seem to be affected by any current anti-ulcer drugs.

Effectiveness of drugs in subsequent attacks

Do the drugs lose their effectiveness when used in the next ulcer attack? This question has received little attention. It is of great importance since ulcer is a chronic relapsing disease; almost every patient who responds to a given drug will receive the same drug again. Mazzacca *et al.* (1988) gave the same treatment

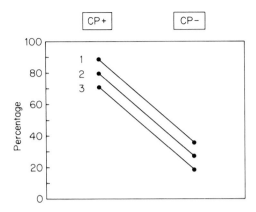

Figure 6.2 Recurrence rate of duodenal ulcer with *C. pylori* either persisting (CP$^+$) or not persisting (CP$^-$) in the antrum after healing the duodenal ulcer with bismuth compounds. (Data from Coghlan *et al.*, 1987 (1), Gilligan *et al.*, 1987 (2), and Marshall *et al.*, 1987 (3))

during two subsequent attacks of duodenal ulcer. In four of 11 patients treated with placebo, in three of 10 patients treated with cimetidine, and in two of 15 patients treated with ranitidine, an adequate response to treatment, as defined by complete healing within 8 weeks, was observed during only one attack and not during the other. In this small series, a drug sometimes had a favourable effect in the first but not the second attack or vice versa. Thus, a good response to treatment does not predict with certainty that the drug will also work a second time, and an inadequate response to treatment should not preclude the administration of the same drug in a future attack. Many more trials of this kind should be conducted.

Applicability of trial results

Are the results of clinical trials applicable to clinical practice? According to a statement of the Lugano Conference, 'it is difficult to apply the results of controlled clinical trials to medical practice because, due to selection, the patients in a controlled clinical trial do not represent the patients usually seen by practising physicians'. This problem is particularly pertinent with respect to trials with antisecretory agents. We have observed a wide variation of placebo healing rates among different trials conducted in different countries (Figure 6.3). A possible explanation for the apparently good placebo healing rate in Switzerland and the slow rate in England might be a selection bias induced by differences in the waiting lists of endoscopy units. When the patient is endoscoped soon after onset of the ulcer symptoms, all ulcers including those with a rapid spontaneous healing rate will still be seen in an active stage; this is the case in Switzerland. When

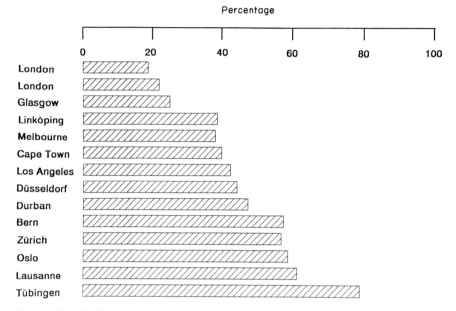

Figure 6.3 Healing rates of duodenal ulcer in patients receiving placebo. The 4-week healing rates are shown as a pecentage. For full details, see Blum (1982)

the interval between symptoms and endoscopy takes several weeks, the ulcers with a good spontaneous healing rate have already healed; only ulcers with a slow healing tendency and an unfavourable response to placebo remain active; this is the case in many parts of the UK.

ROUTINE PREREGISTRATION TRIALS OF ULCER RECURRENCE

In these trials, a new drug is compared with a standard drug or with placebo. During maintenance treatment endoscopy is usually performed when symptoms occur and/or after prefixed time intervals, for example after 6 and 12 months.

In these trials the following questions are asked:

(1) Is there a longer time interval to the first recurrence with a new drug than with a standard drug or with placebo?

(2) Does the new drug produce fewer side-effects than a standard drug or placebo?

(3) Is the recurrence rate affected by 'risk factors' such as smoking?

However, there are several questions which are usually not addressed by routine preregistration trials and which are of great importance.

The nature of the recurrence

Is the recurrence a true breakthrough event or is it due to low compliance? In the few studies where this was studied (Boyd, Wilson and Wormsley, 1983), compliance was important for the appearance of symptomatic but not of asymptomatic recurrences. Many more trials are needed to answer this question.

Maintenance therapy

Does maintenance therapy prevent both symptomatic and asymptomatic recurrences? We have examined whether maintenance treatment with cimetidine prevents symptomatic and asymptomatic recurrences (Tables 6.5 and 6.6). There has been some doubt on the basis of controlled clinical trials whether in fact asymptomatic recurrences are prevented. On the basis of a meta-analysis using the available trials, maintenance treatment with cimetidine prevents not only symptomatic but also asymptomatic recurrences. Overall, the recurrence rate during cimetidine maintenance is 16% for symptomatic and 7% for

Table 6.5 Duodenal ulcer: symptomatic recurrences during maintenance treatment with cimetidine

Author	Year	(months)	Cimetidine		Placebo	
			Recurrences	n	Recurrences	n
Müller	1978	(12)	1	20	16	20
Blackwood	1978	(6)	3	21	12	24
Gray	1978	(6)	7	24	22	27
Dronfield	1979	(6)	5	20	16	22
McCarthy	1979	(11)	13	34	26	37
Berstad	1979	(12)	2	20	14	23
Bardhan	1979	(6)	2	21	3	27
Hetzel	1980	(12)	1	20	16	21
Burland	1980	(12)	28	184	178	333
Bader	1980	(12)	9	52	27	39
Sonnenberg	1981	(12)	7	28	17	27
Capria	1983	(6)	4	20	13	20
Becker	1984	(6)	3	28	12	25
Paoluzi	1985	(6)	2	30	9	26
Bardhan	1986	(12)	6	47	19	43
Total		(11)*	93	569	390	714
			= 16%		= 55%	

(Data from Bauerfeind et al., 1987)
*Weighted mean

Table 6.6 Duodenal ulcer: asymptomatic recurrences during maintenance treatment with cimetidine (placebo controlled trials are listed in chronological order)

Author	Year	(months)	Cimetidine		Placebo	
			Recurrences	n	Recurrences	n
Blackwood	1978	(6)	2	21	9	24
Hansky	1979	(12)	0	20	2	20
Bardhan	1979	(6)	2	21	3	27
Berstad	1979	(12)	0	20	2	23
Hetzel	1980	(12)	4	20	6	21
Walters	1980	(11)	2	34	1	37
Capria	1983	(6)	0	20	0	20
Paoluzi	1985	(6)	3	30	5	26
Bardhan	1986	(12)	4	47	5	43
Total		(8)*	17	233	33	241
			= 7%		= 14%	

(Reproduced from Bauerfeind *et al.*, 1987)
*Weighted mean
Total patients 473, pooled rate difference − 0.038, s.e. 0.024, 95% confidence interval − 0.085 to + 0.010, Z = − 1.54, chi squared for heterogeneity 8.57

asymptomatic recurrences; with placebo the corresponding recurrence rates are 55% and 14%.

Treatment and prevention of recurrences

How are the recurrences treated and how are further recurrences prevented? In most maintenance trials, the patients are not examined again once a recurrence has taken place. However, this is unrealistic since a recurrence signifies when the real medical problem starts. Studies are needed where maintenance trials are not interrupted with the onset of a recurrence (see below).

Quality of life

Does maintenance treatment improve the quality of life? This question is closely related to the previous one. Today, where drugs such as omeprazole lead to 2-week healing rates of 60–80% (Figure 6.4) and to 4-week healing rates of near 100%, it might be argued that treatment of acute attacks has become so efficient that maintenance treatment is not necessary. Furthermore, no complications are observed during curative treatment with antisecretory agents such as histamine antagonists. For example, we have not observed one single complication in 729 patients so far treated with active ulcer drugs such as antisecretory agent sin controlled clinical trials which we helped to organize

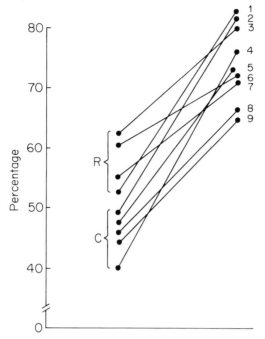

Figure 6.4 Two-week healing rates of duodenal ulcer in trials comparing omeprazole and histamine antagonists. R = ranitidine, C = cimetidine. For full details, see Bauerfeind *et al.* (1988)

(A. L. Blum, unpublished data). Finally, H_2-antagonist-resistant ulcers heal promptly with omeprazole and the recurrence rate can be reduced by the administration of bismuth compounds during the acute ulcer attack (see above). There is no convincing evidence that maintenance treatment reduces the cost of ulcer treatment as compared to mere treatment of ulcer attacks or to surgery (Bardhan, 1980; Sonnenberg and Webersinke, 1986) through adequate calculations including both direct and indirect costs are lacking. It will be necessary to conduct new types of clinical trials (Piper *et al.* 1986) to evaluate whether or not maintenance treatment is of value. The simple observation of a reduction of the recurrence rate is not sufficient in this context.

CONCLUSIONS

Most clinical trials with antisecretory agents are designed for facilitating the process of drug registration. There is an overabundance of these trials while relevant questions which should be answered by trials remain unanswered.

ACKNOWLEDGEMENT

Supported by the Swiss National Fund 3.827-0.86.

REFERENCES

Bardhan, K. D. (1980). Intermittent treatment of duodenal ulcer with cimetidine, *Br. Med. J.*, **281**, 20–2.

Bauerfeind, P., Cilluffo, T., Emde, C. *et al.* (1987*a*). Reduction of gastric acidity with ranitidine or famotidine: early evening dosage is more effective than late evening dosage, *Digestion*, **37**, 217–22.

Bauerfeind, P., Siewert, J. R. and Blum, A. L. (1987*b*). *Ulkus-Almanach,* Vol. 2, *Interdisziplinäre Gastroenterologie.* Springer-Verlag, Berlin.

Bauerfeind, P., Stadler, Ph., Koelz, H. R. *et al.* (1988). Peptische Läsionen: Therapeutische Fortschritte 1987. Therapiewoche 1988, **38**, 867–890.

Bayerdörffer, E., Sommer, A., Kasper, G. and Ottenjann, R. (1987a). *Campylobacter pylori*—Pathogen oder Opportunist bei Ulcera duodeni?, *Z. Gastroenterol.*, **25**, 423.

Bayerdörffer, E., Pirlet, Th., Sommer, A., Kasper, G. and Ottenjann, R. (1987b). Ofloxacin in der Therapie *Campylobacter-pyloridis*-positiver Ulcera duodeni, *Dtsch. Med. Wochenschr.*, **112**, 1407–11.

Bayerdörffer, E., Pirlet, Th., Sommer, A., Kasper, G. and Ottenjann, R. (1988). Ofloxacin in der Therapie 'resistenter' Ulcera duodeni: eine Pilotstudie, *Z. Gastroenterol.*, **26**, 155–9.

Blum, A. L. (1982). Is placebo the ideal anti-ulcer drug? In G. Bianchi-Porro and K. D. Bardhan (eds) *Peptic Ulcer Disease*, Raven Press, New York, pp. 57–61.

Blum, A. L., Popien, J. and Bauerfernd, P. (1988). Decisions in a case of recurrent duodenal ulcer. In T. C. Chalmers (ed.) *Data Analysis For Clinical Medicine*, International University Press, pp. 101–144.

Blum, A. L., Chalmers, T. C., Deutsch, E. *et al.* (1986). Differing attitudes of industry and academia towards controlled clinical trials, *Eur. J. Clin. Invest.*, **16**, 455–60.

Blum, A. L., Chalmers, T. C., Deutsch, F. *et al.* (1987). The Lugano statements on controlled clinical trials, *J. Int. Med. Res.*, **15**, 2–22.

Boyd, E. J. S., Wilson, J. A. and Wormsley, K. G. (1983). Effects of treatment compliance and overnight gastric secretion on outcome of maintenance therapy of duodenal ulcer with ranitidine, *Scand. J. Gastroenterol.*, **18**, 193–200.

Coenen, C. and Brösch, G. (1987). Komplikationsrate während der Akutbehandlung des Magenulkus: Beeinflussung der Incidenz durch Verumtherapie in Plazebokontrollierten Studien, *Z. Gastroenterol.*, **25**, 697–701.

Coghlan, J. G., Gilligan, D., Humphries, H. *et al.* (1987). *Campylobacter pylori* and recurrence of duodenal ulcers—a 12-month follow-up study, *Lancet*, **1**, 1109–11.

Dobrilla, G., Vallaperta, P. and Amplatz, S. (1988). Influence of ulcer healing agents on ulcer relapse after discontinuation of acute treatment: a pooled estimate of controlled clinical trials, *Gut*, **29**, 181–7.

Gilligan, D., Coghlan, G., Humphries, H. *et al.* (1987). *Campylobacter pylori* and recurrence of duodenal ulcers—an eighteen month follow up study, *Gastroenterology*, **92**, 1355 (abstract).

Humphreys, H., Bourke, S., Dooley, C. *et al.* (1988). Effect of treatment on *Campylobacter pylori* in peptic disease: a randomised prospective trial, *Gut*, **29**, 279–83.

Johnston, D. A. and Wormsley, K. G. (1988). Food is bad for ulcers. European Gastro-Club Abstracts, *Hepato-gastroenterology*, **35**, 44.

Kempf, M., Kaufmann, D., Walt, R. P. *et al.* (1988). TV snacks are bad for H₂-receptor-blockade, *Gastroenterology*, **94**, A222.

Kogut, D. G., Agrawal, N., Collen, M. J. and Johnson, J. A. (1988). 300 mg ranitidine administered at 6 p.m. and at 10 p.m. in the treatment of duodenal ulcer disease, *Gastroenterology*, **94**, A233.

McIsaac, R. L., McCanless, I., Summers, K. and Wood, J. R. (1987). Ranitidine and cimetidine in the healing of duodenal ulcer: meta-analysis of comparative clinical trials, *Aliment. Pharmacol. Ther.*, **1**, 369–81.

Marshall, B. J., Goodwin, C. S., Warren, J. R. *et al.* (1987). Long term healing of gastritis and low duodenal ulcer relapse after eradication of *Campylobacter pyloridis*: a prospective double-blind study, *Gastroenterology*, **92** 1518 (abstract).

Mazzacca, G., Sabbatini, F., Piai, G., D'Agostino, L., D'Arienzo, A. and Verre, C. (1988). Failure to heal of duodenal peptic ulcers: a hallmark of the single relapse?, *Gastroenterology*, **94**, A293.

Merki, H., Witzel, L., Hüttemann, W. *et al.* (1988). Single dose treatment with H₂ receptor antagonists: a comparison of an early evening dose vs bedtime administration of ranitidine in the treatment of duodenal ulcer, *Am. J. Gastroenterol.*, **83**, 362–7.

Piper, D. W., Pym, B. M., Toy, S., Gellatly, R., Byth, K. and Seville, P. (1986). The effect of maintenance cimetidine therapy on the medical, social and economic aspects of patients with chronic gastric ulcers: a placebo-controlled prospective study, *Med. J. Aust.*, **145**, 400–3.

Rauws, E. A. J., Langenberg, W., Houthoff, H. J., Zanen, H. C. and Tytgat, G. N. J. (1988). *Campylobacter pyloridis*-associated chronic active antral gastritis, *Gastroenterology*, **94**, 33–40.

Salmon, P. R. (1987). Combination treatment: colloidal bismuth subcitrate with H₂-antagonists, *Digestion*, 37 (Suppl. 2), 42–6.

Schiller, L. R. and Fordtran, J. S. (1986). Ulcer complications during short-term therapy of duodenal ulcer with active agents and placebo, *Gastroenterology*, **90**, 478–81.

Sonnenberg, A. and Webersinke, R. (1986). The costs of medical and surgical treatment of duodenal ulcer disease, *Gastroenterology*, **90**, 1643.

Advances in Drug Therapy of Gastrointestinal Ulceration
Edited by A. Garner and B. J. R. Whittle
© 1989 John Wiley & Sons Ltd

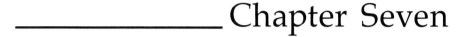

Chapter Seven

Prostaglandins and Mucosal Protection: Laboratory Evidence versus Clinical Performance

C. J. Hawkey

Department of Therapeutics, University Hospital, Nottingham NG7 2UH, UK

INTRODUCTION

Prostaglandin analogues were originally developed for ulcer treatment because of their antisecretory properties, and small trials in the 1970s showed that they could heal gastric and duodenal ulcers. After their clinical prospects had been eclipsed by the advent of H_2-receptor antagonists, interest was revived by observations showing them to mediate numerous defensive processes in the gastroduodenal mucosa. Whilst this has undoubtedly led to better understanding of basic pathophysiological processes, the performance of prostaglandin analogues thus far as ulcer-healing drugs has been disappointing and it is doubtful that healing rates have exceeded that which can be produced by comparable acid inhibition alone.

This chapter reviews the acute actions of prostaglandins in the stomach and duodenum, and their therapeutic performance in clinical practice, and, in the final section, considers reasons for the discrepancy.

EFFECTS OF PROSTAGLANDINS ON THE GASTRIC AND DUODENAL MUCOSA

Acid

Prostaglandins of the E and I series can inhibit acid secretion. Although there has been some debate as to the precise cellular location within the gastric mucosa of histamine, gastrin, acetylcholine and prostaglandin receptors, it now seems clear that, in some species, E prostaglandins bind to high-affinity receptors on the parietal cell (Soll *et al.*, 1986; Tsai *et al.*, 1987). This leads to activation of the inhibitory subunit of adenyl cyclase (which is normally stimulated by histamine), with a lowering of intracellular cyclic AMP and inhibition of acid secretion (Figure 7.1.) Inhibition of endogenous prostaglandins by indomethacin leads to an augmented response to histamine and antral acidification (Levine and Schwartzel, 1984; Befrits, Samuelsson and Johansson, 1984), although 24 h intragastric pH does not change (Walt *et al.*, 1987).

Mucosal defence

One of the more dramatic demonstrations of mucosal protection by prostaglandins involves prevention of microscopic signs of injury caused by absolute ethanol, boiling water, caustic soda and concentrated hydrochloric acid (Figure 7.2) first shown by Robert *et al.* (1979). Non-antisecretory doses of prostaglandins can abolish the grossly evident signs of injury caused by 100% alcohol. Macroscopically these appear as obvious red lesions; microscopically there is deep haemorrhage and necrosis (Lacy and Ito, 1982).

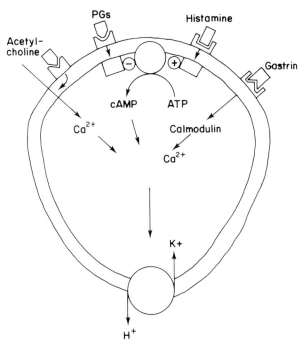

Figure 7.1 Putative control of parietal cell functions. Prostaglandins bind to specific receptors and probably activate the inhibitory subunit of adenyl cyclase

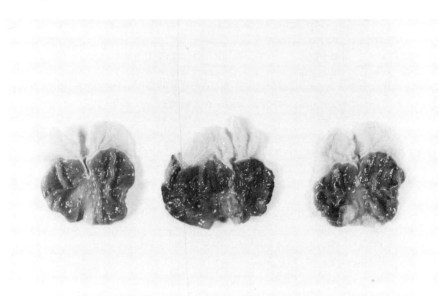

Figure 7.2 Effect of prostaglandin E₁ (300 µg kg⁻¹, p.o.) on macroscopic changes to the rat stomach induced by alcohol. Left, control; middle, 100% ethanol; right, prostaglandin E₁ given 15 min before ethanol

The changes induced by prostaglandins were described as 'cytoprotective', a term which has stimulated a vigorous, continuing and somewhat sterile semantic debate as to whether true cellular protection is involved. Histological studies show that surface epithelial cells are not protected since the mucosa is denuded of epithelium after absolute alcohol whether or not prostaglandin pretreatment is given (Lacy and Ito, 1982). However, the depth of injury appears to be somewhat less in prostaglandin-pretreated animals, and epithelial recovery, occurring in minutes and hours following injury, can be shown by a variety of techniques to be rapid (Silen and Ito, 1985). This early process of recovery involves migration of cells from the gastric crypts to cover the mucosal surface again. This surface restitution may be favoured because such cells are better preserved after prostaglandin pretreatment (Tarnawski *et al.*, 1985). The process of rapid restitution, whilst superficially relevant to ulcer healing, does not involve cell division, occurs at the most superficial level of the epithelium, and has never been shown to be influenced directly by prostaglandins as a result of their effects on the initial depth of mucosal injury. No studies have addressed the question of whether prostaglandins given after injury would accelerate this process.

The mechanisms underlying the reduction in depth of injury mediated by prostaglandins in this model are not fully understood, but may in part be the same as those which prevent deep mucosal haemorrhage and necrosis. Time-lapse studies have shown that the first effect of ethanol is to cause stasis of blood flow in the capillary arcades of the gastric mucosa, followed by engorgement and haemorrhage in the more proximal deeper feeding vessels (Guth, 1986; Pihan *et al.*, 1986). What underlies this property, which may amount to true 'vasculoprotection', is currently not clear.

Numerous other agents have been tested in this model. Several have been shown to prevent the microscopic signs of injury:

(1) *Fatty acid precursors:* Both arachidonic acid and linoleic acid have been shown to enhance prostaglandin production and protect the mucosa against ethanol (Hollander *et al.*, 1982). In these experiments a large dose of fatty acids is given 15 min before ethanol; the question of whether long-term supplementation induces a persisting response has not been investigated.

(2) *Lipoxygenase inhibitors:* The compound BW755C, nordihydroguaretic acid (NDGA) and the fatty acid eicosapentaenoic acid all lead to reduced synthesis of lipoxygenase products of arachidonic acid, and all have been shown to protect against ethanol. However, these drugs all have other actions and more specific 5-lipoxygenase inhibitors have not been protective (Wallace, Beck and Morris, 1988).

(3) *Antibiotics:* Neomycin can prevent ethanol induced injury in rats, but the significance of this is hard to assess.

(4) *Carbenoxolone:* This ulcer-healing drug enhances gastric prostaglandin levels by inhibiting their metabolism and also protects against ethanol damage (Hawkey and Rampton, 1985).

(5) *Mild irritants:* Lower concentrations of ethanol, hydrochloric acid or sodium hydroxide can be shown to stimulate gastric mucosal prostaglandin synthesis and to mimic the effects of exogenous prostaglandins (Robert *et al.*, 1983). This led to the proposal that this process of 'adaptive cytoprotection' was a physiological phenomenon, normally subserved by endogenous prostaglandins stimulated in response to mild injury and fortuitously mimicked by exogenous prostaglandins. However, mild irritants capable of inducing adaptive cytoprotection have not always been shown to stimulate endogenous prostaglandin synthesis, and adaptive cytoprotection has been shown to occur even in the presence of indomethacin sufficient to reduce prostaglandin synthesis by 85% (Hawkey *et al.*, 1988).

(6) *Surface covering:* Histological studies show that mild irritants disrupt the surface epithelium, with formation of a covering of mucus, fibrin and desquamated surface cells (Hawkey *et al.*, 1988) as depicted in Figure 7.3. What is not clear is whether it is the surface cap or the prostaglandin synthesis (which often occurs during the process of desquamation) which is of major importance in this model. It seems likely that both processes play a role in the normal day-to-day protection of the gastroduodenal mucosa. The surface cap following mild or major injury has also been shown to be of importance for epithelial restitution since this is delayed if the cap is removed or subjected to treatment by mucolytic

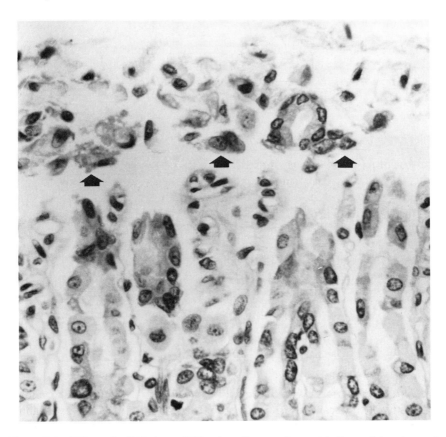

Figure 7.3 Effect of mild irritant (20% ethanol) on surface epithelium of the rat gastric mucosa. Note the desquamated cells and debris. Is the physical effect of this covering or the associated prostaglandin synthesis protective? (Reprinted from Hawkey *et al.* (1988) with permission. ©1988, The American Gastroenterological Association)

agents (Wallace and Whittle, 1986). Agents that increase mucus thickness and viscosity protect the gastric mucosa (Foster *et al.*, 1985).

(7) *Sucralfate, chelated bismuth and antacids:* These agents have all been shown to mimic the effects of mild irritants on mucosal morphology, prostaglandin synthesis and protection against ethanol (Hollander *et al.*, 1985; Hall and Van den Hoven, 1987).

(8) *Mast cell stabilizers:* Agents that stabilize gastrointestinal mucosal mast cells protect against ethanol (Takeuchi, Nishiwaki and Okabe, 1986). Mice congenitally deficient in gastrointestinal mast cells show less severe injury. High concentrations of prostaglandins stabilize mast cells and this has been shown for some analogues such as misoprostol (Reimann *et al.*, 1987).

Agents shown not to be effective in the ethanol model

In animal and human experiments, H_2-receptor antagonists have generally had little or no activity against ethanol-induced damage (Hawkey and Rampton, 1985). The position in respect of proton pump inhibitors is not clear, but some studies have shown protection (Okabe, Miyake and Awane, 1986).

Other models

A different pattern of injury is associated with non-steroid anti-inflammatory drugs (NSAIDs). In rats, indomethacin reduces gastric mucosal blood flow, rendering the mucosa susceptible to injury by mild irritants, such as bile acids, salicylates and food (Whittle, 1977; Satoh, Guth and Grossman, 1982). Aspirin is more directly toxic to the gastric mucosa. The reasons for this are complex and currently under debate. Aspirin combines both an ability to inhibit prostaglandin synthesis and, following hydrolysis, the topical irritancy of salicylates. Although prostaglandin synthesis is inhibited by aspirin, preventing the hydrolysis of acetylsalicylic acid to salicyclic acid may reduce the toxicity of aspirin. The presence of a low pH is also important for maximum injury (Rowe *et al.* 1987).

Gastric mucosal injury by aspirin and other NSAIDs has been studied extensively in acute situations in humans. Prostaglandins can reduce injury measured by DNA exfoliation, endoscopy, bleeding and changes in mucosal potential difference, though most studies have used antisecretory doses and protection can be achieved by antisecretory doses of H_2-receptor antagonists (Hawkey and Rampton, 1985; Hawkey, 1987). For the latter drugs, it is possible that mechanisms in addition to acid inhibition are involved since they have been shown in animals to prevent NSAID and bile acid injury, even when the intragastric pH is kept constant.

With aspirin and other NSAIDs, a process of adaptation to continuing ingestion seems to occur (Graham, Smith and Dobbs, 1983). The mechanism is unclear, as is its relationship to short-term adaptation to alcohol, but the phenomenon is worth investigating since it is possible that a failure of adaptation could underlie the long-term development of clinically significant injury with NSAIDs.

Synopsis

It must be stressed that these models are of limited conceptual relevance to ulcer healing. Moreover, the microscopic changes occurring in response to the extreme stimulus of 100% ethanol have received undue attention. More important to the understanding of basic physiology and possible therapeutic benefits are the individual processes affected by prostaglandins (Table 7.1). These can be classified as follows:

Table 7.1   Mucosal defence mechanisms

Lumen	Acid inhibition
Juxtamucosal	Mucus thickness
Supra-epithelial	Bicarbonate secretion
Epithelial	Phospholipid content
Subepithelial	Ion exchanges
	Vasodilation
	'Vasculoprotection'
Secondary processes	Increased speed of restitution secondary to reduced injury

Reduced access of acid and other small molecules to the surface epithelium

(1) *Mucus and bicarbonate production:* The synthesis and secretion of mucus by the stomach and the thickness of the mucus layer are stimulated by natural and synthetic prostaglandins and inhibited by NSAIDs (Allen and Garner, 1980). An important development has been the recognition that surface epithelial cells secrete bicarbonate. Although several imperfectly understood mechanisms are probably involved, prostaglandins enhance the rate of electrogenic bicarbonate secretion. Bicarbonate secretion is quantitatively much greater in the duodenum than the stomach, and it seems likely that it is an important defence mechanism against acid injury to the duodenum (Hogan and Isenberg, 1988).

(2) *Strengthening of the mucosal barrier:* Several observations in animals and man show that prostaglandins prevent the acid back-diffusion and associated fall in mucosal potential difference caused by aspirin and other agents (Hawkey and Rampton, 1985). Several issues are unclear, however. It is not known whether these changes genuinely occur at the cell surface or at the level of the mucus–bicarbonate barrier. It is of interest that agents which 'break' the mucosal barrier are lipolytic. Whether acid back-diffusion occurs by a transcellular or intercellular (via tight junctions) route is not clear. The permeability of epithelial cell membranes to acid under normal conditions is not known. Changes in mucosal potential difference may mirror injury rather than being fundamental themselves (Hawkey, 1987).

(3) *Surface phospholipids:* Prostaglandins have been reported to increase the phospholipid content of surface epithelial cell membranes, and an opposite effect has been reported for aspirin (Lichtenberger *et al.*, 1983). Increased phospholipids appear to reduce the wettability of the cell surface, in effect making it more waxy, an action which could protect against acid and other water-soluble substances. These data await more widespread confirmation.

Disposal of acid and other small molecules

(1) *Vasodilatation:* Prostaglandins of the E and I series are vasodilators in the gastric mucosa (Whittle, 1977), allowing disposal of substances, including acid, which have gained access to it.

(2) *Ion exchange mechanisms:* Sodium–hydrogen and chloride–bicarbonate exchange mechanisms help to maintain the intracellular and intercellular pH (Machen and Paradiso, 1987).

True 'vasculoprotection'

Although ill-defined, this appears to be important in the ethanol model (Guth, 1986; Pihan *et al.*, 1986). Its role in other less extreme forms of injury and in clinically significant lesions is not clear.

Repair processess

Neither cell motility nor cell division (which are presumably important for ulcer healing) have yet been shown specifically to be stimulated by prostaglandins.

Gastric emptying

Prostaglandins of the E series generally contract longitudinal muscle and relax circular muscle and have been shown to increase gastric emptying in primates. In contrast, prostacyclin delays gastric emptying and inhibits small intestinal transit (Dubois and Conklin, 1987). The role of endogenous prostaglandins in gastric motility in humans is somewhat unclear. Indomethacin has little effect (Chaudhuri and Fink, 1984), but there is surprisingly little data in this area.

Gastrin

Some prostaglandin analogues, notably enprostil and probably arbaprostil, inhibit gastrin release (Mahachai *et al.*, 1985).

Mechanisms that reduce the injury or access of acid to the mucosa are likely to be relevant in determining susceptibility to peptic ulceration. Repair processes may be of more relevance to ulcer healing, and any involvement of prostaglandins in these has not been established.

ABNORMALITIES OF PROSTAGLANDIN SYNTHESIS IN PATIENTS WITH PEPTIC ULCERS

An increasing number of studies have addressed the question of whether prostaglandin synthesis is impaired in patients with gastric or duodenal ulcers. Unfortunately, a consensus is difficult to achieve since all have used widely varying methods. However, a majority of studies of patients with gastric ulcers has shown reduced synthesis of E prostaglandins (Table 7.2; Hawkey and

Table 7.2 Changes in fasting gastric mucosal PGE_2 levels/synthesis and metabolism in patients with gastric ulcer or gastritis

| Author | Tissue | In ulcer disease | | With inflammation | |
		PGE_2 level	Metabolism	PGE_2 level	Metabolism
Wright	Stomach	Lowered			
Konturek	Antrum	Lowered			
Hawkey	Fundus	Lowered slightly		Raised	Degradation
Crampton	Fundus	Lowered	Degradation		
	Antrum	No change	Degradation		
Pugh	Stomach	Lowered			

Rampton, 1985; Hawkey, 1986a,b). The same is not true for duodenal ulcers (compare Tables 7.2 and 7.3). One influential study reported that post-cibal prostaglandin synthesis in the duodenum of patients with healed duodenum ulcers was low in relation to antecibal levels (Figure 7.4) and to the duodenal acid load (Alquist *et al.*, 1983). However, this arose largely because the antecibal levels were higher than normal. In contrast, other studies have variously reported reductions in fasting (antecibal) levels of PGE_2, PGI_2 and PGF_2, or no change from normal (Hawkey, 1986b).

Defective defence mechanisms in ulcer patients which could be prostaglandin mediated

An important finding has been the demonstration of reduced duodenal bicarbonate production by duodenal ulcer patients in remission by Hogan and Isenberg (1986) as shown in Figure 7.5. There are no comparable reports for gastric ulcer patients. The thickness of surface gastric mucus is reduced in duodenal patients but not in gastric ulcer patients (though it may be abnormal) and duodenal mucus has not been investigated.

Table 7.3 Changes in fasting duodenal mucosal prostaglandin levels/synthesis in patients with duodenal ulcers

| Author | Changes in prostaglandin level | | | | |
	PGD_2	PGE_2	$PGF_{2\alpha}$	PGI_2	TXB_2
Alquist	Raised	Raised	Raised	Raised	Raised
Hillier		No change	Lowered	Lowered	No change
Pugh		Lowered			
Crampton		No change			

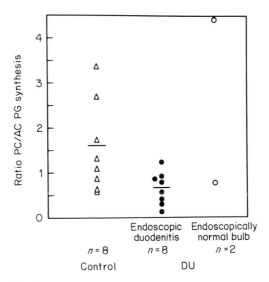

Figure 7.4 Altered ratio of postcibal to anticibal prostaglandin synthesis in duodenal ulcer patients. Note, however, that this reduced ratio is due to elevated anticibal levels (see Table 7.3). (Reprinted from Alquist *et al.* (1983) with permission. ©1983, The American Gastroenterological Association)

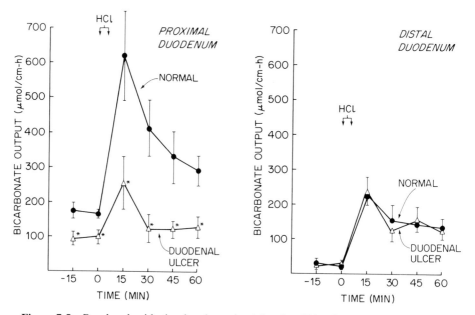

Figure 7.5 Basal and acid stimulated proximal duodenal bicarbonate output in control patients and those with inactive duodenal ulcers. (Reprinted from Isenberg *et al.* (1987) by permission of the *New England Journal of Medicine*)

Influence of predisposing factors on prostaglandin levels

NSAIDs which inhibit gastroduodenal prostaglandin synthesis have been associated clinically at presentation with haematemesis and malaena or peptic ulcer perforation (Somerville, Faulkner and Langman, 1986). The other major identified environmental influence, smoking, is also associated with reduced gastric prostaglandin synthesis or release (McCready, Clark and Cohen, 1985; Quimby *et al.*, 1986) shown in Figure 7.6. Peptic ulcer incidence in the USA and the UK is declining and it has been proposed that the parallel rise in consumption of linoleic acid in vegetable oils, by mediating an increase in prostaglandin synthesis, might be responsible (Hollander and Tarnawaski, 1986). This hypothesis remains to be tested. In contrast there is a rising incidence of ulcer in elderly women, though age and sex *per se* do not appear to be associated with reduced prostaglandin synthesis (Hawkey, 1986b).

PROSTAGLANDIN ANALOGUES AVAILABLE FOR CLINICAL TRIALS

A large number of derivatives of PGE_1, PGE_2 and prostacyclin have been produced and are listed in Table 7.4. The pharmacokinetic and pharmaco-dynamic properties of those analogues for which there are most data are detailed in Table 7.5. With the exception of enprostil, most have a relatively short half-life.

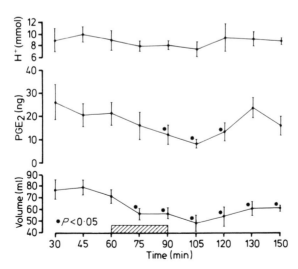

Figure 7.6 Effect of smoking on output of PGE_2 intragastric juice in man. Note the associated reduction in volume. (Reproduced from McCready, Clark and Cohen (1985) by permission of *Gut*)

Table 7.4 Prostaglandin analogues developed for possible use as ulcer-healing agents

Launched		
Enprostil	(Mexico)	Gardrin, Syngard
Misoprostol	(14 countries)	Cytotec
Rosaprostil	(Italy)	Rosal
Clinical trials		*Pharmacology/Phase 1*
Arbaprostil		Enisprost
Dimoxaprost		Epoprostenol
Mexiprostil		FCE-20700
Ornoprostil		GR-55556
Rioprostil		Nileprost
Tiprostanide		Noclaprost
Trimoprostil		RO 31-0521
		U68215
Suspended		
CL-115574		
CS-570		

Acid inhibition

In terms of the dose required to produce a measurable effect on acid, prostaglandin analogues are the most potent antisecretory agents known but their maximum effect is often limited, whether by a therapeutic ceiling or by unacceptable side-effects. Comparative studies are few, but misoprostol 200 μg was of roughly similar potency to cimetidine 200 mg in inhibiting coffee-stimulated

Table 7.5 Pharmacology and therapeutics of main prostaglandin analogues in human subjects

	Acid-inhibiting dose (μg)	Duration of acid inhibition (h)	Inhibition of gastrin release	Mucosal protective dose (μg)	Duodenal ulcer healing
Arbaprostil	50–200		?	110–50	More than placebo
Trimoprostil	750–3000	2–7	—	2000	More than placebo, less than cimetidine
Misoprostol	200–800	2–8	?	25–200	Similar to cimetidine
Enprostil	35–140	6–12	—	?7,35–70	Similar to cimetidine
Rioprostil	300–600		—	?50–100	?Similar to cimetidine

(Data from Hawkey and Rampton, 1985; Hawkey, 1987; Monk and Clissold, 1987; Goa and Monk, 1987; Demol *et al.*, 1986; Muller, Damann and Simon, 1986, 1987.)

acid secretion (Salmon and Barton, 1986). There are only published data on 24 h intragastric acidity for enprostil. In two British studies enprostil 35 μg twice daily or 70 μg nightly produced only modest acid inhibition (Deakin *et al.*, 1986; Walt *et al.*, 1987), whereas in an American study enprostil 35 μg twice daily was more effective than cimetidine (Mahachai *et al.*, 1985).

Enprostil has also been shown to prevent meal stimulated gastrin release (Mahachai *et al.*, 1985).

Mucosal defence

Trimoprostil, misoprostol, enprostil and rioprostil have all been shown to reduce aspirin-induced mucosal injury assessed by bleeding, desquamation, endoscopy or changes in potential difference. Evidence for activity not attributable to changes in acid is relatively limited, but misoprostol has been shown to reduce ethanol injury to the human gastric mucosa to a much greater extent than cimetidine (Agrawal *et al.*, 1986). Doses of misoprostol just below the antisecretory threshold protected against aspirin-induced injury, assessed by bleeding (Monk and Clissold, 1987). Doses of enprostil (7 μg), likely to have a minimal affect on acid, probably gave some protection against aspirin, assessed endoscopically, but this was rather less than seen with higher, antisecretory doses (Goa and Monk, 1987).

Ulcer healing with prostaglandin analogues

Arbaprostil

Although antisecretory doses of arbaprostil heal duodenal ulcers faster than placebo, doses in the cytoprotective range (10 mg or 25 mg four times daily) are ineffective (Euler *et al.*, 1987).

Trimoprostil

Trimoprostil 750 μg four times daily healed significantly fewer duodenal ulcers at 4 weeks than cimetidine 200 mg three times daily, 400 mg nightly (Bardhan *et al.*, 1984).

Misoprostol

Extensive worldwide trials show that ulcer healing and pain relief with misoprostol are dose-dependent and that antisecretory doses of 100 μg four times daily or more are required to enhance the placebo healing rate (Herting and Nissen, 1986). In comparative studies, misoprostol 800 μg/day^{-1} was not significantly different from cimetidine 1200 mg day^{-1} in healing gastric or duodenal ulcers over 4 weeks (Nicholson, 1985; Rachmilewitz, Chapman and Nicholson, 1986).

Enprostil

Doses in the range 35–140 μg day⁻¹ have been shown to heal gastric and duodenal ulcers (Goa and Monk, 1987). However, two comparative studies have shown daily doses of 70 μg to be less effective than ranitidine 300 mg in healing duodenal ulcers, but comparable to cimetidine 800 mg day⁻¹ (Lauritsen *et al.*, 1986; Walt *et al.*, 1987) as shown in Figure 7.7. Maintenance treatment with enprostil 35 μg nightly held fewer duodenal ulcer patients in remission than did ranitidine 150 mg nightly (Lauritsen *et al.*, 1987).

Rioprostil

The only published study has shown rioprostil 600 μg nightly to heal at a rate similar to ranitidine 300 mg nightly (Damman *et al.*, 1986).

Prostacyclin

In one open study, prostacyclin was infused for 5 h day⁻¹ at a rate of 5 ng kg⁻¹ h⁻¹. This was associated with some reduction in duodenal ulcer size (Dembinska-Kiec *et al.*, 1986).

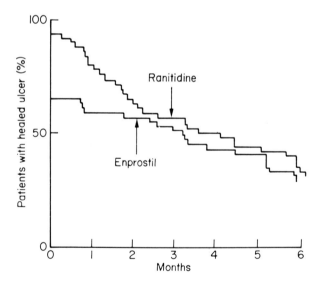

Figure 7.7 Healing and relapse with enprostil 70 μg nightly and ranitidine 300 mg nightly. Note the more rapid initial relapse after healing with ranitidine. This may partially be due to the greater number of ulcers healed, although there may be genuine differences attributable to the initial healing agent

Use in special situations

Like other drugs, prostaglandins will heal the ulcers of patients who continue to take NSAIDs. Likewise, they heal the ulcers of smokers. There is no evidence that they are superior to other drugs in these respects. Enprostil 35 μg nightly has been shown to be inferior to ranitidine 150 mg nightly as maintenance treatment for healed duodenal ulceration (Lauritsen *et al.*, 1987). However, in patients not given maintenance following healing, there is some evidence (see Figure 7.7) that relapse is slower if the initial treatment was misoprostol or enprostil than if it was an H_2-receptor antagonist (O'Keefe *et al.*, 1985; Hawkey *et al.*, 1988). Further work is needed to establish whether this apparent difference is real and, if so, what underlying mechanism is involved.

Adverse reactions

Most prostaglandin analogues have had more side-effects than their comparator in the trials reported above. The most commonly reported is diarrhoea or loose stools. A substantial number of patients are affected, though usually to a relatively mild degree. It is difficult to draw strict comparisons between different prostaglandins because trials have not employed comparable definitions of diarrhoea either explicitly or implicitly. One study has claimed a relatively low incidence of side-effects for rioprostil, but this requires verification by other studies (Damman *et al.*, 1986).

Of particular concern is the ability of prostaglandins to induce abortion by stimulating uterine contraction. When normal clinical doses of misoprostol were given to women at an abortion clinic in the first trimester of pregnancy, about 10% had a completed abortion within 24 h (Monk and Clissold, 1987). It will be important to have similar data for other prostaglandins, but as yet none is in print.

Synopsis

Prostaglandins of the E series inhibit acid secretion probably by activating the inhibitory subunit of adenylate cyclase in the parietal cell. Several classes of prostaglandins protect the mucosa against a variety of insults by several mechanisms, including increased mucus and bicarbonate secretion, vasodilatation and protection of the vascular endothelium. Some of them inhibit gastrin release.

In clinical practice, prostaglandin analogues are a useful addition to the gastroenterologist's therapeutic armamentarium, but they are not a major advance. The failure to heal faster than is predicted by acid inhibition suggests that different mechanisms are involved in ulcer healing and mucosal protection.

REFERENCES

Agrawal, N. M., Godiwala, T., Arimura, A. *et al.* (1986). Comparative cytoprotective effects against alcohol insult: misoprostol versus cimetidine, *Dig. Dis. Sci.*, **31** (Suppl.), 142S-4S.

Allen, A. and Garner, A. (1980). Mucus and bicarbonate secretion in the stomach and their possible role in mucosal protection, *Gut*, **21**, 249-62.

Alquist, D. A., Dozois, R. R., Sinsmeister, A. R. *et al.* (1983). Duodenal prostaglandin synthesis and acid load in health and in duodenal ulcer disease, *Gastroenterology*, **85**, 522-9.

Bardhan, K. D., Whittaker, L., Hinchcliffe, R. F. *et al.* (1984). Trimoprostil vs cimetidine in duodenal ulcer, *Gut*, **25**, A580.

Befrits, R., Samuelsson, K. and Johansson, C. (1984). Gastric acid inhibition by antral acidification mediated by endogenous prostaglandins, *Gastroenterology*, **86**, 1023.

Chaudhuri, T. K. and Fink, S. (1984). Lack of effect of indomethacin on gastric emptying in old men, *J. Am. Geriatr. Soc.*, **32**, 19-20.

Dammann, H. G., Walter, T. A., Muller, P. *et al.* (1986). Rioprostil 600 mg nocte: high duodenal ulcer healing rates, low incidence of side effects, *Gastroenterology*, **90**, 1386.

Deakin, M., Ramage, J., Paul, A. *et al.* (1986). Effect of enprostil, a synthetic prostaglandin F2 on 24 hour intragastric acidity, nocturnal acid and pepsin secretion, *Gut*, **27**, 1054-7.

Dembinska-Kiec, A., Kostka, A. and Kosiniek-Kamysz, A. (1986). Prostacyclin in patients with peptic gastric ulcer — a placebo control study, *Hepato-gastroenterology*, **33**, 262-6.

Demol, P., Schmitz, H. D., Weihrauch, T. R. *et al.* (1986). Prevention of the acetylsalicyclic acid-induced changes of the gastric potential difference by the new synthetic prostaglandin E1 analogue rioprostil, *Arzneimittelforschung*, **36**, 1406-8.

Dubois, A. and Conklin, J. J. (1987). Prostaglandins and gastric emptying. In B. Samuelsson, R. Paoletti and P. W. Ramwell (eds) *Advances in Prostaglandin, Thromboxane and Leukotriene Research*, Vol. 17, Raven Press, New York, pp. 370-2.

Euler, A. R., Tytgat, G., Berenguer, J. *et al.* (1987). Failure of a cytoprotective dose of arbaprostil to heal acute duodenal ulcers: results of multiclinic trial, *Gastroenterology*, **92**, 604-7.

Foster, S. N. E., Allen, A. and Pearson, J. P. (1985). Mechanism for the mucosal protective action of polyacrylate on the gastric mucus barrier, *Gut*, **26**, 24, abstract 1109.

Goa, K. L. and Monk, J. P. (1987). Enprostil: a preliminary review of its pharmacodynamic and pharmacokinetic properties and therapeutics efficacy in the treatment of peptic ulcer disease, *Drugs*, **34**, 539-59.

Graham, D. Y., Smith, J. L. and Dobbs, S. M. (1983). Gastric adaptation occurs with aspirin administration in man, *Dig. Dis. Sci.*, **28**, 1-6.

Guth, P. H. (1986). Gastric blood flow and prostaglandin cytoprotection, *Scand. J. Gastroenterol.*, **21** (Suppl. 125), 86-91.

Hall, D. W., Van den Hoven, W. E. (1987). Gastric mucosa protection and prostaglandin E2 generation in rats by colloidal bismuth subcitrate (DE NOL), *Arch. Int. Pharmacodyn. Ther.*, **286**, 308.

Hawkey, C. J. (1986a). Synthesis of prostaglandin E_2, thromboxane B_2 and prostaglandin catabolism in gastritis and gastric ulcer, *Gut*, **27**, 1484-92.

Hawkey, C. J. (1986b). Endogenous prostaglandins and peptic ulcers. In W. D. W. Rees (ed.) *Proceedings of the 7th BSG.SK&F International Workshop. Peptic Ulcer Disease*, Oxprint, Hatfield, pp. 33-7.

Hawkey, C. J. (1987). Acute human models of gastric mucosal injury, *Aliment. Pharmacol. Ther.*, **1**, 593.

Hawkey, C. J. and Rampton, D. S. (1985). Prostaglandins and the gastrointestinal mucosa: are they important in its function, disease, or treatment?, *Gastroenterology*, **89**, 1162–88.

Hawkey, C. J., Kemp, T. P., Walt, R. P. *et al.* (1988). Evidence that adaptive cytoprotection in rats is not mediated by prostaglandins, *Gastroenterology*, **94**, 948–54.

Herting, R. L. and Nissen, C. H. (1986). Overview of misoprostol clinical experience, *Dig. Dis. Sci.*, **31** (2), 47S–54S.

Hogan, D. L. and Isenberg, J. I. (1988). Gastroduodenal bicarbonate production, *Adv. Intern. Med.*, **33**, 385–408.

Hollander, D. and Tarnawaski, A. (1986). Dietary essential fatty acids and the decline in peptic ulcer disease — a hypothesis, *Gut*, **27**, 239.

Hollander, D., Tarnawski, A., Ivey, K. J. *et al.* (1982). Arachidonic acid protection of rat gastric mucosa against ethanol injury, *J. Lab. Clin. Med.*, **100**, 296–308.

Hollander, D., Tarnawski, A., Drause, W. J. *et al.* (1985). Protective effect of sucralfate against alcohol induced gastric mucosal injury in the rat: macroscopic, histologic ultra structured and functional time sequence analysis, *Gastroenterology*, **88**, 366.

Isenberg, J. I., Selling, J. A., Hogan, D. L. *et al.* (1987). Impaired proximal duodenal mucosal bicarbonate secretion in patients with duodenal ulcer, *New Engl. J. Med.*, **316**, 374–9.

Lacy, E. R. and Ito, S. (1982). Microscopic analysis of ethanol damage to rat gastric mucosa after treatment with a prostaglandin, *Gastroenterology*, **83**, 619–25.

Lauritsen, K., Havelund, T., Laursen, L. S. *et al.* (1987). Enprostil and ranitidine in prevention of duodenal ulcer relapse: one year double blind comparative trial, *Br. Med. J.* **294**, 932–4.

Levine, R. A. and Schwartzel, E. H. (1984). Effect of indomethacin on basal and histamine stimulated human gastric acid secretion, *Gut*, **25**, 718–22.

Lichtenberger, L. M., Graziani, L. A., Dial, E. J. *et al.* (1983). Role of surface-active phospholipid in gastric cytoprotection, *Science*, **219**, 1327–9.

McCready, D. R., Clark, I. and Cohen, M. M. (1985). Cigarette smoking reduces human gastric luminal prostaglandin E2, *Gut*, **26**, 1192–6.

Machen, T. E. and Paradiso, A. M. (1987). Regulation of intracellular pH in the stomach, *Ann. Rev. Physiol.*, **49**, 21–35.

Mahachai, V., Walker, K., Sevelius, H. *et al.* (1985). Antisecretory and serum gastrin lowering effect of enprostil in patients with duodenal ulcer disease, *Gastroenterology*, **89**, 555–61.

Monk, J. P. and Clissold, S. P. (1987). Misoprostol: a preliminary review of its pharmacodynamic and pharmacokinetic properties, and therapeutic efficacy in the treatment of peptic ulcer disease, *Drugs*, **33**, 1–30.

Muller, P., Dammann, H. G. and Simon, B. (1986). Verhindert Die Gleichzeitige Gabe Eines PGE-Analogs Indometacinschaden an der Menschlichen Magenschleimhaut? Eine Endiskopische Dippelblind-Studie, *Z. Rheumatol.*, **45**, 71–3.

Muller, P., Dammann, H. G. and Simon, B. (1987). An alprostadil analogue and human gastric secretion — a double-blind placebo-controlled study of the effects of a tablet and liquid formulation, *Arzneim-Forsch-Drug Res.*, **37**, 972–7.

Nicholson, P. A. (1985). A multicenter international controlled comparison of two dosage regimes of misoprostol and the treatment of duodenal ulcer in out-patients, *Dig. Dis. Sci.*, **30** (Suppl. 11), 171S–7S.

Okabe, S., Miyake, H. and Awane, Y. (1986). Cytoprotective effects of NC-1300 and omeprazole on HCl ethanol-induced gastric lesions in rats, *Jap. J. Pharmacol.*, **42**, 123–33.

O'Keefe, S. J. D., Spitaels, J.-M., Mannion, G. *et al.* (1985). Misoprostol, a synthetic prostaglandin E_1 analogue, in the treatment of duodenal ulcers, *S. Am. J.*, **67**, 321.

Pihan, G., Majzoubi, D. and Szabo, S. (1986). Early microcirculatory stasis in acute gastric mucosal injury in the rat and prevention by 16,16-dimethyl prostaglandin E_2 or sodium thiosulfate, *Gastroenterology*, **91**, 1415–26.

Quimby, G. F., Bonnice, C. A., Burstein, S. H. *et al.* (1986). Active smoking depresses prostaglandin synthesis in human gastric mucosa, *Ann. Intern. Med.*, **104**, 616–9.

Rachmilewitz, D., Chapman, J. W. and Nicholson, P. A. (1986). A multicenter international controlled comparison of two dosage regimens of misoprostol with cimetidine in treatment of gastric ulcer in out-patients, *Dig. Dis. Sci.*, 31 (Suppl. 2), 75S–80S.

Reimann, H. J., Lewin, J., Schmidt, U. *et al.* (1987). Misoprostol prevents damage to the gastric mucosa by stabilizing the mast cells, *Prostaglandins*, **33** (Suppl.), 105–16.

Robert, A., Nezamis, J. E., Lancaster, C. *et al.* (1979). Cytoprotection by prostaglandins in rats: prevention of gastric necrosis produced by alcohol, HCl, NaOH, hypertonic NaCl and thermal injury, *Gastroenterology*, **77**, 433.

Robert, A., Nesamis, J. E., Lancaster, C. *et al.* (1983). Mild irritants present gastric necrosis through 'adaptive cytoprotection' mediated by prostaglandins, *Am. J. Physiol.*, **245**, G113.

Rowe, P. H., Starlinger, M. J., Kasdon, E. *et al.* (1987). Parenteral aspirin and sodium salicylate are equally injurious to the rat gastric mucosa, *Gastroenterology*, **93**, 863.

Salmon, P. R. and Barton, T. (1986). Comparative inhibition of coffee-induced gastric acid secretion employing misoprostol and cimetidine, *Dig. Dis. Sci.*, **31**, 55S–62S.

Satoh, H., Guth, P. H. and Grossman, M. I. (1982). Role of food in gastro-intestinal ulceration produced by indomethacin in the rat, *Gastroenterology*, **83**, 210–15.

Satoh, H., Guth, P. H. and Grossman, M. I. (1983). Role of bacteria in gastric ulceration produced by indomethacin in the rat: cytoprotective action of antibiotics, *Gastroenterology*, **84**, 483–9.

Silen, W. and Ito, S. (1985). Mechanism for rapid re-epithelialization of the gastric mucosal surface, *Ann. Rev. Physiol.*, **47**, 217–29.

Soll, A. H., Chen, M., Amirian, D. *et al.* (1986). Prostanoid inhibition of canine parietal cells, *Am. J. Med.*, **81** (Suppl. 2A), 5–11.

Somerville, K. W., Faulkner, G. and Langman, M. J. S. (1986). Non-steroidal anti-inflammatory drugs and bleeding peptic ulcer, *Lancet*, **i**, 482.

Takeuchi, K., Nishiwaki, H. and Okabe, S. (1986). Cytoprotective action of mast cell stabilizers against ethanol-induced gastric lesions in rats, *Jap. J. Pharmacol.*, **42**, 297–307.

Tarnawski, A., Hollander, D., Stachura, J. *et al.* (1985). Prostaglandin protection of the gastric mucosa against alcohol injury—a dynamic time-related process: role of the mucosal proliferative zone, *Gastroenterology*, **88**, 334–52.

Tsai, B. S., Kessler, L. K., Butchko, G. M. *et al.* (1987). Effect of misoprostol on histamine-stimulated acid secretion and cyclic AMP formation in isolated canine parietal cells, *Dig. Dis. Sci.*, **32**, 1010–16.

Wallace, J. L. and Whittle, B. J. R. (1986). Role of mucus in the repair of gastric epithelial damage in the rat: inhibition of epithelial recovery by mucolytic agents, *Gastroenterology*, **91**, 603–11.

Wallace, J. L., Beck, P. L. and Morris, G. P. (1988). Is there a role for leukotrienes as mediators of ethanol-induced gastric mucosal damage? *Am. J. Physiol.*, **254**, G117–23.

Walt, R. P., Pounder, R. E., Hawkey, C. J. *et al.* (1987). Twenty four hour intragastric acidity and clinical trial of bedtime enprostil 70 μg compared with ranitidine 300 mg in duodenal ulcer, *Aliment. Pharmacol. Ther.*, **1**, 161–6.

Whittle, B. J. R. (1977). Mechanisms underlying gastric mucosal damage induced by indomethacin and bile salts and the actions of prostaglandins, *Br. J. Pharmacol.*, **60**, 455–60.

Advances in Drug Therapy of Gastrointestinal Ulceration
Edited by A. Garner and B. J. R. Whittle
©1989 John Wiley & Sons Ltd

Chapter Eight

Action of Antacids:
More than Bulk Neutralization?

F. Halter and S. K. Lam

Gastrointestinal Unit, University Hospital, Inselspital, Bern, Switzerland and Division of Gastroenterology, Department of Medicine, University of Hong Kong, Queen Mary Hospital, Hong Kong

INTRODUCTION

The use of antacids probably began in the first century with Celsus, who used neutralizing earths for treatment of abdominal distress (see Crohn and Rosenak, 1935). Their use for treatment of peptic ulcer on a scientific basis began in America with the work of Sippy (1910), following the pronouncement by Schwarz in 1910 of his famous dictum, 'no acid no ulcer'. The results of studies performed up to the mid-1970s on the usefulness of antacid treatment were inconclusive, and many expected that the introduction of histamine H_2-antagonists would terminate the antacid era. However, in the last decade, the widespread use of the endoscope as an end-point detector and the method of randomized controlled clinical trials as a decision-maker have established beyond doubt that antacids can promote the healing of duodenal ulcers better than placebo treatment or at a similar rate to cimetidine (Peterson et al., 1977; Ippoliti et al., 1978; Fedeli et al., 1979; Lam et al., 1979; Berstad et al., 1982; Faizallah et al., 1984; Kumar et al., 1984; Lauritsen et al., 1985; Weberg et al., 1985; Bianchi-Porro et al., 1986a; Lux et al., 1986; Becker et al., 1987). These data are summarized in Table 8.1. In addition, one study is available to document the role of antacids in the prevention of recurrence of duodenal ulcer disease (Bianchi-Porro et al., 1986b). The evidence in support of the efficacy of antacids in gastric ulcer is much less convincing (Hollander and Harland, 1973; Isenberg et al. 1983; Pace et al., 1985; Rydning et al., 1986).

Table 8.1 Antacid trials in duodenal ulcer

Study	Antacid form	Daily dose	Daily neutralizing capacity (mmol)	Treatment duration (weeks)	Antacid			Placebo			H₂-antagonists			P value
					n	Healed	%	n	Healed	%	n	Healed	%	
Peterson et al. (1977)	Liquid	15 ml 5×	1008	4	36	28	78	38	17	45	—	—	—	0.005
Lam et al. (1979)	Tablet	2 tab 7×	175	4	26	20	77	24	8	33	—	—	—	0.005
Berstad et al. (1982)	Tablet	2 tab 7×	280	4	37	30	81	38	9	24	—	—	—	0.001
Kumar et al. (1984)	Liquid	7.5 ml 6×	103	4	26	12	46	—	—	—	—	—	—	NS
		15 ml 6×	206	4	27	23	85	24	7	29	—	—	—	0.001
		30 ml 6×	412	4	24	21	87	—	—	—	—	—	—	0.001
Faizallah et al. (1984)	Liquid	30 ml 7×	1050	4	19	6	32	15	2	13	—	—	—	}0.05
		10 ml as needed	107	4	18	12	67	17	6	35	—	—	—	
Weberg et al. (1985)	Tablet	1 tab 4×	120	4	38	28	74	38	11	29	—	—	—	0.001
Ippoliti et al. (1978)	Liquid	30 ml 7×	861	4	32	19	59	—	—	—	33	21	64	NS
Fedeli et al. (1979)	Liquid	30 ml 7×	560	4	24	18	75	—	—	—	27	21	78	NS
Lauritsen et al. (1985)	Liquid	10 ml 7×	600	4	25	21	84	—	—	—	28	25	89	NS
Lux et al. (1986)	Liquid	10 ml 4×	280	4	86	69	80	—	—	—	85	63	75	NS
Bianchi Porro et al. (1986a)	Liquid	15 ml 5×	unknown	4	39	28	72	—	—	—	39	26	67	NS
Becker et al. (1987)	Liquid	10 ml 7×	595	4	34	28	83	—	—	—	33	23	69	NS
				Total	491	363	74	194	60	31	245	179	73	

NS = not significant

   Doses of antacids used in the various studies have varied immensely, with
neutralizing capacities ranging between 1000 and 100 mmol. There has been a
tendency to use smaller and smaller doses in recent years. Figure 8.1 shows the
healing rates at four weeks in different ethnic groups with the different daily
doses of antacid used. It is apparent that despite known differences in acid
secretory capacities in different races (being low, for example, in Chinese and
Indians) there is a steep rise in healing rates even with a small increase in the
antacid dose, reaching a plateau at about 200 mmol (Figure 8.1). Thus, a dose
with a daily neutralizing capacity of 200–400 mmol may prove to be applicable
to all ethnic groups. This would minimize the occurrence of side-effects.
   Recent observations that healing of ulcers can be induced by antacid doses
with low neutralizing capacity have raised the question of whether antacids might
accelerate ulcer healing through other mechanisms. It is therefore of interest
to re-evaluate the pathways through which antacids might heal peptic ulcers.

ACID NEUTRALIZATION?

Studies performed in duodenal ulcer patients by the Fordtran group (Fordtran
and Collyns, 1966; Fordtran, 1973; Fordtran, Morawski and Richardson, 1973)

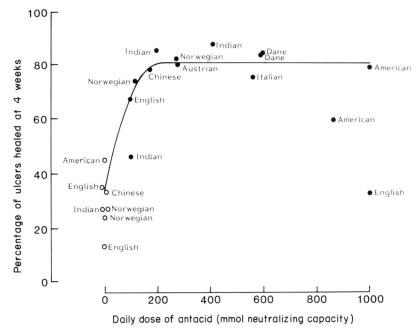

Figure 8.1 Duodenal ulcer healing rates at 4 weeks in different ethnic groups treated
with antacids with various daily neutralizing capacities. Open circles represent placebo
healing rates. Note the steep rise and plateau with small increase in antacid dose

suggested that gastric acidity could be kept at a low level for 4 h if large doses of antacids were given 1 h and 3 h after a meal. It was consequently surmised that such a regimen, if extended over 24 h could very substantially reduce overall gastric acidity of such patients, and this was successfully applied for ulcer treatment in a study by Peterson *et al.* (1977). Application of antacids not earlier than 1 h after a meal is logical, since in the early postprandial phase acid is neutralized by the food contents, and since antacids leave the non-fasting stomach more slowly.

The following factors should be taken into account:

(1) acid buffering by food,
(2) formation of macromolecules — $Al(OH)_3$,
(3) formation of insoluble precipitates — $Al(OH)_3$,
(4) transpyloric loss of unutilized antacid.

Food can counteract the neutralizing capacity of antacids, especially if this is largely derived from $Al(OH)_3$, by reduction of the solubility of this component (Gibaldi, Kanic and Amsel, 1964; Carlson and Malagelada, 1982; Halter, Häcki and Varga, 1982; Halter *et al.*, 1982). This in turn delays the velocity with which antacids interact with acid, leading to a substantial transpyloric loss of non-utilized antacids. Therefore antacids can more effectively neutralize a high intragastric acid load in the absence of food, but this only operates for a limited time due to rapid gastric emptying (Figure 8.2). *In vitro* estimations of the neutralizing capacity of antacids thus tend to substantially overestimate the *in vivo* reactivity of most antacid preparations, especially if they derive their neutralizing capacity largely from $Al(OH)_3$.

Several more recent studies (Halter *et al.*, 1982; Milton-Thompson, 1982; Bauerfeind *et al.*, 1984; Berchtold *et al.*, 1985) in which intragastric pH was measured for up to 24 h have indeed shown that the reduction of intragastric acidity with the Fordtran regimen is much smaller than that resulting from potent histamine H_2-antagonists. The differences were most pronounced following the evening meal. After midnight intragastric pH was similar or, in two studies, even lower than in placebo-treated subjects, the latter observation leading to the suspicion of an acid rebound (Blum, 1984; Merki, unpublished observation). Consequently, antacids do not fit into the model of Hunt *et al.* (1986), who suggested that in duodenal ulcer disease healing rates directly correlate with the decrease of nocturnal acid inhibition.

Unfortunately, in none of the recent ulcer studies has the *in vivo* neutralizing capacity of the antacid in use been measured. It is justified to assume that the doses used in recent trials only marginally inhibit intragastric acid concentration. However, it is premature to conclude that antacids do not induce healing by their effect on gastric pH, as we do not know for what time and at which threshold it is necessary to elevate intragastric pH to induce healing. Nevertheless, it is clear that the long-held theory that pH must be elevated above the pH level

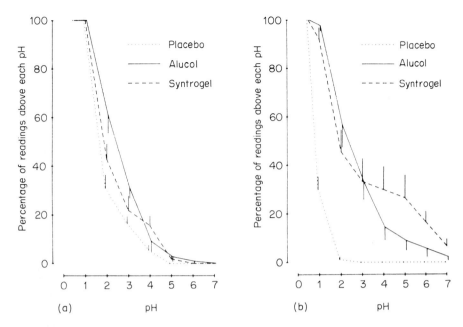

Figure 8.2 Effects of alucol and syntrogel on intragastric pH values during stimulation of acid secretion with food or the H_2-agonist impromidine. For the pH range 1–7, the mean percent readings ± s.e.m. above each pH are recorded throughout (a) the 12 h food study and (b) the 4 h impromidine study

that guarantees pepsin inactivation (pH 3.5) in order to induce peptic ulcer healing is incorrect. Cimetidine, for example, only raises median 24 h pH values from 1.4 to 1.7 (Walt *et al.*, 1983), and during treatment with muscarinic antagonists intragastric pH is only marginally elevated (Etienne and Bron, 1982). Healing of duodenal ulcers can be achieved in the majority of patients with either of these two drugs and it is generally agreed that these drugs heal ulcers solely by interference with acid. One has also to consider that pH studies give no indication of the volume of gastric contents and their discharge rate into the duodenum. Both factors could additively contribute to an underestimate of the reduction of the duodenal acid load.

BILE ACID BINDING

It is well established that antacids can bind conjugated bile and it has been speculated that antacids heal peptic ulcers by preventing the noxious effects of bile acids on the gastric mucosa (Clain, Malagelada and Chadwick, 1977). The attraction of this theory is diminished by the fact that it is likely that duodenogastric reflux is a normal phenomenon which is not increased in peptic ulcer disease (Müller-Lissner *et al.*, 1983). Furthermore, no studies are available to suggest that peptic ulcer healing can be enhanced solely by bile acid binding.

CYTOPROTECTION

Prostaglandins have been shown to reduce damage to the gastric mucosa induced by various noxious agents such as concentrated ethanol, and this phenomenon has been named 'cytoprotection' (Robert *et al.*, 1979). This term is misleading since application of prostaglandins prior to exposure of the gastric mucosa to noxious agents cannot prevent the destruction of the superficial epithelial cells but it can reduce or eliminate the areas of necrotic lesions by minimizing deep mucosal congestion (Lacy and Ito, 1982; Wallace *et al.*, 1982). Following the claim that prostaglandins are cytoprotective to the gastric mucosa, the term 'cytoprotection' has been applied to many drugs, often in an uncritical manner. One has to consider that cytoprotection is much better established in experimental animals than in humans and that any result obtained in animals needs confirmation in man, especially with regard to the healing of peptic ulcers. However, in recent years, some interesting data have accumulated to suggest that cytoprotection could be one of the processes by which antacids increase the resistance of the gastric mucosa.

Studies in experimental animals

Szelenyi and co-workers (Szelenyi, Postius and Engler, 1983; Szelenyi and Postius, 1985; Lanz *et al.*, 1985) were the first to establish that in the rat intragastric instillation of large amounts of $Al(OH)_3$ induces a release of prostaglandins into the gastric juice lasting more than 24 h. Such an effect could not be induced by $Mg(OH)_2$, $CaCO_3$, Al_2O_3 or $AlCl_3$.

Several groups have shown that $Al(OH)_3$, $Al_2(SO_4)_3$ and $AlPO_4$ can protect the gastric mucosa against noxious effects induced by absolute ethanol in a dose-dependent manner, similar to sucralfate (Szelenyi, Postius and Engler, 1983; Szelenyi and Postius, 1985; Lanz *et al.*, 1985; Tarnawski *et al.*, 1985; Domschke *et al.*, 1986; Hollander, Tarnawski and Gergely, 1986). It is possible that aluminium crystals induce superficial damage of the gastric mucosa as observed in histological studies of Tarnawski *et al.* (1984), which may be responsible for antacid-induced prostaglandin release. It can thus not be excluded that the prostaglandin release occurs as a consequence of gastric mucosal damage.

Studies of Domschke *et al.* (1986) have revealed that cytoprotective effects of antacids in experimental animals are mainly confined to the gastric glands while damage to the surface epithelium is not significantly lessened. Accordingly, integrity parameters of the superficial epithelial layer (potential difference, mucus secretion, cell desquamation) do not indicate a protective action of antacids against damage by necrotizing agents. In contrast, significantly diminished microbleeding rates suggest that protection by antacids works at a deeper level within the mucosa. These actions of antacids closely resemble those of protective prostaglandins. Antacids also significantly diminish the rate of gastric microbleeding induced by aspirin. It is therefore likely that antacids may additionally or alternatively act through factors other than prostaglandin synthesis within the gastric mucosa. This is also supported by the observation that antacids appear to have the opposite action to prostaglandins in some respects, e.g. on gastric mucus secretion (Domschke *et al.*, 1986).

Various animal experiments have thus unanimously shown that the $Al(OH)_3$ component of antacids can induce prostaglandin release in the gastric mucosa.

Studies in man

Studies performed in humans are very preliminary and have resulted in inconclusive results. Berstad and Szelenyi (personal communication) could not confirm the data obtained in rat studies in humans. Reimann *et al.* (1984) found that $Al(OH)_3$ but not $CaCO_3$ could stimulate *ex vivo* prostaglandin synthesis in biopsies sampled from the human stomach. This was confirmed by Preclik *et al.* (1987) during prolonged application of Maalox 70. These data do not, however, indicate whether prostaglandin release is involved in ulcer healing or whether it represents an epiphenomenon. There is no evidence available from the immense literature on synthetic prostaglandin analogues in ulcer healing to demonstrate that prostaglandins heal peptic ulcers at doses that do not inhibit acid secretion (Hawkey and Walt, 1986). It should be pointed out that the cytoprotective effects of prostaglandins, such as enhancement of bicarbonate secretion and mucosal blood flow, are dose-dependent phenomena in animals and man (Isenberg *et al.*, 1986). However, the only indirect evidence that mucosal protection might be involved in peptic ulcer healing comes from studies on ulcer healing with sucralfate or colloidal bismuth (Koelz, 1986). It is quite obvious that, at least in an animal model, $Al(OH)_3$ protects the gastric mucosa in a similar fashion to sucralfate, a preparation also containing negatively charged aluminium and which exerts no influence on gastric acidity. It appears, however, that it is the octasulphate and not the aluminium component of sucralfate which protects the acid-exposed oesophageal epithelium in the rabbit (Orlando *et al.*, 1987). Thus it cannot be excluded that antacids may heal peptic ulcers via similar mechanisms to that of sucralfate, such as coating the ulcer crater, changing mucus viscosity or bicarbonate secretion, and maintenance of gastric blood flow (Koelz, 1986). At present it is still easier to defend the acid-neutralizing hypothesis, but it cannot be fully excluded that acid neutralization and cytoprotection additively contribute to the phenomenon which permits even small doses of antacids to heal duodenal ulcers.

CONCLUSIONS

It is now firmly established through a series of controlled trials that antacids can promote duodenal ulcer healing in doses exhibiting a very limited neutralizing capacity both *in vitro* and *in vivo*. Important information has recently been obtained from 24 h pH studies, suggesting that antacids are unable to elevate nocturnal intragastric pH substantially. It is reasonable and timely, therefore, to examine alternative mechanisms of action for antacids. In experimental animals antacids have been shown to release prostaglandins similar to sucralfate. By further analogy with sucralfate, instillation of a small volume of an antacid, prior to administration of concentrated ethanol, protects the mucosa, particularly the deeper layers. Adaptive cytoprotection may be involved, since small crystals and local inflammation have been found in the gastric mucosa following antacid treatment. As the principle of cytoprotection may not apply to humans, the clinical implications of these studies are questionable. It is however, possible that the small amount of acid inhibition and enhancement of the resistance of the gastric mucosa additively contribute to peptic ulcer healing during antacid treatment.

REFERENCES

Bauerfeind, P., Cilluffo, T., Emde, C., Müller-Duysing, W. and Blum, A. L. (1984). Antacids revisited: how do they interact with food *in vivo*?, *Gastroenterology*, **90**, 1340.

Becker, U., Lindorff, K., Andersen, C. and Randlov, P. J. (1987). Antacid treatment of duodenal ulcer, *Acta Med. Scand.*, **221**, 1181–5.

Berchtold, P., Reinhart, W. H., Niederhäuser, U., Koller, U. and Halter, F. (1985). *In vitro* tests overestimate *in vivo* neutralizing capacity of antacids in presence of food, *Dig. Dis. Sci.*, **30**, 522–8.

Berstad, A., Rydning, A., Aaland, E., Kolstad, B., Frislid, K. and Asseth, J. (1982). Controlled clinical trial of duodenal ulcer healing with antacid tablets, *Scand. J. Gastroenterol.*, **17**, 953–9.

Bianchi Porro, G., Lazzaroni, M., Pace, F. and Petrillo, M. (1986a). Long-term low dose antacid versus cimetidine therapy in the treatment of duodenal ulcer recurrence, *Scand. J. Gastroenterol.*, **21**, 1144–6.

Bianchi Porro, G., Parente, F., Lazzaroni, M., Baroni, S. and Panza, E. (1986b). Medium-dose antacids versus cimetidine in the short-term treatment of duodenal ulcer, *J. Clin. Gastroenterol.*, **8**, 141–54.

Blum, A. L. (1984). Ziele bei der Therapie der Ulkuskrankheit, *Schweiz. Med. Wochenschr.*, **114**, 679–82.

Carlson, G. L. and Malagelada, J. R. (1982). Chemistry of the antacids: its relevance to antacid therapy. In F. Halter (ed.) *Antacids in the Eighties*, Urban & Schwarzenberg, Munich, pp. 7–16.

Clain, J. E., Malagelada, J. R. and Chadwick, V. S. (1977). Binding properties *in vitro* of antacids for conjugated bile acids, *Gastroenterology*, **73**, 556–9.

Crohn, B. B. and Rosenak, B. D. (1935). An exhibition of books shown at the Graduate Fortnight illustrating the progress of gastroenterology, *Bull. N.Y. Acad. Med.*, **11**, 74.

Domschke, W., Hagel, J., Ruppin, H. and Kaduk, B. (1986). Antacids and gastric mucosal protection, *Scand. J. Gastroenterol.*, **21** (Suppl. 125), 144–9.

Etienne, A. and Bron, W. (1982). The effect of pirencepine on gastric pH: continuous recording for the selection of the optimal therapeutic dose. In G. Dotevall (ed.) *Advances in Gastroenterology with the Selective Antimuscarinic Compound Pirenzepine*, Stockholm, 17 June 1982, Excerpta Medica, Amsterdam, pp. 81–2.

Faizallah, R., De Haan, H. A., Krasner, N. *et al.* (1984). Is there a place in the United Kingdom for intensive antacid treatment for chronic peptic ulceration?, *Br. Med. J.*, **289**, 869–71.

Fedeli, G., Anti, M., Rapaccini, G. L., De Vitis, I., Butti, A. and Civelo, I. M. (1979). A controlled study comparing cimetidine treatment to an intensive antacid regimen in the therapy of uncomplicated duodenal ulcer, *Dig. Dis. Sci.*, **24**, 758–62.

Fordtran, J. S. (1973). Reduction of acidity by diet, antacids and anticholinergic agents. In M. H. Sleisinger and J. S. Fordtran (eds) *Gastrointestinal Diseases*, 1st edn, WB Saunders, Philadelphia, pp. 718–42.

Fordtran, J. S. and Collyns, J. A. H. (1966). Antacid pharmacology in duodenal ulcer, *New Engl. J. Med.*, **274**, 922–7.

Fordtran, J. S., Morawski, S. G. and Richardson, Ch.T. (1973). *In vivo* and *in vitro* evaluation of liquid antacids, *New Engl. J. Med.*, **288**, 923–8.

Gibaldi, M., Kanic, J. L. and Amsel, L. (1964) Critical *in vitro* factors in evaluation of gastric antacids II, *J. Pharmacol. Sci.*, **53**, 1375–7.

Halter, F., Häcki, W. H. and Varga, L. (1982). Availability of antacids in a meat extract. In F. Halter (ed.) *Antacids in the Eighties*, Urban & Schwarzenberg, Munich, pp. 35–41.

Halter, F., Huber, R., Häcki, W. H., Varga, L. and Bachmann, C. (1982). Effect of food on antacid neutralizing capacity in man, *Eur. J. Clin. Invest.*, **12**, 209–17.

Hawkey, C. J. and Walt, R. P. (1986). Prostaglandins for peptic ulcer, a promise unfulfilled, *Lancet*, **ii**, 1084–6.

Hollander, D. and Harland, J. (1973). Antacids vs placebos in peptic ulcer therapy: a controlled double-blind investigation, *JAMA*, **226**, 1181–5.

Hollander, D., Tarnawski, A. and Gergely, H. (1986). Protection against alcohol-induced gastric mucosal injury by aluminium-containing compounds — sucralfate, antacids and aluminium sulphate, *Scand. J. Gastroenterol.*, **21** (Suppl. 125), 151–3.

Hunt, R. H., Howden, C. W., Jones, D. B., Burget, D. W. and Kerr, G. D. (1986). The correlation between acid suppression and peptic ulcer healing, *Scand. J. Gastroenterol.*, **21** (Suppl. 125), 22–9.

Ippoliti, A. F., Sturdevant, R. A. L., Isenberg, J. I. *et al.* (1978). Cimetidine versus intensive antacid therapy for duodenal ulcer. A multicenter trial, *Gastroenterology*, **74**, 393–5.

Isenberg, J. I., Peterson, W. I., Elashoff, J. D. *et al.* (1983). Healing of benign gastric ulcer with low-dose antacid and cimetidine: a double-blind, randomized, placebo-controlled trial, *New Engl. J. Med.*, **308**, 1319–24.

Isenberg, J. I., Hogan, D. L., Koss, M. H. and Selling, J. A. (1986). Human duodenal mucosal bicarbonate secretion: evidence for basal secretion and stimulation by hydrochloric acid and a synthetic prostaglandin E_1 analogue. *Gastroenterology*, **91**, 370–8.

Koelz, H. R. (1986). Protective drugs in the treatment of gastroduodenal ulcer disease, *Scand. J. Gastroenterol.*, **21** (Suppl. 125), 156–63.

Kumar, N., Vij, J. C., Karol, A. and Anand, B. S. (1984). Controlled therapeutic trial to determine the optimum dose of antacids in duodenal ulcer, *Gut*, **25**, 1199.

Lacy, E. R. and Ito, S. (1982). Microscopic analysis of ethanol damage to rat gastric mucosa after treatment with a prostaglandin, *Gastroenterology*, **83**, 619–25.

Lam, S. K., Lam, K. C., Lai, C. L. *et al.* (1979). Treatment of duodenal ulcer with antacid and sulpiride: a double-blind controlled study, *Gastroenterology*, **76**, 315–22.

Lanz, R., Postius, S., Szelenyi, I. and Brune, K. (1985). PGE_2 release from cultured macrophages induced by antacids and sucralfate, *Gastroenterology*, **88**, 1464.

Lauritsen, K., Bytzer, P., Hansen, J., Bekker, C. and Rask-Madsen, J. (1985). Comparison of ranitidine and high-dose antacid in the treatment of prepyloric or duodenal ulcer: a double-blind controlled trial, *Scand. J. Gastroenterol.*, **20**, 123–238.

Lux, G., Henschel, H., Rohner, H. G. *et al.* (1986). Treatment of duodenal ulcer with low-dose antacids, *Scand. J. Gastroenterol.*, **21**, 1063–8.

Milton-Thompson, G. J. (1982). Monitoring of 24 hour acid secretion during antacid treatment. In F. Halter (ed.) *Antacids in the Eighties*, Urban & Schwarzenberg, Munich, pp. 72–5.

Müller-Lissner, S. A., Fimmel, C. J., Sonnenberg, A. *et al.* (1983). Novel approach to quantify duodenogastric reflux in healthy volunteers and in patients with type I gastric ulcer, *Gut*, **24**, 510–18.

Orlando, R. C., Turjman, N. A., Tobey, N. A., Schreiner, V. J. and Powell, D. W. (1987). Mucosal protection by sucralfate and its components in acid-exposed rabbit esophagus, *Gastroenterology*, **93**, 352–61.

Pace, F., Broker, H. J., Caspary, W. *et al.* (1985). Therapy of stomach ulcer with low-dose antacid gel and cimetidine: a multicenter double-blind study, *Dtsch. Med. Wochenschr.*, **11**, 183–287.

Peterson, W. L., Sturdevant, A. L., Frankl, H. D. *et al.* (1977). Healing of duodenal ulcer with an antacid regimen, *New Engl. J. Med.*, **297**, 341–5.

Preclik, E. F., Stange, G., Gerber, K., Tetze, H., Horn, H. and Ditschuneit, H. (1987). Stimulation of endogenous prostaglandin synthesis by antacids in human gastric and duodenal mucosa, *Gastroenterology*, **92**, 2579.

Reimann, H. J., Schmidt, U., Wendt, P. *et al.* (1984). Die Wirkung von Antazida auf den Gehalt von Gewebshistamin und Prostaglandinen (PGE_2) in der Magenmukosa, *Fortschr. Med.*, **102**, 47–50.

Robert, A., Nezamis, J. E., Lancaster, C. and Hanchar, A. J. (1979). Cytoprotection by prostaglandins in rats: prevention of gastric necrosis produced by alcohol, HCl, NaOH, hypertonic NaCl, and thermal injury, *Gastroenterology*, **77**, 433–43.

Rydning, A., Weberg, R., Lange, O. and Berstad, A. (1986). Healing of benign gastric ulcer with low-dose antacids and fiber diet, *Gastroenterology*, **91**, 56–61.

Schwarz, K. (1910). Ueber penetrierende Magen- und Jejunalgeschwüre, *Beitr. Klin. Chir.*, **67**, 95.

Sippy, B. W. (1910). Gastric and duodenal ulcers, medical cure by efficient removal of gastric juice corrosion, *JAMA*, **64**, 1625.

Szelenyi, I. and Postius, S. (1985). Functional cytoprotection by certain antacids and sucralfate in the rat stomach, *Gastroenterology*, **88**, 1604.

Szelenyi, I., Postius, S. and Engler, H. (1983). Evidence for a functional cytoprotective effect produced by antacids in the rat stomach, *Eur. J. Pharmacol.*, **88**, 403–6.

Tarnawski, A., Hollander, D., Gergely, H. and Stachura, J. (1985). Comparison of antacid, sucralfate, cimetidine and ranitidine in protection of the gastric mucosa against ethanol injury, *Am. J. Med.*, **79** (Suppl. 2C), 19–23.

Tarnawski, A., Hollander, D., Cummings, D., Krause, W. J., Gergely, H. and Zipser, R. D. (1984). Are antacids acid neutralizers only? Histologic, ultrastructural and functional changes in normal gastric mucosa induced by antacids, *Gastroenterology*, **86**, 1276.

Wallace, J. L., Morris, G. P., Krousse, E. J. and Graeves, S. E. (1982). Reduction by cytoprotective agents of ethanol-induced damage to the rat gastric mucosa: a correlated morphological and physiological study, *Can. J. Physiol. Pharmacol.*, **60**, 1686–99.

Walt, R. P., Gomes, M. D., Wood, E. C., Logan, L. H. and Pounder, R. E. (1983). Effect of daily oral omeprazole on 24 hour intragastric activity, *Br. Med. J. (Clin. Res.)*, **287**, 12–14.

Weberg, R., Berstad, A., Lange, O., Schulz, T. and Aubert, E. (1985). Duodenal ulcer healing with four antacid tablets daily, *Scand. J. Gastroenterol.*, **20**, 1041–5.

Advances in Drug Therapy of Gastrointestinal Ulceration
Edited by A. Garner and B. J. R. Whittle
© 1989 John Wiley & Sons Ltd

Chapter Nine

Mechanisms of Action of Non-antisecretory Anti-ulcer Drugs

Rory F. McCloy
University Department of Surgery, Manchester Royal Infirmary, Manchester M13 9WL, UK

The title of this review deliberately avoids the use of the term *cytoprotective* drugs which has frequently been used, inappropriately, to describe drugs which heal ulcers by mechanisms other than suppression or neutralization of acid. A more suitable term would be *cytoreparative* drugs. Cytoprotection implies protection of an intact mucosa against ulcerogenic factors and as such should only be used in a clinical context to describe drugs used for prophylaxis against stress ulcers or to prevent ulcer relapse without affecting acid or acidity. This issue goes deeper than mere semantics since it is now very difficult to define exactly how non-antisecretory anti-ulcer drugs act (Guth, 1987).

In recent years our understanding of the essential elements that comprise the defensive mechanisms in the gastroduodenal mucosa has increased considerably. We now recognize the interplay between different levels of defence. The maintenance of the pre-epithelial mucus–bicarbonate barrier is important as a first line of defence against intraluminal acid and peptic attack (Rees, 1987), whilst at the mucosal level the tight junctions between cells and the surface active phospholipid layer provide deeper protection. These defences are all dependent on an adequate mucosal blood flow and a normal subepithelial microvascular network. Cytoprotective drugs could be expected to act by improving these defence mechanisms.

The local pathophysiological conditions that prevail in an ulcerated mucosa are considerably different. There is an inflammatory exudate with the formation of a mucus cap, into which bicarbonate diffuses through opened paracellular channels (Wallace and Whittle, 1986; Rees, 1987). Back-diffusion of bile salts and hydrogen ions damages the microcirculation of the mucosa and leads to the local release of vasoactive and cytotoxic mediators which compound local

121

ischaemia and induce further tissue damage (Whittle, Oren-Wolman and Guth, 1985). The repair processes start with rapid epithelialization by the process of restitution, followed only later by cell division (Silen and Ito, 1985). The processes by which non-antisecretory ulcer-healing drugs, principally colloidal bismuth and sucralfate, may lead to mucosal repair are likely to be distinct from the mechanisms involved in mucosal defence. Unfortunately, to date, relatively few data are available on the effects of drugs on ulcer healing processes and this review has had to rely on the data pertaining to mucosal defence. The article concentrates on the data with the potential for healing ulcers in man rather than the often confusing and probably irrelevant data on cytoprotection in animal models challenged with gross noxious stimuli.

Our lack of certainty of the clinical importance of improving mucosal defences to heal ulcers, and doubt as to how non-antisecretory ulcer-healing drugs work, was reflected at an international workshop on 'The realities of mucosal defence' held in 1987 (Dent *et al.*, 1989). At the workshop, 67 basic scientists and clinicians from industry, hospitals and universities, all experts in this field, voted on carefully prepared statements. Some of the preliminary results, which fail to demonstrate a clear consensus, are presented during the course of this review.

CARBENOXOLONE SODIUM

Carbenoxolone was the first effective drug to heal peptic ulcers and the first non-antisecretory ulcer-healing drug. It is the hemisuccinate of the natural terpenoid 18β-glycyrrhetic acid (enoxolone) (Parke, 1978). Its modes of action are summarized in Table 9.1. The clinical value of this interesting compound with its unique actions has been limited by its mineralocorticoid side-effects, arising from its potentiation of endogenous aldosterone (Parke, 1978), which

Table 9.1 Modes of action of carbenoxolone sodium

	Reference
Reduction of aggressive factors	
Reduced pepsin secretion	Walker and Taylor (1975)
Improves pyloric sphincter function	Fisher and Lorber (1975)
Improved mucosal resistance	
Increased mucus synthesis	Johnston *et al.* (1975)
Reduced H$^+$ back-diffusion	Domschke, Domschke and Demling (1975)
Increased *N*-acetylneuramic acid-containing glycoproteins in gastric mucus	Domschke, Domschke and Demling (1975)
Decreased gastric mucosal cell exfoliation	Klein, Frotz and Gheorghiu (1975)

result in fluid retention, hypokalaemia and hypertension. Carbenoxolone (Biogastrone, Duogastrone (Winthrop)) no longer occupies an important place in the therapeutic armamentarium against peptic ulcer disease.

LIQUORICE DERIVATIVE

A deglycyrrhizinated preparation of liquorice was developed to overcome the mineralocorticoid effects of carbenoxolone, but there are no hard data available as to its mode of action and few clinical studies. The commercial preparation probably owes its efficacy to the antacid components, in particular the aluminium compound, which are combined with the liquorice derivative (Caved-S (Tillots) deglycyrrhizinated liquorice 380 mg, aluminium hydroxide gel 100 mg, magnesium carbonate 200 mg, sodium carbonate 100 mg).

COLLOIDAL BISMUTH

Recently, tripotassium dicitrato bismuthate (TDB) has been more conveniently referred to as colloidal bismuth subcitrate (CBS). It is commercially available as De-Nol (Brocades) and has a formula which approximates to $Bi_x(OH)_y.(C_6H_5O_7)_z$.

The proposed mechanisms of action of colloidal bismuth are summarized in Table 9.2. Colloidal bismuth reduces the effectiveness of aggressive factors including acid and pepsin in several ways. The compound has been shown to form a complex with gastric mucus glycoprotein *in vitro* (Lee, 1982) which can retard the diffusion of hydrogen ions by 40–90%. However, the diffusion of hydrogen ions is so rapid that this action is unlikely to have a significant effect *in vivo*, especially when the unstirred mucus gel layer in man is only about 0.2 mm thick. Colloidal bismuth selectively adheres to gastric ulcers in both the rat (Koo *et al.*, 1982) and man (Lee, 1982) and this action is likely to be important in concentrating the compound at the site of ulceration. Whilst colloidal bismuth has no significant effect on gastric acid, it does have some weak antipeptic activity (Roberts and Taylor, 1982) though a considerable concentration in the ulcer base would be necessary for this action to be relevant for ulcer healing.

Mucosal resistance can also be improved by colloidal bismuth. The drug has been shown to promote the formation of neutral rather than acid mucus in man (Hollander, Morrissey and Mehta, 1983). Cytoprotective experiments in rats (Konturek *et al.*, 1987b) have shown that endogenous prostaglandins may be stimulated by colloidal bismuth. Studies in the dog and man indicate that the compound can stimulate gastric and duodenal bicarbonate secretion via a

Table 9.2 Modes of action of colloidal bismuth

	References
Reduction of aggressive factors	
Formation of complex with mucus glycoprotein to retard diffusion of H$^+$	Lee (1982)
Selective adherence to ulcer areas	Lee (1982), Koo et al. (1982)
Antipeptic activity	Roberts and Taylor (1982)
Improved mucosal resistance	
Increased neutral mucus	Hollander, Morrissey and Mehta (1983)
Increased prostaglandin biosynthesis	Konturek et al. (1987a)
Increased gastric and duodenal bicarbonate secretion	Konturek et al. (1987b)
Local binding of epidermal growth factor	Konturek (1988)

prostaglandin-mediated mechanism and increase luminal release of prostaglandin E$_2$ (Konturek et al., 1987a). Furthermore, epidermal growth factor, a naturally occurring peptide, could aid in the healing of ulcers by selective accumulation in ulcerated mucosa, and this local accumulation may be increased by colloidal bismuth (Konturek, 1988).

Considerable interest has been focused on the antibacterial actions of bismuth compounds. Colloidal bismuth is bactericidal to *Campylobacter pylori* both *in vitro* and *in vivo* in human studies (Lambert et al., 1985). Bismuth may have an advantage over other antibiotics, many of which have been demonstrated to have *in vitro* but not *in vivo* activity against *C. pylori*, because of its direct action in achieving high local concentrations in gastric mucus. The relevance of this antibacterial activity hinges on the clinical significance of *C. pylori* in the pathogenesis of peptic ulcer disease which is still an open question (Blaser, 1987; Dooley and Cohen, 1988).

There seems little doubt that ulcers healed by colloidal bismuth have a more prolonged ulcer-free period when compared to ulcers healed with H$_2$-receptor antagonists. The combined results of six clinical trials showed that the relapse rate within 1 year was 59% for patients whose ulcers healed on colloidal bismuth and 85% after healing by H$_2$-antagonists (Miller and Faragher, 1986). The mechanisms by which colloidal bismuth achieves this effect have yet to be defined. Temporary eradication of *C. pylori* and persistence of bismuth in the body, especially in the gastric mucosa, may prove to be interrelated actions.

The views of the participants at the Lausanne workshop (Dent et al., 1989) favoured the enhancing of mucosal defences, the protective barrier and antibacterial features of colloidal bismuth as important ulcer-healing actions (Table 9.3).

Table 9.3 Lausanne workshop vote: What mechanisms are responsible for the ulcer healing action of bismuth compounds?

	Agree (%)	Disagree (%)	Uncertain (%)
Mechanisms			
Enhances defences	39	6	45
Forms barrier	36	12	52
Inactivates pepsin	21	18	61
Stimulates mucus	19	19	62
Stimulates mucosal prostaglandins	22	24	46
Antibacterial action	43	10	47
Binds epidermal growth factor	8	27	65
Clinical actions			
Associated with decreased rate of recurrent ulcer compared with H_2-antagonists	60	13	27
Anti-*C. pylori* action responsible for ulcer-free period	27	13	60
Persistence of bismuth in mucosa responsible for delay in ulcer recurrence	22	19	59

SUCRALFATE

The basic aluminium salt of sucrose octasulphate, sucralfate (Antepsin (Ayerst)), with the formula $C_{12}H_{22}O_{11}.[SO_3(Al_2(OH)_5)]_8$, heals ulcers both by reducing aggressive factors and by improving mucosal resistance. These properties are summarized in Table 9.4.

Sucralfate has been reported to delay the diffusion of hydrogen ions *in vitro* by 50% (Nagashima, 1981), but a more clinically relevant action may be the selective binding to experimental ulcer sites in animal models (Nagashima, 1981). Further *in vitro* studies have shown that sucralfate acts against pepsin by a dual mechanism, directly adsorbing the enzyme (Nagashima, Hinohara and Hirano, 1980) and forming complexes with albumin and fibrinogen (Nagashima, 1981), thus decreasing peptic digestion by reducing the available substrate for the enzyme. Sucralfate is also an efficient adsorber of bile salts at acidic pH values (Nagashima, 1981).

Cytoprotective studies with sucralfate in rhesus monkeys (Shea-Donohue *et al.*, 1986) have demonstrated improved mucosal resistance related to increased acidic glycoprotein output by a prostaglandin-independent process. Neutral glycoproteins were unaffected. Sucralfate is known to increase gastric and

Table 9.4 Modes of action of sucralfate

	References
Reduction of aggressive factors	
Delayed diffusion of H^+	Nagashima (1981)
Selective binding to ulcer sites	Nagashima (1981)
Adsorption of pepsin	Nagashima, Hinohara and Hirano (1980)
Antipeptic activity	Nagashima (1981)
Adsorption of bile salts	Nagashima (1981)
Improved mucosal resistance	
Increased acidic mucus	Shea-Donohue et al. (1986)
Increased bicarbonate secretion	Guslandi (1985), Crampton, Gibbons and Rees (1987), Konturek et al. (1987a), Shorrock, Gibbons and Rees (1988), Forssell, McCloy and Olbe (1989)
Increased luminal prostaglandin	Konturek et al. (1987a)
Trophic irritant effect on mucosa	Guslandi (1985)
Local binding of epidermal growth factor	Konturek (1988)

duodenal bicarbonate secretion in animals (Crampton, Gibbons and Rees, 1987) and gastric bicarbonate output in man (Guslandi, 1985; Konturek et al., 1987a; Shorrock, Gibbons and Rees, 1988; Forssell, McCloy and Olbe, 1989). The results of one study examining the effect of sucralfate on human gastric bicarbonate output is shown in Figure 9.1. Although initial studies in man and dog (Konturek et al., 1987a) described a prostaglandin-mediated increase in bicarbonate secretion and luminal prostaglandin E_2 levels, more recent work (Shorrock, Gibbons and Rees, 1988; Forssell, McCloy and Olbe, 1989) suggests that this action of sucralfate may not depend on mucosal prostaglandin biosynthesis. In the rat stomach, sucralfate leads to disruption and exfoliation of some of the surface epithelial cells, mucosal hyperaemia, marked release of mucus, and oedema of the lamina propria and submucosa (Tarnawski et al., 1986). These changes are associated with a drop in gastric mucosal potential difference and a significant increase in luminal release of prostaglandin E_2. Adaptive cytoprotection is a term that has been used to describe these effects, which are likely to be mediated by endogenous mucosal prostaglandins, and are common to many 'mild irritants'. However, mild irritants have the capacity to produce mucosal necrosis and sucralfate cannot produce necrosis even in very high doses. It has been suggested that the term 'mild stimulant' might be more appropriate to describe the local actions of sucralfate (Tarnawski and Hollander, 1987). As with colloidal bismuth, sucralfate may increase the local availability of epidermal growth factor (Konturek, 1988).

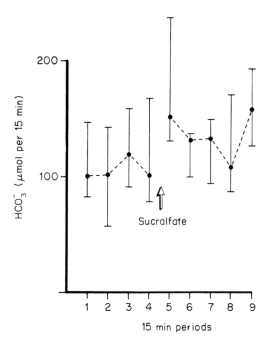

Figure 9.1   Gastric bicarbonate output in response to sucralfate in 7 healthy subjects (median, interquartile ranges). (Forssell, McCloy and Olbe, 1989)

The Lausanne workshop (Dent *et al.*, 1989) voted that the most important ulcer-healing actions of sucralfate were its topical action, provision of a barrier to aggression, and enhancement of mucosal defences (Table 9.5).

The time to recurrence of duodenal ulcer after healing by sucralfate has been shown to be significantly prolonged (Hallerback *et al.*, 1987; Lam *et al.*, 1987). No explanation for this effect has been forthcoming. Sucralfate does not have an antibacterial effect against *C. pylori*. However, whilst it does seem reasonable that sucralfate and colloidal bismuth may not heal precisely the same ulcers as H$_2$-antagonists, both categories of drugs heal approximately 80% of ulcers, so the difference in recurrence rates cannot be attributed to different populations of ulcers. Delayed recurrence of peptic ulcer seems to be a feature of non-antisecretory drugs as a whole (Dobrilla, Vallaperta and Amplatz, 1988), although the published data for single drugs hold good only in the case of colloidal bismuth.

There are several more groups of drugs which could have potent non-antisecretory ulcer-healing properties:

(1) sulfhydryls,
(2) surface-active phospholipids,
(3) meciadanol,

Table 9.5 Lausanne workshop vote: What mechanisms are responsible for the ulcer healing action of sucralfate?

Mechanism	Agree (%)	Disagree (%)	Uncertain (%)
Enhancing mucosal defences	58	6	36
Topical action	72	8	20
Selective adhesion to ulcers	49	16	35
Barrier to aggression	60	8	32
Antipeptic activity	33	22	45
Increased mucosal prosta- glandins by irritant action	39	16	45
Prevents microvascular injury	19	15	66
Local binding of epidermal growth factor	10	24	66

(4) epidermal growth factor,
(5) carotenoids (including vitamin A),
(6) prokinetic agents (metoclopramide, cisapride),
(7) zinc,
(8) antibiotics,

However, there is relatively little published evidence available (Guth, 1987). All the drugs considered in this review have reported healing rates for peptic ulcers comparable to that of H_2-antagonists. The clinical implications for their use have been reviewed elsewhere (McCloy, 1987). The final conclusion of the Lausanne workshop (Dent *et al.*, 1989) was that 'efficient long-term treatment without acid reduction has not been achieved' (57% agree, 27% disagree, 16% don't know).

REFERENCES

Blaser, M. J. (1987). Gastric *Campylobacter*-like organisms, gastritis, and peptic ulcer disease, *Gastroenterology*, **93**, 371–83.

Crampton, J. R., Gibbons, L. and Rees, W. (1987). Effects of sucralfate on gastroduodenal bicarbonate secretion and prostaglandin E_2 metabolism, *Am. J. Med.*, **83** (Suppl. 3B), 14–18.

Dent, J., McCloy, R., Blum, A., Garner, A., Matthews, J. and Rune, S. (1988). Realities of mucosal defence: drugs for the management of peptic disorders. (In preparation)

Dobrilla, G., Vallaperta, P. and Amplatz, S. (1988). Influence of ulcer healing agents on ulcer relapse after discontinuation of acute treatment: a pooled estimate of controlled clinical trials, *Gut*, **29**, 181–7.

Domschke, S., Domschke, W. and Demling, L. (1975). Effect of intravenous prednisolone on net ion fluxes across human gastric mucosa: antagonism by carbenoxolone sodium. In F. Avery Jones and D. V. Parke (eds) *Fourth Symposium on Carbenoxolone*, Butterworths, London, pp. 75–86.

Dooley, C. P. and Cohen, H. (1988). The clinical significance of *Campylobacter pylori*, *Ann. Intern. Med.*, **108**, 70–9.

Fisher, R. S. and Lorber, S. H. (1975). Influence of Biogastrone on pyloric sphincter function in patients with gastric ulcer. In F. Avery Jones and D. V. Parke (eds) *Fourth Symposium on Carbenoxolone*, Butterworths, London, pp. 201–7.

Forssell, H., McCloy, R. and Olbe, L. (1989). Sucralfate stimulates gastric bicarbonate secretion in man. (In preparation)

Guslandi, M. (1985). Sucralfate and gastric bicarbonate, *Pharmacology*, **31**, 298–300.

Guth, P. H. (1987). Mucosal coating agents and other nonantisecretory agents: are they cytoprotective?, *Dig. Dis. Sci.*, **32**, 647–54.

Hallerback, B., Solhaug, J.-H., Carling, L. *et al.* (1987). Recurrent ulcer after treatment with cimetidine or sucralfate, *Scand. J. Gastroenterol.*, **22**, 791–7.

Hollander, D., Morrissey, S. M. and Mehta, J. (1983). Mucus secretion in gastric ulcer patients treated with tripotassium dicitratobismuthate (De-Nol), *Br. J. Clin. Pract.*, **37**, 112–14.

Johnston, B., Lindup, W. E., Shillingford, J. S., Smith, M. and Parke, D. V. (1975). The pharmacological biochemistry of carbenoxolone: its effects on gastric mucus. In F. Avery Jones and D. V. Parke (eds) *Fourth Symposium on Carbenoxolone*, Butterworths, London, pp. 3–21.

Klein, H. J., Frotz, H. and Gheorghiu, Th. (1975). Mechanism of action of carbenoxolone: autoradiographic study of proliferation *in vitro* of epithelial cells from gastric mucosa of carbenoxolone-treated patients. In F. Avery Jones and D. V. Parke (eds) *Fourth Symposium on Carbenoxolone*, Butterworths, London, pp. 161–70.

Konturek, S. J. (1988). Role of epidermal growth factor in gastroprotection and ulcer healing, *Scand. J. Gastroenterol.*, **23**, 129–33.

Konturek, S. J., Bilski, J., Kwiecien, N., Obtulowicz, W., Kopp, B. and Olesky, J. (1987a). De-Nol stimulates gastric and duodenal alkaline secretion through prostaglandin dependent mechanism, *Gut*, **28**, 1557–63.

Konturek, S. J., Radecki, T., Piastucki, I., Brzozowski, T. and Drozdowicz, D. (1987b). Gastrocytoprotection by colloidal bismuth subcitrate (De-Nol) and sucralfate: role of endogenous prostaglandins, *Gut*, **28**, 201–5.

Koo, J., Ho, J., Lam, S. K., Wong, J. and Ong, G. B. (1982). Selective coating of gastric ulcer by tripotassium dicitratobismuthate in the rat, *Gastroenterology*, **82**, 864–70.

Lam, S. K., Hui, W. M., Lau, W. Y. *et al.* (1987). Sucralfate overcomes adverse effect of cigarette smoking on duodenal ulcer healing and prolongs subsequent remission, *Gastroenterology*, **92**, 1193–201.

Lambert, J. R., Hansky, J., Davidson, A., Pinkerd, K. and Stockman, K. (1985). *Campylobacter* like organisms (CLO)—*in vivo* and *in vitro* susceptibility to antimicrobial and antiulcer therapy, *Gastroenterology*, **88**, 1462.

Lee, S. P. (1982). A potential mechanism of action of colloidal bismuth subcitrate: diffusion barrier to hydrochloric acid, *Scand. J. Gastroenterol.*, **17** (Suppl. 80), 17–21.

McCloy, R. F. (1987). Clinical implications. In R. F. McCloy (ed.) *Gastroduodenal Defences*, Current Medical Literature, London, pp. 37–44.

Miller, J. P. and Faragher, E. B. (1986). Relapse of duodenal ulcer: does it matter which drug is used in initial treatment?, *Br. Med. J.*, **293**, 1117–18.

Nagashima, R. (1981). Mechanisms of action of sucralfate, *J. Clin. Gastroenterol.*, **3** (Suppl. 2), 117–27.

Nagashima, R., Hinohara, Y. and Hirano, T. (1980). Selective binding of sucralfate to ulcer lesion. III. Experiments in rats with duodenal ulcer receiving ^{14}C-sucralfate, *Arzneim. Forsch.*, **30**, 88–91.

Parke, D. V. (1978). Some recent advances in the pharmacology of carbenoxolone. In F. Avery Jones, M. J. S. Langman and R. D. Mann (eds) *Peptic Ulcer Healing. Recent Studies on Carbenoxolone*, MTP, Lancaster, pp. 1–8.

Rees, W. D. W. (1987). Mucus–bicarbonate barrier—shield or sieve, *Gut*, **28**, 1553–6.

Roberts, N. B. and Taylor, W. H. (1982). The effect of tripotassium dicitratobismuthate (De-Nol) upon the individual human pepsins, *Scand. J. Gastroenterol.* **17** (Suppl. 78), 305.

Shea-Donohue, T., Steel, L., Montcalm, E. and Dubois, A. (1986). Gastric protection by sucralfate: role of mucus and prostaglandins, *Gastroenterology*, **91**, 660–6.

Shorrock, C. J., Gibbons, L. and Rees, W. D. W. (1988). Effect of sucralfate on human gastric bicarbonate secretion and luminal PGE_2 output, *Gut*, **29**, A710–11.

Silen, W. and Ito, S. (1985). Mechanisms for re-epithelialization of the gastric mucosal surface, *Ann. Rev. Physiol.*, **47**, 217–29.

Tarnawski, A. and Hollander, D. (1987). Cytoprotection of gastric and duodenal mucosa, *Curr. Med. Lit. Gastroenterol.*, **6**, 3–9.

Tarnawski, A., Hollander, D., Krause, W. J., Zipser, R. D., Stachura, J. and Gargely, H. (1986). Does sucralfate affect normal gastric mucosa? Histologic, ultrastructural, and functional assessment in the rat, *Gastroenterology*, **90**, 893–905.

Walker, V. and Taylor, W. H. (1975). Pepsin inhibition *in vivo* and the therapeutic action of carbenoxolone. In F. Avery Jones and D. V. Parke (eds) *Fourth Symposium on Carbenoxolone*, Butterworths, London, pp. 55–69.

Wallace, J. L. and Whittle, B. J. R. (1986). Role of mucus in the repair of gastric epithelial damage in the rat: inhibition of epithelial recovery by mucolytic agents, *Gastroenterology*, **91**, 603–11.

Whittle, B. J. R., Oren-Wolman, N. and Guth, P. H. (1985). Gastric vasoconstrictor actions of leukotriene C_4, PGF_{20}, and thromboxane mimetic U-46619 on rat submucosal microcirculation *in vivo*, *Am. J. Physiol.*, **248**, G580–6.

Advances in Drug Therapy of Gastrointestinal Ulceration
Edited by A. Garner and B. J. R. Whittle
©1989 John Wiley & Sons Ltd

Chapter Ten

Gastroduodenal Mucosal Integrity, Injury and Repair

William Silen
Department of Surgery, Harvard Medical School, Beth Israel Hospital, Boston, Massachusetts, USA

The integrity of the mucosa of the stomach and duodenum is challenged daily by physical and chemical insults. Considering the frequency with which such injurious circumstances occur, the development of chronic ulcerations is relatively rare. The explanation for this discrepancy resides in the remarkable ability of both the gastric and duodenal mucosa (and probably all of the small intestine and colon) to repair with amazing rapidity those superficial injuries incurred during daily life. During the past 7 or 8 years, much has been learned about this remarkable process of rapid repair (also called restitution or reconstitution) and it seems appropriate to review some of these new findings at this time.

MAINTENANCE OF EPITHELIAL INTEGRITY

Description of reconstitution

Rapid repair of the gastroduodenal mucosa (restitution, reconstitution) is that process by which superficial epithelial defects are covered by the migration of uninjured cells over an intact basal lamina (Svanes *et al.*, 1982). There is some evidence that this rapid repair will not occur if the basal lamina is injured or is, for some reason, not intact (Lacy, 1987). The migration of cells from the deeper portions of the mucosa results in a thinner epithelium until such time that cell replication initiated in the progenitor zone restores full thickness of the epithelium—a period of 2 or 3 days

(Lipkin, Sherlock and Bell, 1963). As a result of this migration, oxyntic cells of the gastric fundus come to be placed closer to the luminal surface of the epithelium. The migrating mucous neck and superficial epithelial cells establish normal cell junctions virtually as soon as they contact each other. Restitution has been found to occur *in vivo* in rat stomach after as little as 15 min (Lacy and Ito, 1984a,b) but it may take as long as 4 h *in vitro* in amphibian gastric mucosa (Svanes *et al.*, 1982). However, even the latter extreme is far more rapid than can possibly be accounted for by cell replication. A single sheet of isolated guinea-pig gastric mucosa can rapidly restore epithelial integrity as many as three times in an *ex vivo* chamber, each restitution requiring only 30–60 min (Rutten and Ito, 1983).

Conditions affecting reconstitution

It seems clear that the coverage of superficial defects depends upon the intrinsic motility of surviving epithelial cells. The migrating lamellipodia of the surviving cells contain bundles of microfilaments, usually composed of actin, which are essential for cellular motility. Thus, treatment of superficially injured tissues with cytocholasin B, which inhibits microfilaments, virtually abolishes the process of reconstitution (Critchlow *et al.*, 1985). In addition, epithelial cells will not migrate over a defect in which the basal lamina has been destroyed (Lacy, 1987). Of particular importance in the stomach is that a luminal pH of 2.5 or less also inhibits the re-surfacing of superficial epithelial defects (Svanes *et al.*, 1983; Critchlow *et al.*, 1985). It is not known whether a low pH injures the basal lamina or whether the acidic pH retards restitution by other mechanisms. Studies *in vitro* also suggest that a decreased availability of HCO_3^- inhibits reconstitution (Svanes *et al.*, 1983). Finally, adequate quantities of calcium are required both for migration of cells (perhaps because of the need for Ca^{2+} in microfilamentous function) and for the formation of intercellular junctions (Critchlow *et al.*, 1985). There are no known conditions which accelerate the process of reconstitution.

Implications of rapid repair

The studies of rapid repair described above strongly suggest that the gastric mucosal barrier, a concept proposed by Davenport (1976), is in reality the anatomical integrity of the superficial epithelium. It was originally thought that the disruption and subsequent rapid re-establishment of the gastric mucosal barrier following injury must represent physiological phenomena because of the extreme rapidity with which these processes occurred. In the knowledge of the author, while a systematic study of this question has not been published, instances of 'barrier disruption' by physiological criteria have not been shown or reported in the absence of anatomical injury to the epithelium. It now seems evident that whenever there is disruption of the barrier, there is microscopic evidence of serious injury to the superficial epithelium. The rapid recovery of the barrier can undoubtedly be ascribed to the process of restitution.

It has now been shown that restitution occurs in a variety of epithelia, including the gall bladder, duodenum, colon (Hudspeth, 1975, 1982), and perhaps other tissues. It is likely that in these tissues, too, restitution is responsible for recovery from the minor injuries of daily life.

CAUSES OF CELLULAR DEATH OR INJURY

Surprisingly, the ultimate cause of cell death in epithelial injuries of the stomach and duodenum is not known. Experimentally, it is even difficult to determine whether a given cell is reversibly or irreversibly damaged. Many have lost sight of the fact that a variety of mechanisms are probably responsible for epithelial damage induced by different agents, and therefore attempts to consider them as one are likely to mislead the investigator. Furthermore, some conditions which have been employed experimentally, e.g. 100% ethanol, are so damaging that inferences drawn from these studies cannot be transferred meaningfully to more physiological conditions.

Because of the pivotal role of luminal acid in the development of gastric and duodenal epithelial injury under physiological circumstances, it is natural to assume that acidification of cells is important in the cause of cell death. Yet it has been shown that the luminal plasma membranes of chief cells (Sanders et al., 1985) and antral cells (Ashley et al., 1987) are remarkably impermeable to H^+. Of interest is the finding that the antral mucosa tolerates acidification from the luminal side much more readily and easily than it does acidification from the blood or nutrient side (Ashley et al., 1987). These findings are consistent with the repeated observation that systemic acidosis is extremely damaging to gastric and duodenal mucosa (Cummins, Grossman and Ivey, 1948; Kivilaakso, Fromm and Silen, 1978). The mechanism by which systemic acidosis adversely affects the gastric or duodenal mucosa remains to be elucidated.

Some investigators have suggested that hypoxia is a more important cause of cell death than ischaemia (Bowen, 1981), but this proposal has not been confirmed as yet. Differentiation of the damaging effect of ischaemia and hypoxia will not be easily accomplished. It is possible that the damaging effects of ischaemia may be in large part attributable to the metabolic acidosis produced by inadequate perfusion (Kivilaakso, Fromm and Silen, 1978). Recent studies strongly suggest, however, that oxygen free radicals generated during reperfusion may also play an important role in epithelial injury (Smith et al., 1987).

Certain agents such as bile salts cause dissolution of cell membranes almost immediately upon contact with the epithelium. Other toxic substances such as ethanol induce denaturation of proteins. Studies of injury by these substances have not in the past considered adequately the enormous differences in the effects of such agents upon the stomach. For example, exposure to deoxycholate almost uniformly causes rapid loss of surface epithelial cells while 100% ethanol produces virtually instantaneous fixation of epithelial cells, so that microscopic examination of tissues exposed to 100% ethanol may appear almost uninjured at the same time as the potential difference (PD) across the tissue has dropped to zero and H^+ secretion has ceased irreversibly (Saario et al., 1987, 1988). Whatever the effects of these toxic agents on the epithelial cells, it has been shown that both bile salts and ethanol penetrate the tissue. Since gastric mucosal capillaries are placed in remarkably close apposition to the basement membrane of the epithelial cells, it is not surprising that these blood vessels are injured as rapidly as the epithelial cells themselves (Gannon et al., 1984). Unfortunately, a great deal of confusion has arisen in the literature on this subject because attempts have been made to relate causally the epithelial damage to the vascular injury, when in fact the two might simply be unrelated epiphenomena.

The injurious effects of drugs such as aspirin may be even more complex. There is general unanimity that there are two mechanisms by which aspirin injures the mucosa; a topical effect and a systemic effect. Topically, aspirin enters the mucosa and damages it only if the aspirin is in its undissociated form, i.e. when the luminal pH is at or below its pK_a. The undissociated form enters the cell and dissociates at near-neutral cell pH to release H^+ and acetylsalicylate. Esterases which are known to exist within the gastric mucosa convert the acetylsalicylate to salicylate, the latter being the form which has been shown to interfere with mitochondrial metabolism. It is not known whether it is the H^+ which has been carried into the mucosa or the acetylsalicylate or salicylate anions, or all of these, which are ultimately responsible for cell death. It is clear, however, that in addition to the topical effects of aspirin the drug has a systemic effect since its systemic administration can cause chronic gastric ulcers in cats (Bugat et al., 1976) and mucosal erosions and haemorrhages in rats (Rowe et al., 1987) so long as the lumen of the stomach is acidic. While some have attributed these systemic actions of aspirin to inhibition of cyclo-oxygenase and hence to depletion of mucosal prostaglandins, it has been shown that depletion of mucosal prostaglandins alone is not sufficient provocation for ulceration to develop (Konturek et al., 1981; Ligumisky, Grossman and Kauffman, 1982). It is possible that the toxic systemic effects of aspirin on the gastric mucosa may be related to the injurious effects of salicylate rather than acetylsalicylate since the latter is rapidly converted to salicylate by esterases in the blood, liver and gastric mucosa (Rainsford, 1984). Furthermore, despite the fact that salicylate does not inhibit cyclo-oxygenase, it causes severe topical injury tantamount to that induced by acetylsalicylate, and we have recently demonstrated that salicylate causes severe gastric mucosal injury when given systemically if luminal acid is present (Rowe et al., 1987).

Finally, changes in tonicity may cause severe epithelial injury. For example, 1 mol l^{-1} NaCl produces extensive destruction of the surface epithelial cells of the stomach (Svanes *et al.*, 1982). It is known that changes in cellular volume (i.e. swelling or shrinkage) are strongly influenced by the ubiquitous Na^+,K^+-ATPase and perhaps by Na^+-H^+ exchangers (Spring and Ericson, 1982). The extent to which these homeostatic mechanisms can offset severe changes in tonicity is not known since this question has not been systematically investigated. Obviously in the case of the injury induced by the 1 mol l^{-1} NaCl, the Na^+-K^+ pump and the Na^+-H^+ exchangers are inadequate to prevent extreme damage and cellular disruption.

DETAILED DESCRIPTION OF A SPECIFIC GASTRIC MUCOSAL INJURY

It is useful to consider the physiological and morphological consequences of a specific type of gastric mucosal injury to establish a basis for comparative examination of a variety of damaging agents. For that purpose, I have chosen the injury to *in vitro* amphibian mucosa caused by 1 mol l^{-1} NaCl because this experimental circumstance has been studied in detail and because it is a relatively mild injury from which rapid recovery uniformly occurs. In addition, the *in vitro* nature of this model eliminates the confounding effects of vascular damage. Thus, it is reasonable to consider the processes of injury and subsequent rapid repair as prototypic of pure epithelial damage.

Frog gastric fundic mucosa mounted in an Ussing chamber when exposed on its mucosal surface to a hypertonic challenge, i.e. 1 mol l^{-1} NaCl for 10 min, shows an almost immediate and precipitous decrease in PD and tissue resistance (Svanes *et al.*, 1982). Acid secretion into the lumen ceases abruptly, and is replaced by a large and easily titratable flow of alkaline 'secretion' into the lumen. This titratable alkalinity results from diffusion of HCO_3^--containing nutrient solution from the nutrient or blood side into the lumen through large gaps in the injured epithelium because, if the mucosa is allowed to recover over a period of 4 h in control solutions, the titratable alkaline flow into the lumen is replaced by acid secretion which may return to control levels after 4–6 h (Svanes *et al.*, 1983). During the 4 h of recovery, the PD and resistance also gradually return to control levels. While transmucosal PD itself is influenced by a variety of conditions which do not cause mucosal injury, the PD is a reasonably good indicator of destruction of the epithelium if there is microscopic monitoring and confirmation of mucosal damage. It is also likely that the 'plasma shedding' described by Davenport (1966) *in vivo* after exposure of canine gastric mucosa to acetic or salicyclic acid represents analogous leakage of interstitial fluid into the lumen as well as leakage of albumin-containing plasma from injured capillaries, an effect not observed *in vitro*.

There are remarkably good correlations between the physiological consequences of the 1 mol l^{-1} NaCl injury described above and the morphological changes in the tissue. Immediately after exposure to the hypertonic solution, at a time when the PD and resistance have reached zero and titratable alkalinity appears in the lumen, a thick layer of mucoid debris containing dead, exfoliated cells is seen to cover the denuded lamina propria and wrinkled basal lamina. It is likely that the alkaline milieu of this exfoliated mucoid cover is conducive to rapid epithelial repair because exposure to a luminal pH of 2.5 completely inhibits the process of reconstitution. During the ensuing 4 h, as the PD and resistance gradually return to normal, the surviving mucous neck cells send out lamellipodia which eventually develop contact with each other as these cells migrate over the intact basal lamina and form junctions, re-establishing epithelial continuity. When this process is completed, acid secretion commences once again.

There is some evidence that the thick 'mucoid cap' which forms over the surface of the injured mucosa is in itself protective. Some investigators have suggested that this cap accounts for the phenomenon of 'adaptive cytoprotection' because exposure of the mucosa to a second injury while the mucoid cap is present does not re-damage the mucosa whereas mechanical removal of this cap renders the mucosa susceptible to a second insult (Lacy, 1987). It has also been shown that prostaglandins are not necessary for adaptive cytoprotection (Hawkey *et al.*, 1985) as originally proposed (Robert *et al.*, 1983).

SUMMARY

The gastric mucosa is damaged by a large variety of agents. Injury may be mediated by acidification of the tissue, hypoxia, ischaemia, dissolution of cell membranes, interference with mitochondrial metabolism, denaturation of proteins and liberation of oxygen free radicals. The intimate cellular events associated with death of the cells in each of these types of injury is poorly understood. Because of the diversity of many of these injurious circumstances and their differing effects on the epithelium, these injuries cannot be considered in a unitarian sense. Much more information as to the physiological effects of each type of damage is sorely needed.

The integrity of the gastric and duodenal epithelia in response to the minor injuries of daily life is maintained by the process of rapid repair, also called reconstitution or restitution. Since elucidation of this process, it appears that the gastric mucosal barrier is indeed the physical intactness of the epithelium.

REFERENCES

Ashley, S. W., Soybel, D. I., Moore, D. and Cheung, L. Y. (1987). Intracellular pH (pH$_i$) in gastric surface epithelium is more susceptible to serosal than mucosal acidification, *Surgery*, **102**, 371–9.

Bowen, J. C. (1981). The oxygen microelectrode as an indicator of nutrient blood flow to gastric epithelium. In J. W. Harmon (ed.) *Basic Mechanisms of Gastrointestinal Mucosal Cell Injury and Protection*, Williams & Wilkins, Baltimore, pp. 67–76.

Bugat, R., Thompson, M. R., Aures, D. and Grossman, M. I. (1976). Gastric mucosal lesions produced by intravenous infusion of aspirin in cats, *Gastroenterology*, **71**, 754–9.

Critchlow, J., Magee, D., Ito, S., Takeuchi, K. and Silen, W. (1985). Requirements for restitution of the surface epithelium of frog stomach after mucosal injury, *Gastroenterology*, **88**, 237–49.

Cummins, G. M., Grossman, M. I. and Ivey, A. C. (1948). An experimental study of the acid factor in ulceration of the gastrointestinal tract in dogs, *Gastroenterology*, **10**, 714–26.

Davenport, H. W. (1966). Fluid produced by the gastric mucosa during damage by acetic and salicylic acids, *Gastroenterology*, **50**, 487–99.

Davenport, H. W. (1976). Physiological parameters of the gastric mucosal barrier, *Dig. Dis. Sci.*, **21**, 141–3.

Gannon, B., Browning, J., O'Brien, P. and Rogers, P. (1984). Mucosal microvascular architecture of the fundus and body of human stomach, *Gastroenterology*, **86**, 866–75.

Hawkey, C. J., Kemp, R. T., Walt, R. P., Baskar, N. K., Davies, J. and Filipowicz, B. (1985). Adaptive cytoprotection: evidence against mediation by prostaglandins, *Gut*, **26**, A1147.

Hudspeth, A. J. (1975). Establishment of tight junctions between epithelial cells, *Proc. Natl. Acad. Sci. USA*, **72**, 2711–13.

Hudspeth, A. J. (1982). The recovery of local transepithelial resistance following single-cell lesions, *Exp. Cell Res.*, **138**, 331–42.

Kivilaakso, E., Fromm, D. and Silen, D. (1978). Relationship between ulceration and intramural pH of gastric mucosa during hemorrhagic shock, *Surgery*, **84**, 70–7.

Konturek, S. J., Radecki, T., Brzozowski, T., Piastucki, I., Zmuda, A. and Dembrinska-Kiec, A. (1981). Aspirin-induced gastric ulcers in cats: prevention by prostaglandins, *Dig. Dis. Sci.*, **26**, 1003–112.

Lacy, E. R. (1987). Gastric mucosal defense after superficial injury, *Clin. Invest. Med.*, **10**, 189–200.

Lacy, E. R. and Ito, S. (1984a). Rapid epithelial restitution of the rat gastric mucosa after ethanol injury, *Lab. Invest.*, **51**, 573–83.

Lacy, E. R. and Ito, S. (1984b). Ethanol-induced insult to the superficial rat gastric epithelium: a study of damage and rapid repair. In A. Allen, G. Flemstrom, A. Garner, W. Silen and L. A. Turnberg (eds) *Mechanisms of Mucosal Protection in the Upper Gastrointestinal Tract*, Raven Press, New York, pp. 49–56.

Ligumisky, M., Grossman, M. I. and Kauffman, G. L. (1982). Endogenous gastric mucosal prostaglandins: their role in mucosal integrity, *Am. J. Physiol.*, **242**, G337–41.

Lipkin, M., Sherlock, P. and Bell, B. (1963). Cell proliferation kinetics in the gastrointestinal tract of man. II. Cell renewal in stomach, ileum, colon and rectum, *Gastroenterology*, **45**, 721–9.

Rainsford, K. D. (1984). *Aspirin and the Salicylates*, Butterworths, London.

Robert, A., Lancaster, C., Hanjar, A. J. and Nezamins, J. E. (1983). Mild irritants prevent gastric necrosis through 'adaptive cytoprotection' mediated by prostaglandin formation, *Am. J. Physiol.*, **245**, G113–21.

Rowe, P. H., Starlinger, M. J., Kasdon, E., Hollands, M. J. and Silen, W. (1987). Parenteral aspirin and sodium salicylate are equally injurious to the rat gastric mucosa, *Gastroenterology*, **93**, 863–71.

Rutten, M. J. and Ito, S. (1983). Morphology and electrophysiology of guinea pig gastric mucosal repair *in vitro*, *Am. J. Physiol.*, **244**, G171–82.

Saario, I., Carter, K., Rosen, S. and Silen, W. (1987). Effects of ethanol on the *in vitro* frog gastric mucosa: electrophysiology and acid secretion, *Gastroenterology*, **92**, 1607.

Saario, I., Rosen, S., Carter, K. and Silen, W. (1988). Effect of ethanol on frog gastric mucosa: electrophysiologic and morphologic correlations, *Gastroenterology*, **94**, 638–46.

Sanders, M. J., Ayalon, A., Roll, M. and Soll, A. H. (1985). The apical surface of canine chief cell monolayers resists H^+ back diffusion, *Nature*, **313**, 52–4.

Smith, S. M., Grisham, M. B., Manci, E. A., Granger, D. N. and Kvietys, P. R. (1987). Gastric mucosal injury in the rat: role of iron and xanthine oxidase, *Gastroenterology*, **92**, 950–6.

Spring, K. R. and Ericson, G. C. (1982). Epithelial cell volume modulation and regulation, *J. Membr. Biol.*, **69**, 167–76.

Svanes, K., Ito, S., Takeuchi, K. and Silen, W. (1982). Restitution of the surface epithelium of *in vitro* frog gastric mucosa after damage with hyperosmolar sodium chloride: morphologic and physiologic characteristics, *Gastroenterology*, **82**, 1409–26.

Svanes, K., Takeuchi, K., Ito, S. and Silen, W. (1983). Effect of luminal pH and nutrient bicarbonate concentration on restitution after gastric surface cell injury, *Surgery*, **94**, 494–500.

Advances in Drug Therapy of Gastrointestinal Ulceration
Edited by A. Garner and B. J. R. Whittle
© 1989 John Wiley & Sons Ltd

_____ Chapter Eleven

Peptic Activity and the Mucus–Bicarbonate Barrier

Adrian Allen, Andrew C. Hunter, Andrea J. Leonard,
Jeffrey P. Pearson and Lynda A. Sellers
_Department of Physiological Sciences, Medical School,
The University, Newcastle upon Tyne NE2 4HH, UK_

Acid and pepsin are endogenous aggressors secreted in the gastric juice, and defence mechanisms have presumably evolved to protect the gastroduodenal mucosa from autodigestion. Much of this chapter will be concerned with the role the adherent mucus barrier plays as part of the natural gastroduodenal mucosal defence mechanisms against pepsin and acid and, ultimately, against peptic ulceration. In discussing the role of the mucus barrier in gastroduodenal mucosal defence, it is important to note the distinction between endogenous aggressors, e.g. acid and pepsin, and exogenous damaging agents, e.g. ethanol and non-steroidal anti-inflammatory drugs, administered by man to himself or experimental animals. The natural mucosal defensive response to acid and pepsin may well be different from that of the exogenous aggressors. This is certainly the case for gastroduodenal mucus which is part of the natural barrier to pepsin and acid but does not protect the mucosa against acute damage by agents such as ethanol (Allen _et al._, 1986). Mucus does have some role in formation of the protective gelatinous coat formed subsequently over the repairing epithelium following acute ethanol damage. However, this gelatinous coat is largely fibrin gel, necrotic cells with mucus forming only a minor component (Sellers _et al._, 1987a).

STRUCTURE OF THE GASTRODUODENAL MUCUS BARRIER

Mucus is ubiquitous throughout the gastrointestinal tract and is its major organic secretion in terms of output by weight and biosynthetic requirements. The primary gastroduodenal mucus secretion is a water-insoluble gel which adheres to the epithelial surfaces. This adherent mucus is seen on unfixed mucosal sections as a thin layer of translucent gel of mean thickness 180 μm and 80 μm in man and rat respectively (Kerss, Allen and Garner, 1982; Allen *et al.*, 1986). Two other phases of mucus can be identified:

(1) Presecreted intracellular mucus stores which give the mucus-secreting epithelia their characteristic pattern of neutral and acidic mucin staining.

(2) Viscous soluble mucus which can be removed with the luminal contents by washing the mucosal surfaces.

However, it is the adherent gel phase that provides the stable protective barrier over the mucosal surfaces. This mucus gel is physically distinct from the soluble mucus in the lumen. The latter is freely mobile and unlikely to afford protection against the gastric juices with which it is mixed. Soluble mucus is likely to be important as a lubricant in protecting the mucosal surface from mechanical abrasion during the digestive processes.

Fundamental to its protective function against the gastric juices is the thickness of the adherent mucus gel layer and its continuity over the mucosa. A simple method for measuring gastroduodenal mucus gel thickness is by observation of unfixed, transverse, sections of mucosa (Kerss, Allen and Garner, 1982). Under these conditions the mucus layer is seen as continuous, varying in thickness from 50 to 450 μm (median 180 μm) for human antral stomach and 10 to 300 μm (median 80 μm) for rat stomach and duodenum. Mucus thickness can also be measured indirectly on an everted mucosa using a slit lamp and pachymeter, but thickness dimensions by this method are consistently about twice those from direct observation of unfixed sections (Bickel and Kauffman, 1981). An explanation for this difference in thickness values is that the pachymeter method is measuring, in part, unstirred solution which remains attached to the mucus gel (Allen *et al.*, 1983).

Little, if any, extracellular mucus is apparent on a typical histologically fixed and stained gastroduodenal mucosal section from undamaged mucosa (Morris and Wallace, 1981; Morris, Harding and Wallace, 1984). Some workers, on the basis of such observations, have questioned the existence of a continuous barrier over an undamaged mucosa. In support of their conclusions, the network of mucus threads seen on electron micrographs is also cited. However, such conclusions are invalid since fixatives, such as ethanol and glutaraldehyde, used for histological processing cause shrinkage and dehydration of the mucus gel (McQueen, Allen and Garner, 1984; Bell *et al.*, 1985). A similar criticism can be made of electron microscopy preparation methods which also dehydrate the mucus gel. This is confirmed by studies which show that, if the extracellular adherent mucus gel is first fixed *in situ* by techniques such as freeze vapour substitution or with mucus antibodies, a continuous layer over the mucosal surface is seen on histological sections and electron micrographs (Sakata and Englehart, 1981; Rozee *et al.*, 1982; Bollard *et al.*, 1986). Furthermore, the binding and internalization of catonized ferritin to gastric epithelia *in vitro* take place only after the adherent mucus cover lying over the epithelial surfaces has been removed (Sturrock and Hopwood, 1986).

A cause of confusion has been the contrast between the lack of extracellular adherent mucus on fixed histological sections of undamaged mucosa compared with the thick gelatinous or 'mucoid' coat observed on similarly processed sections of mucosa following acute damage by ethanol. Although substantial numbers of necrotic cells and the presence of fibrin have been observed within the gelatinous coat covering the ethanol-damaged mucosa, it has been designated by some as mucus (Morris, Harding and Wallace, 1984; Wallace and Whittle, 1986). This mucoid coat has now been shown to be primarily a fibrin gel with exfoliated cells and some mucus and, unlike the original adherent mucus layer over the undamaged mucosa, it is not lost during histological fixation (Sellers *et al.*, 1987a). Evidence is now strongly in favour of a continuous adherent mucus gel barrier over the undamaged gastroduodenal mucosa.

The special features of the adherent gastroduodenal mucus barrier are as follows:

(1) It adheres to epithelial surfaces.
(2) It is a continuous layer of mean thickness 180 μm in man.
(3) It flows and reseals over 30–120 min.
(4) Its gel-forming component is mucin glycoprotein.
(5) It is insoluble in water, 2 mol l^{-1} NaCl and bile, and at pH 1–8.
(6) It is dehydrated by ethanol and glutaraldehyde.
(7) Mucolysis is caused by proteolytic enzymes (e.g. pepsin) and thiol agents (e.g. *N*-acetylcysteine, mercaptoethanol).

Rheological studies on isolated mucus gel and studies *in vivo* demonstrate substantial physical stability (Bell *et al.*, 1985). Mucus structure is unchanged following exposure to isotonic saline over 24 h, solutions of pH 1–8, bile or 2 mol l^{-1} saline. Mucus gel is resistant to mechanical disruption although it has the special characteristic that it will flow over a relatively long period of time (about an hour) and reseal when sectioned. It also adheres strongly to cell surfaces. These properties facilitate the maintenance of a continuous and effective protective, adherent mucus barrier over the mucosal surface.

Mucus gels are effectively solubilized by either proteolytic enzymes, e.g. pepsin, or by disulphide bond breaking agents, e.g. *N*-acetylcysteine or mercaptoethanol (Snary, Allen and Pain, 1970; Allen, 1978; Bell *et al.*, 1985). These procedures result in cleavage of the polymeric mucins which form the gel matrix. This has important implications *in vivo* in the stomach and, when the pH is low, in the duodenum, since pepsin in the lumen progressively erodes the mucus barrier to produce soluble degraded mucus glycoprotein. A dynamic balance exists across the adherent gastroduodenal mucus barrier where mucus lost by peptic solubilization and mechanical erosion at its luminal surface is replaced by secretion of new mucus from the mucosa. Since a continuous, adherent layer of mucus gel is seen on the undamaged mucosa, it follows that mucus secretion normally replenishes that lost by erosion. However, as discussed below, in cases of excess proteolytic activity *in vivo* (from pepsin and other sources) this dynamic balance may be swung in favour of adherent mucus erosion with the resultant breaching of the gastroduodenal mucus barrier.

THE MUCUS–BICARBONATE BARRIER AND ACID

The role for adherent mucus in protection of the underlying epithelia against luminal acid appears to be the maintenance of a stable unstirred layer at the mucosal surface. The H^+ ions in the lumen can diffuse rapidly through the mucus gel layer, which is 95% water, but are neutralized by bicarbonate ions from the gastroduodenal mucosa (Figure 11.1) (Allen and Garner, 1980; Flemström and Turnberg, 1984). The role of the unstirred layer within the mucus is to act as a mixing barrier, preventing the relatively small quantities of epithelial bicarbonate from being swamped by the large amount of acid in the luminal juice. Evidence supporting this mucus–bicarbonate barrier is:

(1) the extensive characterization of gastroduodenal mucosal bicarbonate secretion *in vivo* and *in vitro* (Allen and Garner, 1980; Flemström and Garner, 1982);

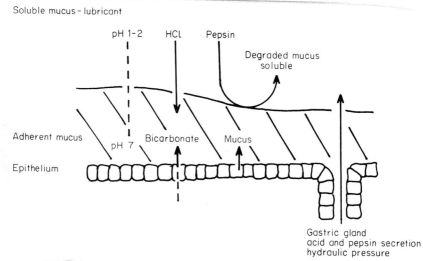

Figure 11.1 The mucus barrier on the undamaged gastric mucosa; protection against endogenous aggressors, acid and pepsin. (Modified from Allen *et al.* (1986))

(2) the demonstration of pH gradients at the gastroduodenal mucosal surface from an acid pH in the lumen to a near neutral pH at the mucosal surface in man and other mammals *in vivo* and amphibian *in vitro* (Williams and Turnberg, 1981; Ross and Turnberg, 1983; Kivilaakso and Flemström, 1984);

(3) the properties and continuity of the adherent mucus gel over the mucosal surface, discussed above.

In the duodenum, the basal and acid-stimulated bicarbonate secretion would appear sufficient to maintain neutrality at the mucosal surface at the lowest luminal pH values measured *in vivo*. In the stomach, however, maximal bicarbonate secretion is not sufficient for surface neutralization of acid when the luminal pH falls to below pH 2. Under these conditions of high acidity, the surface pH gradient has been shown to be dissipated (Ross and Turnberg, 1983). Periods of high luminal acidity (below pH 2) regularly occur during a 24 h cycle in the gastric lumen in man. Neutralization of these high luminal concentrations of acid can be maintained in both the interstitial and intracellular compartments by perfusion with bicarbonate-rich plasma and operation of epithelial membrane Na^+/H^+ and Cl^-/HCO_3^- exchanges (Machen and Paradiso, 1987). The actual cellular mechanisms for mucosal protection against luminal acid below pH 2 in the gastric lumen remain to be elucidated. However, even at pH 1, the adherent mucus gel remains intact and will support surface neutralization of acid, whatever the source of alkali.

It has been proposed that mucus protects against acid by functioning as a diffusion barrier to H^+. The rate of diffusion of H^+ through isolated mucus gel *in vitro* has been shown to be about four-fold slower than through an equivalent layer of unstirred solution (Williams and Turnberg, 1980). This rate of diffusion of H^+ is still fast and acid in the lumen will rapidly equilibrate, in a matter of minutes, across the adherent mucus gel layer. Evidence *in vivo* shows that acid, in the presence of insufficient bicarbonate, can rapidly penetrate through the mucus layer. This has been demonstrated by the formation of acute mucosal lesions in man following histamine stimulation (Katz, Siegel and Glass, 1969). Also, in rat stomach, increased back-diffusion of acid in response to mucosal damaging agents such as aspirin occurs rapidly, within 2–3 min (Davenport, 1979). Such observations demonstrate that the adherent mucus layer is most unlikely to provide an effective physical permeability barrier to prevent acid in the lumen from reaching the epithelium. It has been proposed that phospholipid monolayers within the mucus layer act as a diffusion barrier to H^+ (Lichtenburger *et al.*, 1983). Since H^+ rapidly penetrates the mucus gel, such a phospholipid monolayer would appear to have little physiological significance.

MUCUS AND PROTECTION AGAINST PEPSIN

'No acid, no ulcer' has long been an accepted dictum and is exemplified by the therapeutic success of the histamine H_2-receptor antagonists. However, at higher pH values, pepsin activity will be inhibited and the success of H_2 blockers may well in part be a reflection of this inhibition. There is good evidence that excess luminal pepsin activity *per se* can be a potent mucosal damaging agent in its own right. Thus, there are a number of reports *in vitro* and *in vivo* in which the gastroduodenal mucosa becomes damaged following exposure to pepsin and hydrochloric acid but not acid pH 1 alone (Nagashima and Samloff, 1985). Pepsin-induced gastric damage in the anaesthetized rat is a good model for studying the interaction of pepsin and the mucus barrier *in vivo* (Leonard and Allen, 1986). Instillation of acid (pH 1) alone into pylorus ligated stomach for 2 h does not cause damage to the adherent mucus or epithelium. However, addition of pepsin ($1-2$ mg ml^{-1}) to the acid instillate (over 2 h) results in a progressive disruption of the adherent mucus gel layer and the release of soluble degraded mucus glycoprotein. This is associated with the development of small focal haemorrhagic erosions in the epithelium and bleeding into the lumen (Figure 11.2). Such studies show that excess luminal pepsin (about two- to three-fold above the maximally stimulated levels) will progressively destroy the mucus barrier at its luminal surface at a rate faster than that at which it can be replaced by mucosal secretion. Once through the mucus barrier, pepsin is seen to readily digest the epithelium. There is indirect evidence for increased degradation of the adherent mucus barrier in man *in vivo* following stimulation of pepsin. In gastric washouts from duodenal ulcer patients, there is an approximately three-fold rise in both pepsin activity and soluble degraded luminal mucus glycoprotein following insulin stimulation (Younan, Pearson and Allen, 1982). This insulin-induced increase in luminal degraded glycoprotein is absent in vagotomized patients, where no rise in luminal pepsin is observed following insulin.

Evidence strongly favours the adherent mucus layer as a barrier which normally prevents luminal pepsin from digesting the underlying epithelium. This statement is based on two main observations. Firstly, the gastroduodenal mucus gel is a physical diffusion barrier to large molecular weight proteins such as pepsin (mol. wt 32 000–40 000) (Allen, 1988). Experiments *in vitro* show that the smaller sized protein myoglobin (mol. wt 17 500) does not penetrate a mucus gel layer 1 mm thick after 24 h. Secondly, since a continuous layer of adherent mucus gel is observed *in vivo*, it must physically exclude diffusion of pepsin across it to the underlying epithelium.

During secretion, acid at concentrations below pH 1 will be attained in the lumen of the gastric gland and here newly secreted pepsinogen will be rapidly converted to pepsin. There is no mucus–bicarbonate barrier in these glands and the apical surfaces of these cells must be resistant to their own secretions. This has been demonstrated experimentally by the culture of monolayers of

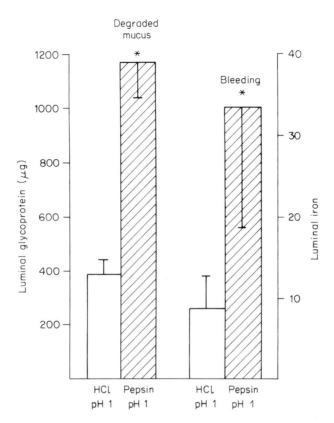

Figure 11.2 Pepsin damage in stomach of anaesthetized rat; degradation of mucus barrier and mucosal bleeding. Either HCl pH 1 □ or pepsin 2 mg ml^{-1} pH 1 ▨ was instilled over 2 h into the pylorus ligated stomach of an anaesthetized rat. Degradation of the mucus barrier was monitored by the content of degraded glycoprotein in the lumen (PAS method); mucosal damage was monitored by the content of blood in the lumen measured as increased iron content. Mucosal haemorrhage with loss of blood into the lumen, absent in the pH 1 control, was always present following pepsin pH 1 although the amount of bleeding was variable between different animals. Iron in the control pH 1 represents a loss of iron from mucosal surface not associated with bleeding: mucosal scapings from one stomach contained less than 50% of the iron in the control value.
(Data adapted from Leonard and Allen (1986) and unpublished observations)

pepsinogen-secreting chief cells which can adequately resist acidification of their apical surfaces at least to pH 2 (Sanders *et al.*, 1985). In contrast, the surface epithelium of the stomach and duodenum is not resistant to high concentrations of pepsin and acid, as demonstrated in animal models of damage. Furthermore, acid and pepsin are clearly essential ingredients for the natural peptic ulceration process to occur. It is not yet known whether there is an intrinsic resistance to acid and pepsin by the apical surfaces of the mucus-secreting epithelia in the absence of the adherent mucus barrier and neutralizing bicarbonate (including that from plasma). Another unresolved question is how pepsin and acid are rapidly secreted through an apparently continuous mucus layer from the deep-seated gastric glands into the lumen. A hypothesis is that the volume of acid and pepsin secretion creates a hydraulic pressure which propels these secretions through the overlying mucus gel into the lumen. In support of this, studies with acid-sensitive dyes show that acid secretion through the mucus layer is restricted to areas above the gastric crypts (Holm and Flemstrom, 1988). Current methods for observing adherent mucus cannot show whether intermittent holes occur in the mucus gel cover over the entrance to the gastric glands during secretion.

MUCUS STRUCTURE

A knowledge of the structure of the mucus gel is a prerequisite for understanding changes in the mucus barrier in peptic ulcer disease. The principal gel-forming components of mucus secretions are large molecular weight (several million) glycoproteins or mucins. Mixed within the mucus are other gastrointestinal secretions, for example enzymes and secretory immunoglobulin IgA, microorganisms, sloughed off cells and ingested food at various stages of digestion. However, gel with the same physical structure and rheological properties as the native mucus barrier can be reproduced by concentration of the purified mucin alone (Bell *et al.*, 1985). This demonstrates that there is no need to implicate non-mucus components, protein, lipid or nucleic acid, in determining the structure of the mucus gel barrier. The detailed structure of mucins and their physical properties are complex and the reader is referred to specialist reviews (Allen, 1988; Neutra and Forstner, 1987).

A key structural feature of mucins is their polymeric form, which is made up of several glycoprotein subunits (molecular weight 5×10^5) joined together by disulphide bridges (Snary, Allen and Pain, 1970; Allen, 1978). Each glycoprotein subunit consists of a central protein core with many closely packed carbohydrate side-chains attached (Figure 11.3). The carbohydrate chains are composed of several sugar residues (up to 19 in length in gastric mucus) and many will carry a negative charge due to the presence of ester sulphate and sialic acid residues. Each glycoprotein subunit can be divided into two structural regions on the basis of the location of the carbohydrate chains attached to the protein core. These are:

(1) glycosylated regions where carbohydrate chains form a closely packed sheath around the central protein core protecting it from proteolytic attack;

(2) non-glycosylated regions of the protein core which have little or no carbohydrate attached and are therefore accessible to proteolytic attack by pepsin and other proteases.

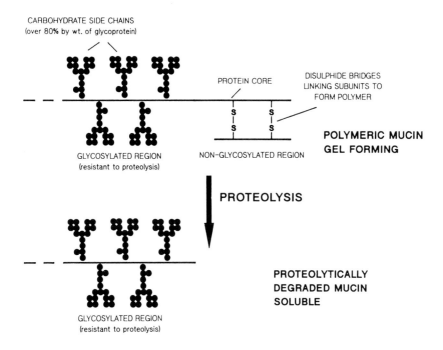

CARBOHYDRATE SIDE CHAINS
(over 80% by wt. of glycoprotein)

PROTEIN CORE

DISULPHIDE BRIDGES
LINKING SUBUNITS TO
FORM POLYMER

POLYMERIC MUCIN
GEL FORMING

GLYCOSYLATED REGION
(resistant to proteolysis)

NON–GLYCOSYLATED REGION

PROTEOLYSIS

PROTEOLYTICALLY
DEGRADED MUCIN
SOLUBLE

GLYCOSYLATED REGION
(resistant to proteolysis)

Figure 11.3 A diagrammatic representation of the structure of gastric mucin demonstrating the site of proteolysis and associated breakdown of the polymeric mucin

The non-glycosylated regions of the protein core are also the site of disulphide bridges which join the glycoprotein subunits together to form the polymeric mucin structure. Proteolysis digests the non-glycosylated regions of the protein core and hence that part containing the disulphide bridges that join the glycoprotein subunits together. The resulting degraded subunits consist of the glycosylated region which is resistant to further proteolytic digestion. There is no detectable loss of carbohydrate during proteolysis and, since it constitutes over 80% by weight of the mucin, the proteolytically degraded mucin is still quite large (approaching 5×10^5 molecular weight).

Mucus gels are formed by non-covalent interactions between polymeric mucin molecules at relatively high concentrations, for example 50 mg ml^{-1} for gastric and duodenal mucus (Bell *et al.*, 1985). The nature of these gel-forming interactions has yet to be fully resolved, but rheological evidence points to an involvement of the carbohydrate side-chains. An interdigitation of the carbohydrate side-chains between adjacent mucin molecules, and a more specific lectin type of interaction have both been proposed as models (Bell *et al.*, 1984; Silberberg, 1987). For gel formation to take place, the mucin must be in its polymeric form (Bell *et al.*, 1985; Allen, 1978). This is why proteolytic enzymes such as pepsin or thiol reagents which degrade the mucin polymeric structure will dissolve mucus gels. A direct correlation has been shown to exist between the ratio of the amounts of polymeric mucin to lower size mucin subunit (or proteolytically degraded mucin) in the mucus secretion and the measured strength and overall stability of the gel (Sellers *et al.*, 1987b).

Changes in the structure of the mucus barrier and pepsin types in peptic ulcer disease

Structural studies show that the polymeric form of mucins is essential for gel formation and it is therefore a prerequisite in maintaining the integrity of the protective mucus barrier. An important question is whether there is a deficiency in the mucin polymeric structure in adherent gastric mucus gel from patients with peptic ulcer disease. The amount of polymeric mucin in adherent mucus from surgically removed antral gastrectomy samples can be measured by gel filtration chromatography where 67%, 50% and 35% polymeric mucin is present in adherent mucus from control (non-ulcerated mucosa removed for cancer of the pancreas), duodenal ulcer and gastric ulcer patients respectively (Younan *et al.*, 1982b) (Table 11.1). From such structural studies it is clear that the adherent mucus barrier which covers the mucosa of gastric ulcer and, to a lesser extent, duodenal ulcer patients, will be a weaker and poorer quality gel than that covering non-ulcerated mucosa. Further evidence for a disrupted adherent gastric mucus layer in peptic ulcer patients is apparent from observation of unfixed mucosal sections (Allen *et al.*, 1986). Over the antrum from non-ulcerated stomachs, a layer of translucent, adherent mucus gel was observed, while that from gastric ulcer patients, although still continuous, was markedly more heterogeneous and granular in appearance due to mixing of mucus with cellular material.

There are various possibilities which might explain this breakdown in the structure of the adherent antral mucus in peptic ulcer patients. Evidence favours

Table 11.1   Changes in polymeric mucin in adherent antral mucus in peptic ulcer disease

Disease	Gel-forming polymer (% total glycoprotein)	Gel strength	Mucus thickness
Pancreatic cancer (histologically normal antrum)	66.6 ± 5.1		180 μm
Duodenal ulcer	49.8 ± 3.3	↑	120 μm
Gastric ulcer	34.9 ± 2.8		Heterogeneous mixture of tissue and mucus

Data from Younan *et al.* (1982), Allen *et al.* (1986) and W. J. Cunliffe, unpublished results. Results from at least six different patients were included in each value and all values for peptic ulcer disease were significantly different from corresponding controls ($P < 0.05$)

an increased rate of adherent mucus degradation once it has been secreted, although a fault in the initial secretory and biosynthetic mechanisms is possible. At least three sources for increased proteolytic activity and therefore degradation of the mucus barrier in peptic ulceration can be identified. Firstly, it could arise from increased release of intracellular proteases (lysosomal) derived from exfoliated cells given that the rate of cell turnover is known to be higher for the gastritic mucosa (Lipkin, 1987). Another possibility is that it originates from *Campylobacter pylori*, a species of bacterium which is intimately associated with gastric mucosa (Rathbone, Wyatt and Heatley, 1986) and recently claimed to possess mucolytic activity (Slomiany *et al.*, 1987). The third and, in the context of this review, the most interesting explanation is that it results from changes in the pattern of secreted pepsin types which are known to occur in peptic ulcer disease.

Gastric juice contains different pepsins, which can be separated from each other by electrophoresis (Taylor, 1982). Pepsin 3 is the major pepsin in man, whereas pepsin 1 accounts for only 3.6% of total pepsin activity in non-symptomatic controls. However, in gastric and duodenal ulcer patients, pepsin 1 accounts on average for 23% and 16.5% respectively of the total pepsin activity present (Walker and Taylor, 1980; Roberts, Sheers and Taylor, 1981). This is significant because the ulcer-associated pepsin (pepsin 1) has been shown to digest mucus more readily than pepsin 3, both at the pH optimum, pH 2.0 (two-fold greater activity) and particularly at higher pH values, pH 4, where the difference is even more marked (six-fold greater activity) as shown in Figure 11.4 (Pearson

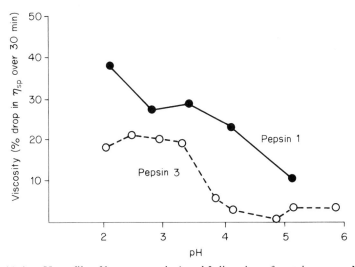

Figure 11.4 pH profile of human pepsin 1 and 3 digestion of gastric mucus. Mucolytic activity of enzyme samples was assessed by measuring the percentage fall in specific viscosity (η_{sp}) over 30 min at 37 °C. The viscosity values were corrected for any endogenous enzyme activity in the mucus glycoprotein sample. ○ Pepsin 3, ● pepsin 1. (Data from Pearson *et al.* (1986))

et al., 1986). Similarly, gastric juice from duodenal ulcer patients digests mucus more readily than that from non-symptomatic controls, both at the optimum pH of 2 and markedly at higher pH values, e.g. pH 4. Thus the raised concentration of pepsin 1 in the gastric juice of peptic ulcer patients would be expected to result in an increased degradation of the adherent mucus barrier under conditions of higher pH likely to prevail in the duodenal bulb (pH 4 and above) as well as the lower pH in the stomach. Pepsin 1 also displays increased (five-fold) collagenolytic activity by comparison with pepsin 3 (Etherington, Roberts and Taylor, 1980) and this might impair the repair process once the mucus barrier is breached. In summary, a structural weakness in the mucus barrier occurs in peptic ulcer disease which correlates with an increased pepsin activity in the gastric juice of these patients.

MUCUS AND EPITHELIAL REPAIR

Exogenous mucosal damaging agents such as alcohol, non-steroidal anti-inflammatory drugs and hypertonic saline are all sufficiently small in size to rapidly diffuse through the adherent gastroduodenal mucus gel and in the case of high ethanol concentrations will cause its dehydration (Allen *et al.*, 1986). In animal models of damage, such agents rapidly penetrate the gastroduodenal mucus barrier causing epithelial damage, cell exfoliation and, in more severe cases, vascular damage, haemorrhage and visible lesions. Following acute epithelial damage (except at the sites of haemorrhage), rapid repair occurs by the process of re-epithelialization (Morris and Wallace, 1981; Lacy, 1985; Silen and Ito, 1985; Wallace and Whittle, 1986). Two mechanisms have been identified by which re-epithelialization can be protected from acid, pepsin and further exposure to the damaging agent. Firstly, plasma exudation will provide neutralizing bicarbonate as well as washing the damaging agent away from the mucosal surface. Secondly, following acute ethanol damage in the rat, a thick, gelatinous coat, often referred to as a mucoid coat, forms over the repairing epithelium (Figure 11.5).

The thick gelatinous or mucoid coat associated with epithelial repair is quite different in properties and composition from the original adherent mucus layer characteristic of the undamaged mucosa (Sellers, Allen and Bennett, 1987). The gelatinous coat is substantially thicker (median thickness 700 μm compared to 80 μm) and visibly far more granular and much less viscous in appearance than the adherent mucus layer. Histological studies using peroxidase–antiperoxidase stain for fibrin show that this gelatinous coat is composed principally of acellular bands of fibrin gel with overlying layers of necrotic cells and small amounts of mucus. The formation of this gelatinous coat may be facilitated by the original adherent mucus gel providing a template for the deposition of the fibrin gel. This is suggested by the effect of mucus gel on plasma coagulation times

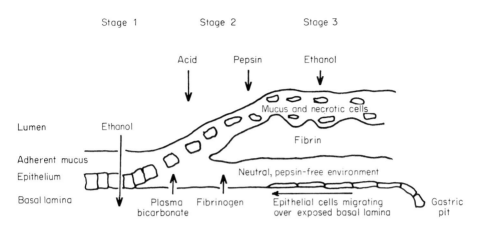

Figure 11.5 Mucus ethanol damage and subsequent epithelial repair: diagram of formation of protective fibrin based gelatinous coat. Stage 1: ethanol penetrates mucus barrier, causing exfoliation and epithelium and vascular damage. Stage 2: plasma containing bicarbonate and fibrinogen flows out; fibrin formation occurs underneath the remaining mucus and necrotic cells. Stage 3: re-epithelialization protected from acid, pepsin and now ethanol by fibrin-based gelatinous coat. (From Allen *et al.* (1986))

in vitro. In the presence of Ca^{2+}, citrated plasma took 100 s to clot, but clotting was virtually instantaneous in the presence of mucus (Sellers, Allen and Bennett, 1987). A 'fluffy' gelatinous coat has also been observed covering the repairing epithelium following acute damage with hypertonic (1 mol l^{-1}) saline (Silen and Ito, 1985), but it has yet to be shown whether this involves fibrin deposition.

PHYSIOLOGICAL AND PHARMACOLOGICAL CONSIDERATIONS OF THE MUCUS BARRIER

An increase in thickness of the adherent mucus gel barrier over the undamaged mucosa would be expected to enhance its protective efficacy against acid and pepsin. A thicker adherent mucus gel will provide a more extensive unstirred layer to support surface neutralization of acid. In protection against pepsin, the crucial factor would appear to be the maintenance of continuity of the mucus layer. Therefore, the thicker the mucus gel cover, the less likely it is to become discontinuous from erosion by peptic mucolysis. Median thickness of the mucus barrier has been shown to be increased up to three-fold by neural stimulation (cholinergic), hormonal stimulation (secretin), and paracrine stimulation (prostaglandins) (Allen and Carroll, 1985). It should be emphasized that when assessing the protective capabilities of the mucus barrier it is the adherent mucus gel layer that is the primary consideration. Many other agents have been assumed to stimulate mucus 'secretion' by virtue of an increase in the output of soluble luminal mucus. However, soluble mucus has no obvious protective function against the gastric juice with which it is mixed. Furthermore, soluble mucus in the lumen contains pepsin-degraded adherent mucus, as well as that produced by direct secretion. It has been shown experimentally that soluble mucus content is not related to the thickness of the protective adherent mucus barrier (Allen and Carroll, 1985). It is also important to distinguish between changes in the rate of mucin biosynthesis from changes in the rate of secretion of the adherent mucus gel. For example, the anti-ulcer agent carbenoxolone sodium has been shown to increase the rate of mucus biosynthesis, but does not increase adherent mucus gel thickness (McQueen, Allen and Garner, 1984).

In designing suitable alternative peptic ulcer therapy to H_2-blockers, there is a need for good experimental ulcer models. Much attention has been given to understanding the ethanol damage model, the phenomenon of 'cytoprotection' and the process of re-epithelialization. In the ethanol model, adherent mucus does not protect the mucosa and has a minor role in formation of the mucoid cap covering the repairing epithelium. The adherent mucus barrier does, however, have a leading role in protection against pepsin and a strong supporting role in protection against acid. This is demonstrated in the model of rat gastric damage induced by pepsin, which shows a different mucosal response than that seen with ethanol. Thus, excess pepsin causes mucosal damage by progressively hydrolysing the adherent mucus gel layer to reach the underlying epithelium, causing focal haemorrhagic damage. This is in contrast to excess ethanol which rapidly penetrates the mucus barrier and causes total epithelial exfoliation. Furthermore, no protective mucoid cap is formed in association with pepsin damage (Allen et al., 1987). The pepsin-induced damage model may well prove a more appropriate ulcer model than that induced by ethanol. A suitable line for future therapeutic investigation would be the development of selective inhibitors of pepsin secretion which do not modify acid secretion. Agents that inhibit pepsin activity and preferably bind to the mucus barrier, for example sucralfate and polyacrylates (Nagashima and Samloff, 1985; Foster, Allen and Pearson, 1985), merit further investigation.

REFERENCES

Allen, A. (1978). Structure of gastrointestinal mucus glycoproteins and the viscous and gel-forming properties of mucus, Br. Med. Bull., 34, 28–33.

Allen, A. (1988). Mucus secretions. In J. Forte (ed.) American Handbook of Physiology, volume on Gastric, Pancreatic Hepatobiliary and Salivary Secretion. (In press)

Allen, A. and Carroll, N. J. H. (1985). Adherent and soluble mucus in the stomach and duodenum, Dig. Dis. Sci., 30, 558–628.

Allen, A. and Garner, A. (1980). Gastric mucus and bicarbonate secretion and their possible role in mucosal protection, Gut, 21, 249–62.

Allen, A., Hutton, D. A., McQueen, S. and Garner, A. (1983). Dimensions of gastroduodenal surface pH gradients exceed those of adherent mucus gel layers, *Gastroenterology*, **85**, 463–76.

Allen, A., Hutton, D. A., Leonard, A. J., Pearson, J. P. and Sellers, L. A. (1986). The role of mucus in protection of the gastroduodenal mucosa, *Scand. J. Gastroenterol.*, **21** (Suppl. 125), 71–7.

Allen, A., Bennett, M. K., Leonard, A. J. and Sellers, L. A. (1987). Pepsin and ethanol damage: two different mechanisms of response by the rat gastric mucosa, *J. Physiol.*, **391**, 69.

Bell, A. E., Allen, A., Morris, E. R. and Ross-Murphy, S. B. (1984). Functional interactions of gastric mucus glycoprotein, *Int. J. Biol. Macromol.*, **6**, 309–15.

Bell, A. E., Sellers, L. A., Allen, A., Cunliffe, W. J., Morris, E. R. and Ross-Murphy, S. B. (1985). Properties of gastric and duodenal mucus: effect of proteolysis, disulfide reduction, bile, acid, ethanol and hypertonicity on mucus gel structure, *Gastroenterology*, **88**, 269–80.

Bickel, M. and Kauffman, G. L. (1981). Gastric mucus gel thickness: effects of distension, 16,16-dimethyl prostaglandin E_2 and carbenoxolone, *Gastroenterology*, **80**, 770–5.

Bollard, J. E., Vanderwee, M. A., Smith, G. W., Tasman-Jones, C., Gavin, J. B. and Lee, S. P. (1986). Preservation of mucus *in situ* in rat colon, *Dig. Dis. Sci.*, **31**, 1338–44.

Davenport, H. W. (1979). Mucosal barrier to hydrogen ion back diffusion. In R. Fisher (ed.) *Peptic Ulcer Disease*, Biomedical Information Corp., New York, pp. 77–88.

Etherington, D. J., Roberts, N. B. and Taylor, W. H. (1980). The collagen degrading activity of purified human pepsins 1 and 3, *Clin. Sci.*, **58**, 30.

Flemström, G. and Garner, A. (1982). Gastroduodenal HCO_3 transport: characteristics and proposed role in acidity regulation and mucosal protection, *Am. J. Physiol.*, **242**, G183–93.

Flemström, G. and Turnberg, L. A. (1984). Gastroduodenal defense mechanisms, *Clin. Gastroenterol.*, **13**, 327–55.

Foster, S. N. D., Allen, A. and Pearson, J. P. (1985). Mechanism for the mucosal protective action of polyacrylates on the gastric mucus barrier, *Gut*, **26**, A11009.

Holm, L. P. and Flemström, G. (1988). *In vivo* microscopy of gastric surface acidity, *Acta Physiol. Scand.* (In press)

Katz, D., Siegel, H. I. and Glass, G. B. J. (1969). Acute gastric mucosal lesions produced by augmented histamine test, *Am. J. Dig. Dis.*, **14**, 447–55.

Kerss, S., Allen, A. and Garner, A. (1982). A simple method for measuring thickness of the mucus gel layer adherent to rat, frog and human gastric mucosa: influence of feeding, prostaglandin, *N*-acetylcysteine and other agents, *Clin. Sci.*, **63**, 187–95.

Kivilaakso, E. and Flemström, G. (1984). Surface pH gradient in gastroduodenal mucosa, *Scand. J. Gastroenterol.*, **19**, 50–52.

Lacy, E. R. (1985). Gastric mucosal resistance to a repeated ethanol insult, *Scand. J. Gastroenterol.*, **20** (Suppl. 10), 63–72.

Leonard, A. and Allen, A. (1986). Gastric mucosal damage by pepsin, *Gut*, **27**, A1236–7.

Lichtenburger, L. H., Graziani, L. A., Dial, E. J., Butler, B. D. and Hills, B. A. (1983). Role of surface-active phospholipids in gastric glycoprotein, *Science*, **219**, 1327–9.

Lipkin, M. (1987). Proliferation and differentiation of gastrointestinal cells in normal and diseased states. In L. R. Johnson *et al.* (eds) *Physiology of the Gastrointestinal Tract*, 2nd edn, Raven Press, New York, pp. 255–84.

Machen, T. and Paradiso, A. M. (1987). Regulation of intracellular pH in the stomach, *Ann. Rev. Physiol.*, **49**, 21–5.

McQueen, S., Allen, A. and Garner, A. (1984). Measurements of gastric and duodenal mucus gel thickness. In A. Allen, G. Flemström, A. Garner, W. Silen and L. Turnberg (eds) *Mechanisms of Mucosal Protection in the Upper Gastrointestinal Tract*, Raven Press, New York, pp. 215–21.

Morris, G. P. and Wallace, J. L. (1981). The roles of ethanol and of acid in the production of gastric mucosal erosions in rats, *Virchows Arch.*, **46**, 239–51.

Morris, G. P., Harding, R. J. and Wallace, J. L. (1984). A functional model for extracellular gastric mucus in the rat, *Virchows Arch.*, **38**, 23–38.

Nagashima, R. and Samloff, I. M. (1985). Aggressive factors II: pepsins. In F. Brooks *et al.* (eds) *Peptic Ulcer Disease*, Churchill Livingstone, Edinburgh, pp. 181–214.

Neutra, M. R. and Forstner, J. F. (1987). Gastrointestinal mucus: synthesis, secretion, function. In L. R. Johnson (ed.) *Physiology of the Gastrointestinal Tract II*, Raven Press, New York, pp. 975–1009.

Pearson, J. P., Ward, R., Allen, A., Roberts, N. B. and Taylor, W. (1986). Mucus degradation by pepsin: comparison of mucolytic activity of human pepsin 1 and pepsin 3: implications in peptic ulceration, *Gut*, **27**, 243–8.

Rathbone, B. J., Wyatt, J. I. and Heatley, R. V. (1986). *Campylobacter pyloridis* — a new factor in peptic ulcer disease?, *Gut*, **27**, 635–41.

Roberts, N. B., Sheers, R. and Taylor, W. H. (1981). Pepsin 1 secretion in normal human subjects, *Clin. Sci.*, **61**, 37.

Ross, I. N. and Turnberg, L. A. (1983). Studies of the 'mucus–bicarbonate' barrier on rat fundic mucosa: the effects of luminal pH and a stable prostaglandin analogue, *Gut*, **24**, 1030–3.

Rozee, K. R., Cooper, D., Lam, K. and Costerton, J. W. (1982). Microbial flora of the mouse ileum mucus layer and epithelial surface, *Appl. Environ. Microbiol.*, **43**, 1451–63.

Sakata, T. and Englehart, W. V. (1981). Luminal mucin in the large intestine of mice, rats and guinea pigs, *Cell Tissue Res.*, **219**, 629–35.

Sanders, M. J., Ayalon, A., Roll, M. and Soll, A. H. (1985). The apical surface of canine chief cell monolayers resists H^+ back diffusion, *Nature*, **313**, 82–4.

Sellers, L. A., Allen, A. and Bennett, M. K. (1987a). Formation of a fibrin based gelatinous coat over repairing rat gastric epithelium following acute ethanol damage: interaction with adherent mucus, *Gut*, **28**, 835–43.

Sellers, L. A., Allen, A., Morris, G. P. and Ross-Murphy, S. B. (1987b). Mechanical characterisation and properties of gastrointestinal mucus gel, *Biorheology*, **24**, 615–23.

Silberberg, A. (1987). A model for mucus glycoprotein structure, *Biorheology*, **24**, 605–14.

Silen, W. and Ito, S. (1985). Mechanisms for rapid re-epithelialisation of the gastric mucosal surface, *Ann. Rev. Physiol.*, **47**, 217–29.

Slomiany, B. J., Sarosiek, J., Marty, V. L. N. *et al.* (1987). *Campylobacter pyloridis* degrades mucin and undermines gastric mucosal integrity, *Biochem. Biophys. Res. Commun.*, **144**, 307–14.

Snary, D., Allen, A. and Pain, R. H. (1970). Structural studies on gastric mucoproteins: lowering of molecular weight after reduction with 2-mercaptoethanol, *Biochem. Biophys. Res. Commun.*, **40**, 844–51.

Sturrock, N. and Hopwood, D. (1986). The effects of mucus on the binding of cationized ferritin by human and animal gastrointestinal epithelium, *Histochemistry*, **85**, 255–8.

Taylor, W. H. (1982). Biochemistry and pathological physiology of pepsin 1, *Adv. Clin. Enzymol.*, **2**, 79–81.

Walker, V. and Taylor, W. H. (1980). Pepsin 1 secretion in chronic peptic ulceration, *Gut*, **21**, 766–71.

Wallace, J. L. and Whittle, B. J. R. (1986). Role of mucus in the repair of gastric epithelial damage in the rat: inhibition of epithelial recovery by mucolytic agents, *Gastroenterology*, **91**, 603–11.

Williams, S. E. and Turnberg, L. A. (1980). Retardation of acid diffusion by pig gastric mucus: a potential role in mucosal protection, *Gastroenterology*, **79**, 299–304.

Williams, S. E. and Turnberg, L. A. (1981). Studies of the 'protective' properties of gastric mucus: evidence for a mucus–bicarbonate barrier, *Gut*, **22**, 94–6.

Younan, F., Pearson, J. P. and Allen, A. (1982). Gastric mucus degradation *in vivo* in peptic ulcer patients and the effects of vagotomy. In E. N. Chantler, J. B. Elder and M. Elstein (eds) *Mucus in Health and Disease II*, Plenum Press, New York, pp. 253–73.

Younan, T., Pearson, J. P., Allen, A. and Venables, C. W. (1982). Changes in the structure of the mucous gel on the mucosal surface of the stomach in association with peptic ulcer disease, *Gastroenterology*, **82**, 827–31.

Advances in Drug Therapy of Gastrointestinal Ulceration
Edited by A. Garner and B. J. R. Whittle
©1989 John Wiley & Sons Ltd

_____ Chapter Twelve

Neural Regulation of Gastroduodenal Secretion and Mucosal Protection

G. Flemström and S.-O. Granstam
Department of Physiology and Medical Biophysics, Uppsala University, S-751 23 Uppsala, Sweden

The demonstration of an alkaline surface layer in the stomach and duodenum, its potential role in acid protection and its dependence on mucosal bicarbonate secretion makes it of considerable interest to study the regulation of this secretion. The presence of acid in the duodenal lumen is a potent stimulant of alkaline secretion, and previous studies have provided evidence that local mucosal production of prostaglandins as well as humoral factors are important in the mediation of this response (Flemström, 1987). More recently, it has been shown that mucosal bicarbonate secretion is also under neural influence. The aim of this chapter is to summarize recent studies of the neurohumoral influence on gastroduodenal mucosal bicarbonate secretion and to discuss its possible use in therapy of ulceration.

VAGAL INFLUENCE

Sham-feeding is a stimulant of gastric and duodenal bicarbonate secretion in humans (Feldman, 1985; Forssell, Stenquist and Olbe, 1985; Ballesteros _et al._, 1988) and in conscious dogs (Konturek and Thor, 1986). The stimulation of gastric alkaline secretion in humans is abolished by the antimuscarinic agent benzilonium bromide as illustrated in Figure 12.1 but unaffected by the cyclo-oxygenase inhibitor indomethacin. This indicates cholinergic transmission of the gastric response. Electrical stimulation in the peripheral direction of the cut vagal nerves in cats and rats increases both gastric and duodenal bicarbonate secretion (Fändriks, 1986a; Jönson _et al._, 1986; Nylander _et al._, 1987). The duodenal response is abolished by hexamethonium but only partially reduced

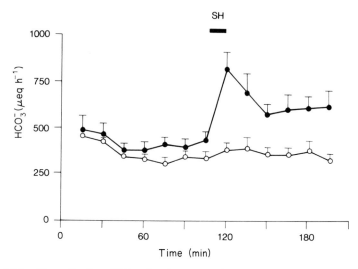

Figure 12.1 Sham-feeding (SH) stimulates gastric bicarbonate secretion in healthy volunteers ($n = 16$) and pretreatment with benzilonium bromide ($n = 6$) abolishes this response. Data are shown as means ± s.e.m. (Data from H. Forssell with permission)

by atropine. The duodenal response to sham-feeding in humans and dogs is similarly only partially reduced by atropine, further indicating that a proportion of vagal transmission in the duodenum is non-cholinergic.

Infusion of the muscarinic agonist carbachol causes only a small ($\sim 20\%$) increase in duodenal bicarbonate secretion in the rat (Flemström *et al.*, 1985). It is without effect in the rabbit (Granstam, Flemström and Nylander, 1987) and cat (Fändriks, 1986a) duodenum *in vivo* and frog duodenum *in vitro* (Flemström, 1987). The selective M_1 agonist, McN-A-343, has similarly only a small stimulatory action on bicarbonate secretion in the duodenum in the rat (Flemström, Säfsten and Jedstedt, 1987). In contrast, carbachol (or bethanechol) is a relatively potent stimulant of alkaline secretion in the stomach of the guinea-pig (Garner and Flemström, 1978) and human (Feldman and Schiller, 1982) and in gastric mucosa *in vitro* (Mattsson, Carlsson and Carlsson, 1984). The gastric response to carbachol is abolished by atropine. Atropine (and tetrodotoxin) have also been reported to inhibit the stimulation of bicarbonate secretion by prostaglandin 16,16-dimethyl PGE_2 in dog gastric mucosa, suggesting some interaction between cholinergic and prostaglandin stimulation (Miller *et al.*, 1983).

Mucosal intrinsic neural activity has been demonstrated to influence gastric bicarbonate secretion in humans (Forssell and Olbe, 1987a,b). Distension of the gastric fundus stimulated bicarbonate secretion, and the response in patients following selective proximal vagotomy was very similar to that in healthy volunteers. Benzilonium bromide abolished the response to distension while indomethacin was without effect, indicating cholinergic mediation of the intramural reflex. Basal gastric secretion of bicarbonate determined 2 months after vagotomy was 30% higher than that before the denervation. This may suggest that the vagal nerves also possess fibres with an inhibitory action on gastric bicarbonate secretion. In the duodenum of conscious dogs, it has been observed that the rate of 'basal' bicarbonate secretion varies in phase with the myoelectric activity (Konturek and Thor, 1986).

SYMPATHETIC INFLUENCE

The sympathetic influence on bicarbonate secretion has been investigated by infusing adrenergic drugs and studying secretion in splanchnicotomized and/or adrenal-ligated animals. The α_2-agonist clonidine has been shown to inhibit basal duodenal secretion in cats and rats and to inhibit gastric bicarbonate secretion in rats (Nylander and Flemström, 1986; Fändriks, Jönsson and Nylander, 1987). The α_1-agonist phenylephrine, in contrast, increases duodenal alkaline secretion in the rat and the effects of clonidine and phenylephrine were inhibited by the antagonists yohimbine and prazosin, respectively. Drugs acting at β-adrenoceptors are without effect on duodenal bicarbonate secretion in the rat and on gastric and duodenal bicarbonate secretion in the cat.

The rise in both duodenal and gastric bicarbonate secretion on electrical vagal stimulation in the cat is enhanced by splanchnicotomy and/or ligation of adrenal glands. Administration of the α_2-antagonist yohimbine or the adrenolytic agent guanethidine (Figure 12.2) similarly enhances the vagally mediated stimulation (Fändriks, 1986b; Fändriks, Jonsson and Nylander, 1987; Nylander et al., 1987). Potentiation of the vagal effect by adrenal ligation alone has been demonstrated in duodenum in rats (Jönsson et al., 1986). The loss of endogenous glucocorticosteroids was compensated for in these animals. An increase in sympathetic activity elicited by minor bleeding (5 and 10% of total blood volume) reduced duodenal alkaline secretion in rats by 18 and 31%, respectively. Thoracic epidural anaesthesia, splanchnicotomy or administration of yohimbine almost abolished this decrease (Jönsson and Fändriks, 1986, 1987). The combined results indicate that gastric and duodenal bicarbonate secretion, as well as the vagally mediated stimulation of these secretions, are under α_2-adrenergic inhibitory regulation.

The adrenergic inhibition is of particular interest in view of the observed amelioration of stress ulceration in animals by adrenergic blockade (Menguy and Masters, 1978). Furthermore, water immersion stress is reported to decrease duodenal mucosal alkaline secretion in rats simultaneously with increasing mucosal susceptibility to damage by acid (Takeuchi, Furukawa and Okabe, 1986). An increase in plasma concentration of noradrenaline has been reported in patients with duodenal ulcer disease (Järhult et al., 1983). It should also be

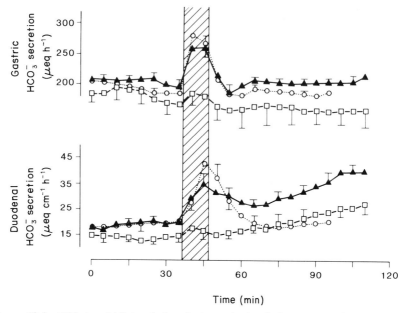

Figure 12.2 Effects of bilateral electrical vagal stimulation on gastric and duodenal mucosal bicarbonate secretion in anaesthetized cats. The stimulation (10 Hz, width 5 ms, 5–8 V) is indicated by the shaded area. All experiments were performed in animals with ligated adrenal glands. Data are shown as means ± s.e.m. of secretion in cats with intact sympathetic neural supply (squares), in splanchnicotomized cats (rings) and in guanethidine-treated cats (triangles) ($n \geqq 5$). Note the enhancement of the vagal response by splanchnicotomy or guanethidine. (Adapted from Fändriks, 1986b). Reproduced by permission of *Acta Physiologica Scandinavica*

noted that splanchnic nerve stimulation inhibits the release of vasoactive intestinal peptide from the intestine in the pig (Fahrenkrug *et al.*, 1978). This polypeptide is a very potent stimulant of duodenal mucosal alkaline secretion. The effects of some catecholamines on gastric bicarbonate secretion have also been tested *in vitro*. Noradrenaline inhibits secretion by isolated frog (Figure 12.3) and guinea-pig gastric mucosa, suggesting an action directly on the secreting cells or possibly on neural tissue remaining in the *in vitro* preparation (Flemström, 1978; Fromm *et al.*, 1976).

CENTRAL NERVOUS INFLUENCE

The stimulation of gastroduodenal mucosal alkaline secretion by sham-feeding provides evidence that such secretion is under the influence of the central nervous system. Other evidence for the presence of a central influence is provided by the findings that intrahypothalamic or intracerebroventricular administration

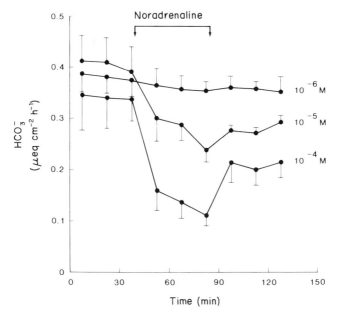

Figure 12.3 Norepinephrine inhibited bicarbonate secretion by frog (*Rana temporaria*) fundic mucosa *in vitro*. None of the concentrations caused significant changes in tissue electrical resistance or transmucosal electrical potential difference. The histamine H_2-receptor antagonist metiamide (10^{-3} mol l^{-1}) was present throughout the experiments to inhibit acid secretion. Data are shown as mean $\pm$ s.e.m. ($n \geqq 6$). (Adapted from Flemström, 1978). Reproduced by permission of *Acta Physiologica Scandinavica*

of some peptides influences both gastric and duodenal bicarbonate secretion. Intrahypothalamic injection of corticotropin-releasing factor (CRF) causes an increase of gastric bicarbonate secretion in the rat (Gunion, Tache and Kauffman, 1985). Intracerebroventricular, but not intravenous, infusion of thyrotropin-releasing hormone (TRH) stimulates the duodenal secretion in this species as illustrated in Figure 12.4. The stimulatory action of centrally administered TRH is abolished by cervical vagotomy or hexamethonium, further indicating the central action mediated by the vagal nerves (Flemström and Jedstedt, 1988). Intracerebroventricular infusion of CRF has a similar stimulatory action in the duodenum while intracerebroventricular administration of bombesin inhibits the duodenal secretion after transient stimulation.

The tricyclic compound pirenzepine binds to muscarinergic (M_1) receptors in ganglia and in some areas in the brain. Intravenous administration of this drug stimulates duodenal mucosal alkaline secretion in the rat (Säfsten and Flemström, 1986). The stimulation is abolished by vagotomy, which may suggest a central action mediated via vagal nerves. An alternative explanation is that

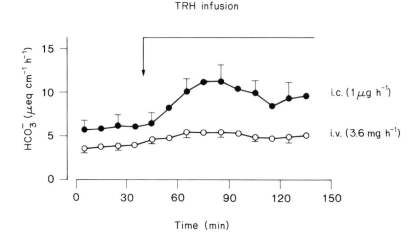

Figure 12.4 Intracerebroventricular infusion of thyrotropin-releasing hormone (TRH) increased duodenal mucosal bicarbonate secretion in the anaesthetized rat, whereas intravenous infusion of the much larger dose of the peptide was without effect. Data are shown as means ± s.e.m. ($n = 8$)

pirenzepine antagonizes muscarinergic transmission in the sympathetic ganglia, thereby inhibiting the postganglionic adrenergic activity.

It may be of interest in this context that acupuncture, a procedure that releases endogenous opioid peptides, is reported to stimulate gastric alkaline secretion in the conscious dog (Zhou and Chey, 1982). Intravenous injection of very small amounts (20 ng kg^{-1}) of the opioid peptides β-endorphin, methionine-enkephalin and leucine-enkephalin increases duodenal mucosal bicarbonate secretion in the rat duodenum. Pretreatment with the μ-receptor antagonist naloxone prevented this stimulation, suggesting that the effect is mediated via opiate μ-receptors (Flemström, Jedstedt and Nylander, 1986). The same opioid peptides are, however, without effects when infused intracerebroventricularly, suggesting a peripheral site of action.

SUMMARY AND PERSPECTIVES

Secretion of bicarbonate by the gastric mucosa probably provides a first line of mucosal defence against luminal acid by alkalinizing the viscoelastic mucus gel adherent to the surface. The duodenal mucosal alkaline secretion is very probably a major mechanism of duodenal defence against acid discharged from the stomach and this secretion has also been reported to be deficient in patients with duodenal ulcer disease (Isenberg et al., 1987). Both secretions are increased by vagally mediated stimuli and are under α_2-adrenergic inhibitory influence.

This may suggest that drugs decreasing the sympathetic tone could increase mucosal resistance and contribute to prevention of ulceration. The findings that intrahypothalamic or intracerebroventricular administration of some peptides stimulates duodenal and gastric mucosal bicarbonate secretion suggest the possibility of influencing mucosal protection by drugs affecting the central nervous system.

REFERENCES

Ballesteros, M. A., Hogan, D. L., Koss, M. A., Chen, H. S. and Isenberg, J. I. (1988). Vagal stimulation of human duodenal bicarbonate secretion acts by non-cholinergic mechanisms, *Gastroenterology*, **94**, 1720.

Fahrenkrug, J., Galbo, H., Holst, J. J. and Schaffalitzky de Muckadell, O. B. (1978). Influence of the autonomic nervous system on the release of vasoactive intestinal polypeptide from the porcine gastrointestinal tract, *J. Physiol. Lond.*, **280**, 405–22.

Fändriks, L. (1986a). Vagal and splanchnic neural influences on gastric and duodenal bicarbonate secretions, *Acta Physiol. Scand.*, **128** (Suppl. 555), 1–39.

Fändriks, L. (1986b). Sympatho-adrenergic inhibition of vagally induced gastric motility and gastroduodenal HCO_3^- secretion in the cat, *Acta Physiol. Scand.*, **128**, 552–62.

Fändriks, L., Jönsson, C. and Nylander, O. (1987). Effects of splanchnic nerve stimulation and of clonidine on gastric and duodenal HCO_3^- secretion in the anesthetized cat, *Acta Physiol. Scand.*, **130**, 251–8.

Feldman, M. (1985). Gastric H^+ and HCO_3^- secretion in response to sham feeding in humans, *Am. J. Physiol.*, **248**, G188–91.

Feldman, M. and Schiller, L. S. (1982). Effect of bethanechol (urecholine) on gastric acid and non-parietal secretion in normal subjects and duodenal ulcer patients, *Gastroenterology*, **83**, 262–6.

Flemström, G. (1978). Effect of catecholamines, Ca^{2+} and gastrin on gastric HCO_3^- secretion, *Acta Physiol. Scand.* (Suppl.), *Gastric Ion Transport*, pp. 81–90.

Flemström, G. (1987). Gastric secretion of bicarbonate. In L. R. Johnson, J. Christensen, M. J. Jackson, E. D. Jacobson and J. H. Walsh (eds) *Physiology of the Gastrointestinal Tract*, 2nd edn, Raven Press, New York, pp. 1011–29.

Flemström, G. and Jedstedt, G. (1988). TRH and CRF influence central nervous control of duodenal mucosal bicarbonate secretion in the rat *in vivo*, *Acta Physiol. Scand.*, **132**, 1317.

Flemström, G., Jedstedt, G. and Nylander, O. (1986). Beta-endorphin and enkephalins stimulate duodenal mucosal alkaline secretion in the rat *in vivo*, *Gastroenterology*, **90**, 368–72.

Flemström, G., Kivilaakso, E., Briden, S., Nylander, O. and Jedstedt, G. (1985). Gastroduodenal bicarbonate secretion in mucosal protection: possible role of vasoactive intestinal peptide and opiates, *Dig. Dis. Sci.*, **30** (Suppl.), 63S–8S.

Flemström, G., Säfsten, B. and Jedstedt, G. (1987). Muscarinic influence on the bicarbonate secretion by rat duodenum *in vivo*, *Gastroenterology*, **92**, 1391.

Forssell, H. and Olbe, L. (1987a). Effect of proximal gastric vagotomy on basal and vagally stimulated gastric bicarbonate secretion, *Scand. J. Gastroenterol.*, **22**, 949–55.

Forssell, H. and Olbe, L. (1987b). Effect of fundic distension on gastric bicarbonate secretion in man, *Scand. J. Gastroenterol.*, **22**, 627–33.

Forssell, H., Stenquist, B. and Olbe, L. (1985). Vagal stimulation of human gastric bicarbonate secretion, *Gastroenterology*, **89**, 581–6.

Fromm, D., Schwartz, J. H., Robertson, R. and Fuhro, R. (1976). Ion transport across isolated antral mucosa of the rabbit, *Am. J. Physiol.*, **231**, 1783–9.

Garner, A. and Flemström, G. (1978). Gastric HCO₃⁻ secretion in the guinea pig, *Am. J. Physiol.*, **234**, E535–45.

Granstam, S. O., Flemström, G. and Nylander, O. (1987). Bicarbonate secretion by the rabbit duodenal mucosa *in vivo*: effects of prostaglandins, vagal stimulation and some drugs, *Acta Physiol. Scand.*, **131**, 377–85.

Gunion, M. W., Tache, Y. and Kauffman, G. L. (1985). Intrahypothalamic corticotropin-releasing factor (CRF) increases gastric bicarbonate content, *Gastroenterology*, **88**, 1407.

Isenberg, J. I., Selling, J. A., Hogan, D. L. and Koss, M. A. (1987). Impaired proximal duodenal mucosal bicarbonate secretion in duodenal ulcer patients, *New Engl. J. Med.*, **316**, 374–9.

Järhult, J., Angerås, U., Farnebo, L. O., Graffner, H. and Hamberger, B. (1983). Elevated plasma levels of noradrenalin in duodenal ulcer, *World J. Surg.*, **7**, 385–9.

Jönson, C. and Fändriks, L. (1986). Bleeding decreases duodenal HCO₃⁻ secretion by a nervous mechanism, *Acta Physiol. Scand.*, **127**, 273–4.

Jönson, C. and Fändriks, L. (1987). Bleeding inhibits vagally-induced duodenal HCO₃⁻ secretion via activation of the splanchnic nerves in anaesthetized rats, *Acta Physiol. Scand.*, **130**, 259–64.

Jönson, C., Nylander, O., Flemström, G. and Fändriks, L. (1986). Vagal stimulation of duodenal HCO₃⁻ secretion in anaesthetized rats, *Acta Physiol. Scand.*, **128**, 65–70.

Konturek, S. J. and Thor, P. (1986). Relation between duodenal alkaline secretion and motility in fasted and sham-fed dogs, *Am. J. Physiol.*, **251**, G591–6.

Mattsson, H., Carlsson, K. and Carlsson, E. (1984). Omeprazole is devoid of effect on alkaline secretion in isolated guinea pig antral mucosa. In A. Allen, G. Flemström, A. Garner, W. Silen and L. A. Turnberg (eds) *Mechanisms of Mucosal Protection in the Upper Gastrointestinal Tract*, Raven Press, New York, pp. 141–6.

Menguy, R. and Masters, Y. F. (1978). Mechanism of stress ulcer: influence of alpha-adrenergic blockade on stress ulceration and gastric mucosal energy metabolism, *Am. J. Dig. Dis.*, **23**, 493–7.

Miller, T. A., Henagan, J. M., Watkins, L. A. and Loy, T. M. (1983). Prostaglandin induced bicarbonate secretion in the canine stomach: characteristics and evidence for a cholinergic mechanism, *J. Surg. Res.*, **35**, 105–12.

Nylander, O. and Flemström, G. (1986). Effects of alpha-receptor agonists and antagonists on duodenal surface epithelial HCO₃⁻ secretion in the rat *in vivo*, *Acta Physiol. Scand.*, **126**, 433–41.

Nylander, O., Flemström, G., Delbro, D. and Fändriks, L. (1987). Vagal influence on gastroduodenal HCO₃⁻ secretion in the cat *in vivo*, *Am. J. Physiol.*, **252**, G522–8.

Säfsten, B. and Flemström, G. (1986). Stimulatory effect of pirenzepine on mucosal bicarbonate secretion in rat duodenum *in vivo*, *Acta Physiol. Scand.*, **127**, 267–8.

Takeuchi, K., Furukawa, O. and Okabe, S. (1986). Induction of duodenal ulcers in rats under water-immersion stress conditions: influence of stress on gastric acid and duodenal alkaline secretion, *Gastroenterology*, **91**, 554–63.

Zhou, L. and Chey, W. Y. (1982). Electric acupuncture stimulates non-parietal cell secretion in dog, *Life Sci.*, **34**, 2233–8.

Advances in Drug Therapy of Gastrointestinal Ulceration
Edited by A. Garner and B. J. R. Whittle
Published by John Wiley & Sons Ltd
©1989 Wellcome Foundation

_____ Chapter Thirteen

Pro-ulcerogenic Eicosanoids and Related Lipid Mediators in Gastric Mucosal Damage

Brendan J. R. Whittle and Juan V. Esplugues
*Department of Pharmacology, Wellcome Research Laboratories,
Beckenham, Kent BR3 3BS, UK*

INTRODUCTION

Activation of the enzyme phospholipase A_2 releases membrane-bound phospholipids that are capable of being metabolized by distinct biochemical pathways into a subsequent range of biologically potent lipid mediators including the eicosanoids and the phospholipid, platelet-activating factor (PAF-acether).

Eicosanoids are the products of the fatty acid, arachidonic acid, that are formed through action of the cyclo-oxygenase and the lipoxygenase enzymes. Following its liberation from membrane-bound phospholipids, arachidonic acid is converted into prostanoids by the action of cyclo-oxygenase and into lipoxygenase products, including the leukotrienes, by the action of the 5-, 12-, or 15-lipoxygenase enzymes (Figure 13.1).

Cyclo-oxygenase converts arachidonic acid into unstable intermediate endoperoxides, and it is at this biosynthetic step that aspirin, indomethacin and similar non-steroid anti-inflammatory drugs act to inhibit the formation of prostanoids. These labile endoperoxides are subsequently converted into various prostaglandins, the nature and profile of which depend on the tissue under investigation (Moncada and Vane, 1979). Thus, prostaglandin E_2 (PGE_2) and prostacyclin (PGI_2) are formed by a wide variety of tissues and cells, including gastric mucosal tissue. These prostanoids can inhibit gastric acid secretion, stimulate gastric bicarbonate and mucus secretion, affect mucosal sodium and chloride ionic flux, and induce vasodilatation in the mucosal microcirculation

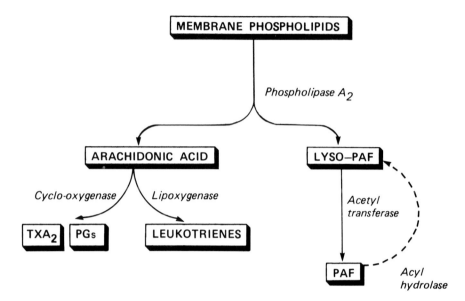

Figure 13.1 Formation of endogenous lipid mediators from cellular membrane phospholipids following activation of phospholipase A_2

and prevent the vascular stasis induced by damaging agents (see Whittle and Vane, 1987). These prostanoids and their synthetic analogues protect the gastric mucosa from necrotic damage, an action which may be brought about by their effects on several of the above parameters (see Robert, 1981; Hawkey and Rampton, 1985; Whittle and Vane, 1987).

However, not all cyclo-oxygenase metabolites are protective in the gastrointestinal tract. Thus, the cyclo-oxygenase product thromboxane A_2 (Figure 13.2) has been demonstrated to exert potent pro-ulcerogenic actions and may be involved in the pathogenesis of gastric damage (Whittle, Kauffman and Moncada, 1981). Thromboxane A_2 (TXA_2) is a highly active, unstable metabolite, enzymatically formed from the endoperoxides. The chemical half-life of TXA_2 in aqueous solution at 37 °C is less than 30 s, readily decomposing to thromboxane B_2 (TXB_2), which has minimal biological activity. TXA_2, which is synthesized in substantial quantities by platelets, is a powerful stimulant of platelet aggregation. TXA_2 constricts vascular smooth muscle *in vitro* while it is a potent vasoconstrictor agent in most vascular beds that have been studied *in vivo* (Whittle and Moncada, 1983a). The enzyme involved in the biosynthesis of these thromboxanes has been characterized and can be selectively inhibited by several experimental compounds, notably derivatives of imidazole (Moncada and Vane, 1979). The vasoconstrictor properties of this eicosanoid could underlie a potential role of TXA_2 as a mediator of mucosal ulceration, and such a possibility has been explored in several experimental models, which will be described below.

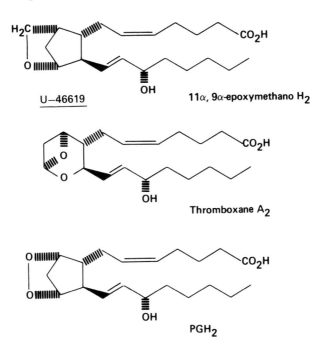

Figure 13.2 Chemical structure of the endogenous eicosanoids, PGH_2 and thromboxane A_2, and of the synthetic chemically stable epoxy-methano derivative of PGH_2, U-46619, which acts as a thromboxane mimetic

A further family of arachidonate metabolites arises from the actions of the lipoxygenase enzymes as shown in Figure 13.1. The 5-, 12- and 15-lipoxygenase enzymes convert arachidonic acid to the corresponding 5-, 12- or 15-hydroperoxy intermediates (the HPETEs; hydroperoxy eicosatetraenoic acids), which then can form the corresponding hydroxy derivatives (the HETEs). Unlike the cyclo-oxygenase enzyme, the activity of the lipoxygenase enzymes is generally not inhibited by non-steroid anti-inflammatory agents. Further biologically potent products of the 5-lipoxygenase pathway are the leukotrienes, so called because their formation was originally described in leukocytes and they have a triene bond in their structure (Samuelsson, 1983). These leukotrienes are derived from the intermediate 5-HPETE via the formation of the epoxide, leukotriene A_4 (LTA_4). Enzymic hydrolysis of LTA_4 yields the potent chemotactic and pro-inflammatory substance LTB_4, whereas the peptidoleukotriene LTC_4, which is formed by the addition of glutathione, is enzymically degraded to LTD_4 and LTE_4. The leukotrienes LTC_4, LTD_4 and LTE_4 have bronchoconstrictor, vascular and permeability-inducing properties, and constitute the principle earlier defined as slow-reacting substance of anaphylaxis. The vasoactive and pro-inflammatory actions of these leukotrienes could therefore contribute to the pathogenesis of gastric mucosal damage that results from such conditions as ischaemia and gastritis.

PAF-acether is an endogenous, low molecular weight phospholipid which can be formed and released by a variety of cell types including platelets, neutrophils, basophils, macrophages, monocytes and endothelial cells (see Braquet et al., 1987). The release of PAF-acether has been implicated as a mediator of inflammation and in the pathophysiology of several disease processes including asthma, anaphylaxis and allergy. Furthermore, PAF-acether induces a range of pathophysiological events which resemble shock states (Bessin et al., 1983). These actions include increased vascular permeability, haemo-concentration, hypotension and circulatory collapse, neutrophil aggregation, and lysosomal enzyme release (Doebber, Wu and Shen, 1984; Braquet et al., 1987). This profile of the biological actions of PAF-acether thus makes it a potential candidate as a mediator of gastrointestinal damage, in conditions of both shock and inflammation.

THROMBOXANES IN MUCOSAL DAMAGE

Biosynthesis

Thromboxanes have been shown to be biosynthesized in gastric mucosal tissue from several species. Thus, a radiolabelled metabolite with the same chromatographic mobility as TXB_2, is formed in microsomal fractions prepared from bovine and dog mucosa (Zamecnik et al., 1977; Le Duc and Needleman, 1979; Ali and McDonald, 1980). The capability of gastric mucosal homogenates prepared from rat, rabbit, dog, pig, guinea-pig and man to synthesize TXB_2, has been demonstrated following incubation with the radiolabelled endoperoxide, PGH_2 or arachidonic acid (Ahlquist et al., 1982; Whittle and Boughton-Smith, 1984). Its endogenous biosynthesis has also been determined by specific radioimmunoassay for TXB_2 following incubation and subsequent extraction of gastric tissue (Wallace and Whittle, 1985; Hawkey, 1986). Using short-term culture of biopsy specimens of human gastric mucosa, the release of TXB_2 has likewise been determined by radioimmunoassay (Rachmilewitz et al., 1984).

It is not yet clearly established which cells within the mucosa contain the thromboxane synthetase enzyme. Indeed, any platelets entrapped in the gastric microcirculation would be a potentially rich source of such products and may contribute to the overall synthetic capacity of the tissue to generate TXB_2. The synthesis of TXB_2 by primary cultures of epithelial cells obtained from the rat gastric mucosa has, however, been demonstrated (Hiraishi et al., 1986).

Vascular actions of arachidonic acid

Since TXA_2 is so highly labile, the effects of this moiety can only be determined following *de novo* generation. The action of TXA_2 on gastric mucosal integrity has been investigated *in vivo*, using the chambered fundic mucosa of the dog stomach *in situ*.

Intra-arterial injection of the precursor arachidonic acid into a delay coil, to allow its incubation with the flowing arterial blood for 30 s before reaching the stomach, induced pronounced vasoconstriction (Kauffman and Whittle, 1982). This vasoconstrictor response, which was abolished by indomethacin, reflected the biotransformation of arachidonic acid by the blood-borne platelets to TXA_2, which was detected by radioimmunoassay as the breakdown product, TXB_2. This was further confirmed by use of the specific thromboxane synthetase inhibitor, 1-benzylimidazole, which abolished this arachidonate-induced vasoconstriction (Whittle, Kauffman and Moncada, 1981). Others have likewise observed that direct infusion of high doses of arachidonic acid to the exteriorized canine stomach can reduce blood flow (Walus, Gustaw and Konturek, 1980).

Under conditions in which the gastric mucosa was bathed with isotonic saline or an acid solution, a 30 min period of arachidonate infusion to generate TXA_2 in gastric arterial blood did not lead to any macroscopically apparent damage to the mucosa. However, when the mucosa was exposed to acid–taurocholate mixture, in a concentration itself inducing only minimal macroscopic damage, extensive mucosal damage developed during the 30 min intra-arterial infusion of arachidonic acid (Whittle, Kauffman and Moncada, 1981). Thus, localized areas of blanching, followed by engorgement and stasis, was clearly observed during this local TXA_2 generation. These areas were often the initial or predominant sites for necrosis and punctate bleeding, which became apparent within 10–15 min. Sloughing of the mucosal epithelial tissue led to extensive bleeding from the exposed underlying tissue following termination of the TXA_2 generation.

Ulcerogenic actions of a thromboxane mimetic

The extreme lability of TXA_2 and the complexities of generating it locally obviously limits the extent and nature of the pharmacological investigations that can be conducted. Studies using the chemically stable endoperoxide analogue, 11α, 9α-epoxymethano-PGH_2 (U-46619; Figure 13.2), which has been characterized pharmacologically as a thromboxane mimetic acting at thromboxane-sensitive sites, have therefore been conducted to extend these observations further. As with locally generated TXA_2, intra-arterial infusion of U-46619 to the canine stomach *in situ* induced pronounced vasoconstriction and, in the presence of topical acidified taurocholate, induced distinct areas of haemorrhagic necrosis (Whittle and Moncada, 1983b).

In our more recent studies in the rat, a novel technique for the close-arterial administration of substances via a cannula inserted into the left gastric artery has been utilized (Esplugues and Whittle, 1988a). Intra-arterial infusion of U-46619 for 10 min, in doses having no effect on systemic arterial blood pressure, induced extensive damage in both the antral and corpus regions of the gastric mucosa, as assessed macroscopically by planimetry. Interestingly, antral damage was apparent macroscopically as deep penetrating ulcers. In the presence of a dilute concentration of intraluminal ethanol, intra-arterial infusion of lower doses of U-46619 induced haemorrhagic and necrotic mucosal damage (Figures 13.3 and 13.4).

These ulcerogenic actions of U-46619 were abolished by pretreatment with the selective thromboxane antagonist BM 13177 (Esplugues and Whittle, 1988a). This indicates that the damage induced by U-46619 was not a non-specific action, but was the result of interaction with thromboxane receptor sites in the mucosa, possibly located in the microvasculature.

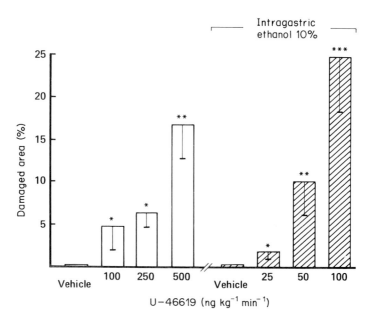

Figure 13.3 Macroscopically assessed gastric mucosal damage following local intra-arterial infusion of the thromboxane mimetic U-46619 (100–500 ng kg^{-1} min^{-1} for 10 min), or by lower doses of U-46619 (25–100 ng kg^{-1} min^{-1}) in the presence of 2 ml intragastric ethanol (10%). Results, shown as the percentage of total area exhibiting damage, are the mean ± s.e.m. of 3–9 experiments for each group, where statistical significance from the corresponding vehicle-infused control is *$P<0.05$, **$P<0.01$, ***$P<0.001$. (Data adapted from Esplugues and Whittle (1988a))

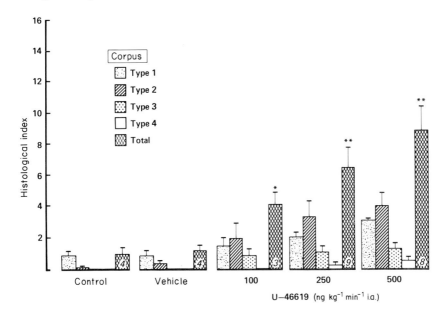

Figure 13.4 Histological evaluation of the effects of local intra-arterial infusion of the thromboxane mimetic U-46619 (100–500 ng kg^{-1} min^{-1} for 10 min) on the gastric corpus mucosa of the rat *in vivo*. The data are shown in terms of the histological score for various types of damage (type 1 to 4) and the total histological index in the gastric corpus mucosa. Results are shown as mean ± s.e.m. of *n* values. For clarity, significant differences from vehicle group is given for total histological index only, where *P < 0.05, **P < 0.01

Histological assessment of damage

For histological assessment of the damage, determined 20 min after terminating the local intra-arterial infusion of the thromboxane mimetic in the rat, two samples of the corpus and one sample of the antrum were excised from standardized regions of the stomach, which had been immersed in neutral buffered formalin. These were embedded in paraffin, and sections (4 μm) stained with haematoxylin and eosin were examined under a light microscope. The 1 cm length of each histological section was divided into five fields and each further divided into four equal subsections. Each subsection was histologically assessed in a randomized manner for epithelial cell damage (a score of 1 being assigned), glandular disruption, vasocongestion or oedema in the upper mucosa (a score of 2), haemorrhagic damage in the mid to lower mucosa (a score of 3) and a deep necrosis or ulceration (a score of 4). Each subsection was evaluated on a cumulative basis, and the overall mean value of the scores for each of the 5–6 fields was taken as the histological index for that section.

In control experiments, close intra-arterial infusion of isotonic saline for periods of 30–80 min caused no damage to the mucosal tissue, as assessed by both macroscopic and histological techniques. On histological inspection, following local intra-arterial infusion of U-46619, vascular congestion throughout the corpus mucosa was observed, which was particularly marked in the upper region of the mucosa. Disruption of the epithelial cells and glands was also noted (Figures 13.5). Histological damage in the antral region of the mucosa was as intense as in the corpus region, the characteristics of this damage being comparable in both regions (Figure 13.5). These damaging actions of U-46619 were dose related in both the corpus (Figure 13.6) and the antral regions (Figure 13.7).

Microvascular actions of the thromboxane mimetic

To investigate the microvascular actions of the thromboxane mimetic, its actions on the rat gastric microcirculation were studied using an *in vivo* microscopy technique to determine gastric submucosal arteriolar and venular responses (Whittle, Oren-Wolman and Guth, 1985).

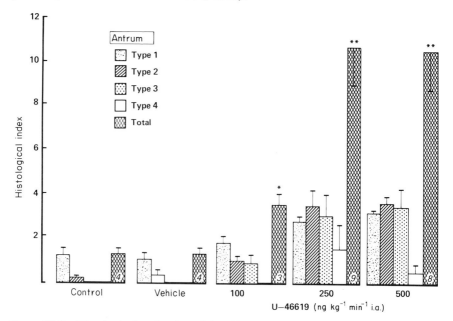

Figure 13.5 Histological evaluation of the effects of local intra-arterial infusion of the thromboxane mimetic U-46619 (100–500 ng kg^{-1} min^{-1} for 10 min) on gastric antral mucosa of the rat *in vivo*. The data are shown in terms of the histological score for various types of damage (type 1 to 4) and the total histological index in the gastric antral mucosa. Results are shown as mean ± s.e.m. of *n* values. For clarity, significant differences from vehicle group is given for total histological index only, where *$P<0.05$, **$P<0.01$

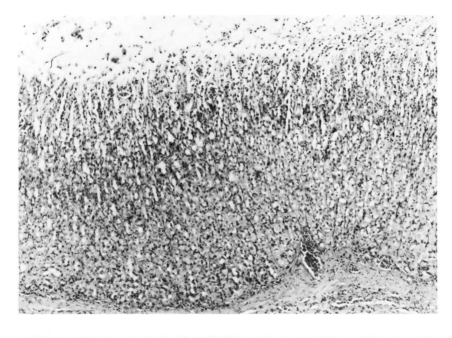

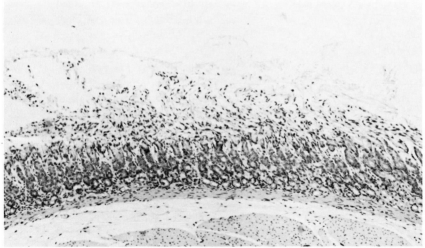

Figure 13.6 Histological appearance of the corpus (upper panel) and antral (lower panel) regions of the rat gastric mucosa following close-arterial infusion of the thromboxane mimetic, U-46619 ($500 \, ng \, kg^{-1} \, min^{-1}$ for 10 min). Extensive epithelial exfoliation and glandular disruption, vasocongestion and extravasation of erythrocytes is apparent in both the corpus and antral sections. The 4 μm sections were stained with haematoxylin and eosin following routine preparation and embedding in paraffin wax. The section is derived from the studies of Esplugues and Whittle (1988a)

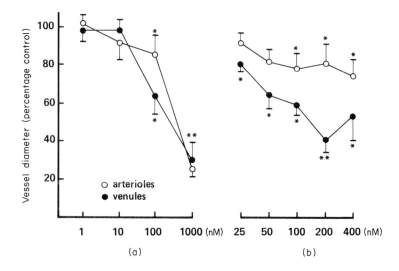

Figure 13.7 The vasoconstrictor effects of the local application of (a) thromboxane mimetic U-46619 (1–100 nmol l^{-1}) and (b) leukotriene C_4 (25–400 nmol l^{-1}) on the gastric submucosal arterioles ($\bigcirc$–$\bigcirc$) and venules ($\bullet$–$\bullet$) of the anaesthetized rat. Results are shown as percentage change in vessel diameter from control value, mean ± s.e.m. of 6–11 experiments, where *$P<0.05$, **$P<0.01$. (Data adapted from Whittle, Oren-Wolman and Guth (1985))

Topical application of U-46619 to the exposed submucosal vasculature reduced vessel diameter in both arterioles and venules (Figure 13.7). Pronounced focal vasoconstriction was observed in the venules, leading to stasis of blood flow with entrapped pools of blood within the constricted segments (Whittle, Oren-Wolman and Guth, 1985). Such actions on the microcirculation would lead to distinct areas of ischaemia, sites that would be susceptible to subsequent damage and ulceration. More recently, intravenous infusion of U-46619 has likewise been demonstrated to reduce gastric mucosal blood flow, as determined by laser Doppler techniques (Currington *et al.*, 1987).

Protective actions of thromboxane synthase inhibitors

To investigate the role of endogenous TXA_2 in the pathogenesis of gastric ulceration, the protective actions of selective thromboxane synthase inhibitors have been investigated in various experimental models of mucosal damage.

Oral or subcutaneous administration of 1-benzylimidazole reduced the incidence and severity of the gastric haemorrhage erosions seen after acid–ethanol treatment (Whittle, 1984). In further studies, this thromboxane synthase inhibitor also inhibited gastric lesions induced by indomethacin. Since the dose of indomethacin used was sufficient to inhibit cyclo-oxygenase, and therefore itself would reduce TXA_2 formation, the mechanisms of the protective action of benzylimidazole under these conditions are not fully clear (Whittle, 1984).

Other studies with selective thromboxane synthase inhibitors in experimental models also give support to the concept that TXA_2 is involved in the pathogenesis of gastric damage. Thus, the non-imidazole agent OKY-1581 reduced bile-salt-induced gastric necrosis in the rat, although it failed to inhibit that induced by ethanol (Konturek et al., 1983). Furthermore, oral administration of the imidazole derivative dazmegrel, in doses reducing TXB_2 synthesis by the rat gastric mucosa, likewise reduced macroscopically assessed mucosal damage induced by acidified bile salts (Walt et al., 1987). In preliminary studies, the thromboxane synthase inhibitor dazoxiben, as well as thromboxane antagonists, was shown to reduce ethanol-induced gastric lesions (Price et al., 1985).

Mechanisms of thromboxane damage

Studies with TXA_2 and its stable mimetic have demonstrated potent vasoconstrictor actions on the mucosal microvasculature. The resultant mucosal ischaemia would account for the damage subsequently observed and would also predispose the mucosa to injury by weak irritants such as dilute ethanol. However, thromboxane may, in addition, activate or aggregate platelets or other blood cells in the microcirculation, leading to the occlusion of the microvessels. Furthermore, such actions would lead to the release of further tissue-destructive mediators including TXA_2 itself, lipoxygenase products, lysosomal or hydrolase enzymes and free radicals. In addition, TXA_2 and its mimetic could exert direct cytolytic actions on the gastric microvasculature or mucosal cells (Esplugues and Whittle, 1988a).

LIPOXYGENASE METABOLITES IN GASTRIC DAMAGE

Biosynthesis

A product derived from the arachidonate 12-lipoxygenase pathway, 12-HETE, has been detected in human gastric tissue using gas chromatography–mass spectrometry techniques (Bennett et al., 1981). Similarly, a radiolabelled product co-migrating with 12-HETE has been detected by thin-layer chromatography following incubation of homogenates of canine or guinea-pig gastric mucosa with radiolabelled arachidonate (Ahlquist et al., 1982). Other hydroxy acids may also be formed, since 11- and 15-HETE can co-chromatograph with 12-HETE. Conversion of radiolabelled arachidonate to HETEs has also been detected in homogenates of both rabbit and dog gastric mucosa (Whittle and Boughton-Smith, 1984).

More recently, the formation of sulphidopeptide leukotrienes by gastric mucosal tissue has been identified using radioimmunoassay techniques (Peskar *et al.*, 1986). These original observations that LTC_4 was formed by segments of rat gastric mucosa under basal conditions or following challenge *in vivo* with ethanol have been confirmed by others (Boughton-Smith and Whittle, 1987; Wallace, 1987). The identity of the immunoreactive LTC_4 has been confirmed by high-pressure liquid chromatography techniques (Peskar *et al.*, 1986; Boughton-Smith and Whittle, 1988a). Likewise, fragments of human gastric and jejuno-ileal mucosa have been shown to release both LTB_4 and a mixture of LTC_4 along with its metabolites LTD_4 and LTE_4 (Dreyling *et al.*, 1986).

The cellular source of these lipoxygenase products has not been characterized, nor is it known whether mucosal tissue itself can generate such products. Like the thromboxanes, the HETEs may be derived from platelets trapped in the microcirculation (Hamberg, 1976). Circulating inflammatory white cells are also a potent source of lipoxygenase products, and their possible contribution following acute challenge and tissue damage has also to be considered. However, recent studies have demonstrated that elevated levels of both LTB_4 and LTC_4 can be formed from the rat gastric mucosa following ethanol challenge *in vitro*. Indeed, the levels formed were similar to that observed following *in vivo* challenge, suggesting that these leukotrienes were derived from mucosal cells rather than as the result of acute infiltration of circulating cells (Boughton-Smith and Whittle, 1988a). It is not yet known whether these cells are specific to the gastric mucosa or are resident or entrapped inflammatory cells.

Vascular actions of leukotrienes

Using the *in vivo* gastric microscopy technique, local application of LTC_4 to the submucosal tissue induced pronounced constriction in both the arterioles and venules (Figure 13.7). In the venules, the segmental constriction lead to a stasis of blood flow (Whittle, Oren-Wolman and Guth, 1985). Such microvascular changes are comparable to those described following local mucosal application of ethanol (Guth, Paulsen and Nagata, 1984; Szabo *et al.*, 1985). Indeed, a recent study (Oates and Hakkinen, 1988) has characterized submucosal venular constriction following ethanol challenge of a similar nature to that observed with LTC_4, giving support to the concept that local LTC_4 release contributes to the microvascular events associated with ethanol-induced damage.

Local intra-arterial infusion of LTC_4 to the canine chambered stomach *ex vivo* induced a dose-dependent fall in both gastric mucosal blood flow (determined by hydrogen gas clearance) and total gastric blood flow (Pawlik *et al.*, 1987). As found in the rat following submucosal application (Whittle, Oren-Wolman and Guth, 1985), intra-arterial infusion of LTB_4 had minimal vasoactive effects in the canine gastric circulation.

These gastric microvascular changes, particularly the local vasoconstrictor effects in the submucosal microcirculation, identify LTC_4 as a potential endogenous pro-ulcerogenic mediator. Indeed, the stasis of blood flow could induce the further release of vasoactive mediators from the entrapped cells in the blood, as well as tissue-destructive hydrolase and lysosomal enzymes. Furthermore, infusion of LTC_4 as well as LTD_4 into the coeliac artery has been recently demonstrated to augment the damage induced by intragastric instillation of ethanol in the rat, with histological examination of the tissue indicating extensive disruption of the microcirculation (Pihan and Szabo, 1988).

Effects of lipoxygenase inhibitors

The role of lipoxygenase metabolites in gastric damage has been further explored by use of inhibitors of the lipoxygenase enzymes. The first such agent to be utilized, BW 755C, is known to inhibit both cyclo-oxygenase and lipoxygenase enzymes in many tissues and inflammatory cells (Higgs et al., 1980), yet in the gastric mucosa it fails to inhibit prostanoid formation. BW 755C was thus considered to be a useful probe for elucidating the involvement of lipoxygenase products. Oral administration of BW 755C was found to reduce dose-dependently the mucosal damage induced by acidified ethanol in the rat (Wallace and Whittle, 1985). In addition, subcutaneous administration of BW 755C also had a protective effect against challenge with acidified ethanol, while the cyclo-oxygenase inhibitor indomethacin substantially augmented the damage (Figure 13.8).

The non-specific lipoxygenase inhibitor nordihydroguiaretic acid (NDGA) likewise reduced ethanol-induced gastric damage (Peskar et al., 1986), as did the 5-lipoxygenase inhibitor REV 5901 (Nielsen, Beninati and Chang, 1987). This latter inhibitor, as well as L651 392, a further 5-lipoxygenase inhibitor, has also been shown to reduce indomethacin-induced lesions in cholinomimetic-treated mice (Rainsford, 1987). More recently, studies in the rat with L651 392 have demonstrated inhibition of ethanol-induced gastric damage at low doses, yet it had no such protective effect at higher doses that inhibited LTC_4 formation (Wallace, Beck and Morris, 1988).

The findings with several of these agents are complicated by their lack of specificity in vivo or by their poor bioavailability in vivo, which may lead to variability in their degree of lipoxygenase inhibition. We have, however, conducted experiments with a series of potent, more selective 5-lipoxygenase inhibitors which are active in vivo following oral administration (Tateson et al., 1988; Bhattacherjee et al., 1988). These acetohydroxamic acids, exemplified by BW A4C, induce a dose-dependent reduction in the formation of LTC_4 and LTB_4 by gastric mucosal tissue following ethanol challenge. However, these agents had no significant effect on the extent of ethanol-induced mucosal damage, even in doses that induced maximal 5-lipoxygenase inhibition

(Boughton-Smith and Whittle, 1988b). Although, in parallel studies, administration of BW 755C did reduce such macroscopic damage induced by ethanol, there was a dissociation from the concurrent inhibition of mucosal 5-lipoxygenase. These findings therefore suggest that BW 755C may inhibit mucosal damage either by inhibiting the formation of products from the 12- or 15-lipoxygenase pathways, against which BW A4C is poorly effective, or by alternative mechanisms such as through its antioxidant activity and ability to scavenge free radicals (Boughton-Smith and Whittle, 1988b).

The inability of these potent, selective inhibitors of 5-lipoxygenase to prevent the mucosal damage induced by ethanol challenge suggests that LTB_4 and LTC_4 are not the primary mediators in this acute model. However, such findings do not rule out the involvement of these leukotrienes in the pathogenesis of more chronic gastric damage or ulceration.

PAF-ACETHER IN GASTRIC DAMAGE

Biosynthesis

PAF-acether is a low molecular weight phospholipid characterized by an ether linkage at the 1′ position (usually with a fatty acid chain of 16 or 18 carbons) and an acetyl group at the 2′ position of a phosphatidylcholine giving the structure of 1-O-alkyl-2-O-acetyl-sn-glyceryl-2-phosphocholine (see Braquet et al., 1987). Its immediate precursor, lyso-PAF, is released from membrane-bound phospholipids by the action of the same enzyme which releases arachidonic acid, phospholipase A_2. Lyso-PAF, which has little or no intrinsic biological activity, is metabolized into PAF-acether by the action of acetyl-CoA transferase, and is subsequently broken down to lyso-PAF by the action of the enzyme acyl hydrolase (Figure 13.1).

The formation of PAF-acether by segments of the rat gastrointestinal tract has been determined following extraction and thin-layer chromatography, by specific bioassay, utilizing its potent ability to aggregate suspensions of rabbit washed platelets (Whittle et al., 1987).

Effects of intravenously administered PAF-acether in the rat

Intravenous infusion of PAF-acether in low doses induces extensive damage to the rat gastric mucosa, being the most potent gastric ulcerogen so far described (Rosam, Wallace and Whittle, 1986). The mucosal damage was macroscopically characterized as extensive hyperaemia and vasocongestion, with areas of haemorrhagic damage. On histological evaluation, microvascular engorgement and congestion was the predominant feature, with epithelial and glandular destruction, with focal areas of necrosis that extended throughout the depth of the mucosal and submucosal microvasculature. The presence of white-cell aggregates within these vessels was also observed, particularly at the base of the mucosal glands and submucosal vessels (Rosam, Wallace and Whittle, 1986).

Close-arterial administration of PAF-acether in the rat

Local intra-arterial infusion of PAF-acether for 10 min in the rat, using the technique described earlier, resulted in a dose-dependent increase in macroscopically assessed damage to the gastric mucosa (Figure 13.8). The macroscopic appearance of this damage was comparable to that described following

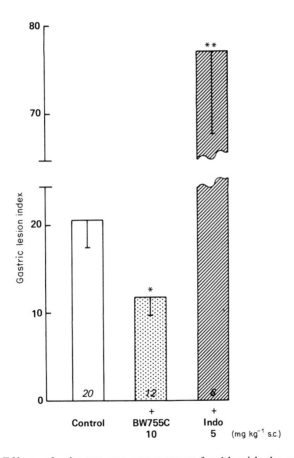

Figure 13.8 Effects of subcutaneous pretreatment for 1 h with the cyclo-oxygenase inhibitor indomethacin (5 mg kg^{-1}) or the lipoxygenase inhibitor BW 755C (10 mg kg^{-1}) on the gastric mucosal damage induced by acidified ethanol (40% in 100 mmol l^{-1} HCl) in the rat. Results are shown as the lesion index, mean ± s.e.m. of n experiments, where
*$P < 0.05$, **$P < 0.01$

intravenous infusion and was characterized by extensive hyperaemia and haemorrhage, being located in the corpus region (Esplugues and Whittle, 1988b).

PAF-acether induced a dose-related increase in the histological index of damage (Figure 13.9). Histological examination indicated congestion in the mucosal and submucosal microvasculature throughout the antral and corpus regions, which was accompanied by extensive damage to surface epithelium, dilatation of the gastric glands, and subepithelial oedema where the epithelium had remained intact.

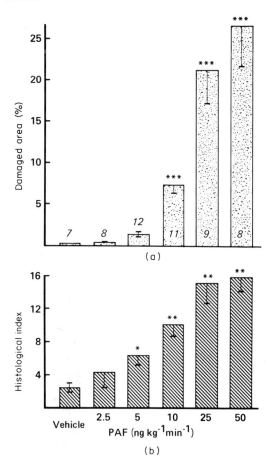

Figure 13.9 Gastric damage induced by PAF-acether following local intra-arterial infusion (2.5–50 ng kg^{-1} min^{-1} for 10 min) on the rat stomach *in vivo*. The degree of damage was assessed (a) macroscopically as the percentage of the total mucosal area that exhibited damage and (b) histologically as a histological index. Results are expressed as mean ± s.e.m. of *n* experiments. Significant difference from the control intra-arterial infusion of vehicle is given as *$P < 0.05$, **$P < 0.01$, ***$P < 0.001$. (Results adapted from Esplugues and Whittle (1988b))

The threshold local doses of PAF-acether for induction of macroscopic or histological damage in both antral and corpus regions following close-arterial infusion produced minimal systemic hypotension, indicating a dissociation between systemic cardiovascular actions and gastric damage (Esplugues and Whittle, 1988b). The predominant histological feature of congestion and engorgement of the mucosal microvessels following both local and intravenous administration of PAF-acether suggested that vascular stasis may be an important mechanism underlying the mucosal damage.

Microvascular actions of PAF-acether in the rat

To investigate whether the microcirculatory stasis could have resulted from direct vasoconstriction in the submucosal arterioles and venules, the *in vivo* microscopy technique has been utilized in the rat. No change in the diameter of these submucosal vessels could be detected during intravenous administration of PAF-acether in doses that induced mucosal damage (Whittle *et al.*, 1986). However, slowing of blood flow could clearly be observed during administration of PAF-acether, with stasis of flow being observed in 50% of arterioles and 58% of the venules with the highest dose investigated (Whittle *et al.*, 1986).

Using hydrogen-gas clearance as a further index of gastric mucosal blood flow, a dose-dependent reduction in blood flow was determined during the intravenous infusion of PAF-acether. With the highest doses of PAF-acether investigated, clearance reached an abrupt plateau within 4 min, indicating that blood flow had ceased (Whittle *et al.*, 1986).

To investigate whether changes in blood flow could be detected in the mucosal capillaries, red blood cell velocity was determined, again using *in vivo* microscopy techniques. Intravenous infusion of PAF-acether induced a significant fall in capillary blood flow within 2–3 min of the start of infusion, with sluggish flow and sludging of blood cells along the capillary walls being observed. At the highest dose of PAF-acether used, capillary blood flow fell to non-detectable levels within 5 min of the start of infusion, and no flow could be detected during the remainder of the infusion period. Stasis of flow in the capillaries could clearly be observed on the video recordings (Whittle *et al.*, 1986).

Effects in the canine gastric mucosa

The effects of intravenous or local gastric intra-arterial infusion of PAF-acether have also been investigated in the dog, utilizing the chambered gastric mucosa *in situ* (Whittle, Kauffman and Wallace, 1987). During intravenous infusion of PAF-acether, an initial fall in gastric vascular resistance was followed by a rise above the resting value (Figure 13.10), an effect which was also observed following local intra-arterial infusion. Following termination of the PAF-acether, vascular resistance continued to increase, accompanied by a darkened

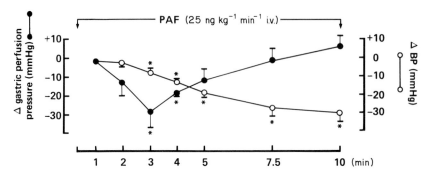

Figure 13.10 Effect of an intravenous infusion of PAF-acether (25 ng kg^{-1} min^{-1} for 10 min) on gastric vascular perfusion pressure (●) as a measure of vascular resistance and on systemic arterial blood pressure (○) in the anaesthetized dog. The initial fall in vascular resistance was followed by a rebound to values greater than the control, while blood pressure gradually fell during the period of PAF-acether infusion. Macroscopically, the initial flushed appearance of the mucosa was followed by a darkened vasocongested appearance. Results, shown as Δ mmHg, are the mean ± s.e.m. of three experiments, where significant difference from the control is shown as *$P < 0.05$. (Data adapted from Whittle, Kauffman and Wallace (1987))

vasocongested appearance of the chambered mucosal surface. On histological examination, extensive vascular congestion extended into the submucosa, with extravasation of erythrocytes, prominent subepithelial oedema and haemorrhage.

Mechanisms of mucosal damage

Deposition of blood cells along the walls of the rat gastric microvessels was observed during the periods of sluggish blood flow in the gastric microcirculation induced by PAF-acether (Whittle *et al.*, 1986). These cells were not identified as platelets and indeed, despite its name, PAF-acether is only weakly active in stimulating platelet aggregation in the rat. Furthermore, extensive mucosal damage can be induced by PAF-acether in platelet-depleted rats (Rosam, Wallace and Whittle, 1986).

However, the presence of neutrophil aggregates was observed on histological examination of the rat gastric mucosa and systemic neutropenia has been detected after infusion of ulcerogenic doses of PAF-acether (Wallace and Whittle, 1986a). These aggregates, by initially occluding the smaller capillaries, may thus contribute to the reduction in mucosal blood flow. Such effects would be enhanced by the concurrent marked haemoconcentration resulting from the extensive systemic extravasation of plasma protein that follows administration of PAF-acether in ulcerogenic doses (Wallace and Whittle, 1986a). Thus, the changes in the rheological properties of the blood as a consequence of such haemoconcentration, coupled with the presence of aggregated cells, could account for the sluggish flow and eventual stasis observed in the gastric microcirculation. In the dog, the pronounced changes in the gastric microcirculatory parameters are also suggestive of direct vascular spasm or the accumulation of microaggregates in the mucosal microvasculature, reducing blood flow.

PATHOGENESIS OF GASTRIC ULCERATION

Evidence has been provided for the ability of the endogenous lipid mediators, TXA_2, the leukotrienes and PAF-acether to induce pronounced damage to the gastric mucosa. These agents thus offer therapeutic targets for the development of novel strategies to interfere with the pathogenesis of mucosal damage and ulceration.

Although TXA_2 does not appear to be involved with the primary haemostatic events that terminate bleeding in the gastric mucosa (Whittle, Kauffman and Moncada, 1986) the studies with *de novo* synthesized TXA_2 and the thromboxane mimetic support the possibility that locally generated TXA_2 could be involved in the induction of gastric damage and ulceration. The finding that low intra-arterial doses of U-46619 could not only substantially damage the rat gastric mucosa, but could greatly augment that induced by normally mild topical irritants in both rat and dog further characterizes TXA_2 as a local mediator of tissue disruption. Thus, in pathological conditions, particularly in stress or shocked states resulting from haemorrhage or bacterial infection, which can lead to platelet activation or disseminated intravascular coagulation, the associated gastrointestinal injury may reflect the local formation and release of TXA_2. Clinical studies with selective inhibitors of thromboxane synthesis or receptor antagonists would be required to investigate these possibilities.

The lipoxygenase products 5-, 12- and 15-HPETE, being lipid peroxides, have the potential to induce damage to gastric mucosal cells or the endothelial lining of the gastric microcirculation. Such products, on conversion to the corresponding HPETEs, liberate free radicals which can likewise induce local cellular damage. The involvement of such arachidonate moieties in gastric tissue damage requires further exploration. More attention has focused on the role of the leukotrienes in the pathogenesis of mucosal damage, following characterization of the pro-ulcerogenic profile of LTC_4 on the gastric microcirculation, and identification of its release from the gastric mucosa following acute challenge with ethanol (Whittle, Oren-Wolman and Guth, 1985; Peskar *et al.*, 1986). However, the recent findings that potent, selective 5-lipoxygenase inhibitors fail to attenuate ethanol-induced damage suggest that LTC_4 is not the primary mediator of such acute mucosal disruption (Boughton-Smith and Whittle, 1988b; Wallace, Beck and Morris, 1988). This does not exclude the contribution of LTC_4 or LTB_4 in other forms of mucosal damage, and indeed it would be more appropriate for such mediators to be involved in chronic phases of peptic ulceration, as well as the associated inflammatory response at the ulcer crater. Furthermore, these leukotrienes could contribute not only to inflammatory conditions of the lower intestine such as ulcerative colitis or Crohn's disease, but also to diseases such as gastritis and oesophagitis. Inhibitors of the lipoxygenase enzymes may therefore be of clinical benefit for these utilities, while their effects on the healing or relapse of gastroduodenal ulceration may warrant investigation.

The extremely potent mucosal disruptive actions of PAF-acether throughout the gastrointestinal tract make this endogenous mediator also of pathological interest. Indeed, it has been proposed that the release of PAF-acether makes a major contribution to the associated gastrointestinal damage in endotoxin or septic shock (Gonzalez-Crussi and Hsueh, 1983; Wallace and Whittle, 1986b; Wallace et al., 1987). The endogenous release of PAF-acether may also contribute to the enhanced gastrointestinal motility observed in endotoxaemia (Esplugues and Whittle, 1988c). Furthermore, an interaction between the endogenous release of both PAF-acether and TXA_2 in the induction of intestinal damage during endotoxin shock has recently been proposed (Whittle et al., 1988). Experimental studies with specific antagonists of PAF-acether have demonstrated that such endotoxin-induced gastrointestinal damage can be substantially ablated (Wallace and Whittle, 1986b; Wallace et al., 1987). Studies on the clinical effectiveness of such selective PAF-antagonists in attenuating the characteristics of septic shock, including hypotension, haemoconcentration, intravascular coagulation and gastrointestinal disruption are thus anticipated.

PAF-acether, like TXA_2 and the leukotrienes, may contribute to micro-vascular disturbances and ischaemic episodes which are associated with many gastrointestinal diseases. Likewise, the pro-inflammatory properties of PAF-acether may contribute to inflammatory conditions of the gut, and perhaps interact synergistically with the other inflammatory mediators. Furthermore, the local mucosal release of PAF-acether, along with such mediators as the leukotrienes, induced by bacterial toxin, may account for or contribute to the gastric damage that is associated with colonization with Campylobacter pylori. Much recent clinical gastroenterological research has been directed to elucidating the role of this bacterium in the pathogenesis of peptic ulceration and the events leading to relapse after antisecretory therapy, although the mechanisms by which such organisms contribute to damage in the gastroduodenal mucosa is not clear. The local release of pro-inflammatory mediators may be involved in such actions and indeed a local inflammatory response could make a contribution to the ulcerative process. If so, the development of selective pharmacological agents that interfere with the synthesis or actions of PAF-acether, the leukotrienes and other lipoxygenase products, as well as the thromboxanes, may offer novel therapeutic approaches for the treatment of gastrointestinal disease.

REFERENCES

Ahlquist, D. A., Duenes, J. A., Madson, T. H., Romero, J. C., Dozois, R. R. and Malagelada, J. R. (1982). Prostaglandin generation from gastroduodenal mucosa: regional and species differences, *Prostaglandins*, **24**, 115–25.

Ali, M. and McDonald, J. W. D. (1980). Synthesis of thromboxane B_2 and 6-keto-prostaglandin $F_{1\alpha}$ in bovine gastric mucosal and muscle microsomes, *Prostaglandins*, **20**, 245–54.

Bennett, A., Hensby, C. N., Sanger, G. J. and Stamford, I. F. (1981). Metabolites of arachidonic acid formed by human gastrointestinal tissue and their actions on the muscle layers, *Br. J. Pharmacol.*, **74**, 435–44.

Bessin, P., Bonnet, J., Apffel, A. *et al.* (1983). Acute circulatory collapse caused by platelet-activating factor (PAF-acether) in dogs, *Eur. J. Pharmacol.*, **86**, 403–13.

Bhattacherjee, P., Boughton-Smith, N. K., Follenfant, R. L. *et al.* (1988). The effects of a novel series of selective inhibitors of arachidonate 5-lipoxygenase on anaphylactic and inflammatory responses, *Ann. N.Y. Acad. Sci.*, **524**, 307–20.

Boughton-Smith, N. K. and Whittle, B. J. R. (1987). Prostaglandin inhibition of ethanol-induced release of gastric mucosal leukotrienes, *Gastroenterology*, **90**, 53P.

Boughton-Smith, N. K. and Whittle, B. J. R. (1988a). Inhibition by 16,16-dimethyl PGE_2 of ethanol-induced gastric mucosal damage and leukotriene formation, *Prostaglandins*, **35**, 945–57.

Boughton-Smith, N. K. and Whittle, B. J. R. (1988b). Failure of the inhibition of rat gastric mucosal 5-lipoxygenase by novel acetohydroxamic acids to prevent ethanol-induced damage, *Br. J. Pharmacol.*, **95**, 101–8.

Braquet, P., Shen, T. Y., Touqui, L. and Vargaftig, B. B. (1987). Perspectives in platelet-activating factor research, *Pharmacol. Rev.*, **39**, 97–145.

Currington, A., Pipkin, G., Price, C. A. and Swayne, G. T. (1987). The effect of U-46619 on rat gastric blood flow using laser Doppler velocimetry, *Br. J. Pharmacol.*, **90**, 233P.

Doebber, J. W., Wu, W. S. and Shen, T. Y. (1984). Platelet activating factor intravenous infusion in rats stimulates vascular lysosomal hydrolase secretion independent of blood neutrophils, *Biochem. Biophys. Res. Commun.*, **125**, 980–7.

Dreyling, K. W., Hoppe, U., Peskar, B. A., Morgenroth, K., Kozuschek, W. and Peskar, B. M. (1986). Leukotriene synthesis by human gastrointestinal tissues, *Biochim. Biophys. Acta*, **878**, 184–93.

Esplugues, J. V. and Whittle, B. J. R. (1988a). Close-arterial administration of the thromboxane mimetic U-46619 induces damage to the rat gastric mucosa, *Prostaglandins*, **35**, 137–48.

Esplugues, J. V. and Whittle, B. J. R. (1988b). Gastric mucosal damage induced by local intra-arterial administration of PAF in the rat, *Br. J. Pharmacol.*, **93**, 222–8.

Esplugues, J. V. and Whittle, B. J. R. (1988c). Mechanisms underlying PAF-induced rat gastric motility *in vivo*, *J. Physiol.*, **398**, 99P.

Gonzalez-Crussi, F. and Hsueh, W. (1983). Experimental model of ischemic bowel necrosis: the role of platelet-activating factor and endotoxin, *Am. J. Pathol.*, **112**, 127–35.

Guth, P. H., Paulsen, G. and Nagata, H. (1984). Histologic and microcirculatory changes in alcohol-induced lesions in the rat: effect of prostaglandin cytoprotection, *Gastroenterology*, **87**, 1083–90.

Hamberg, M. (1976). On the formation of thromboxane B_2 and 12L-hydroxy-5,8,10,14-eicosatetraenoic acid (12 ho-20:4) in tissues from the guinea pig, *Biochim. Biophys. Acta*, **431**, 651–4.

Hawkey, C. J. and Rampton, D. S. (1985). Prostaglandins in the gastrointestinal mucosa: are they important in its function, disease or treatment?, *Gastroenterology*, **89**, 1162–88.

Hawkey, C. J. (1986). Synthesis of prostaglandin E_2 and thromboxane B_2 and prostaglandin catabolism in gastritis and gastric ulcer, *Gut*, **12**, 1484–92.

Higgs, G. A., Eakins, K. E., Mugridge, K. G., Moncada, S. and Vane, J. R. (1980). The effects of non-steroid anti-inflammatory drugs on leukocyte migration in carrageenin-induced inflammation, *Eur. J. Pharmacol.*, **66**, 81–6.

Hiraishi, H., Terano, A., Ota, S. *et al.* (1986). Prostaglandin production in cultured gastric mucosal cells: role of cAMP on its modulation, *Prostaglandins*, **32**, 259–73.

Kauffman, G. L. and Whittle, B. J. R. (1982). Gastric vascular actions of prostanoids and the dual effect of arachidonic acid, *Am. J. Physiol*, **242**, G582–7.

Konturek, S. J., Brzozowski, T., Piastucki, I., Radecki, T. and Dembinska-Kiec, A. (1983). Role of prostaglandin and thromboxane biosynthesis in gastric necrosis produced by taurocholate and ethanol, *Dig. Dis. Sci.*, **28**, 154–60.

Le Duc, L. E. and Needleman, P. (1979). Regional localization of prostacyclin and thromboxane synthesis in dog stomach and intestinal tract, *J. Pharm. Exp. Ther.*, **211**, 181–8.

Moncada, S. and Vane, J. R. (1979). Pharmacology and endogenous roles of prostaglandin endoperoxides, thromboxane A_2, and prostacyclin, *Pharmacol. Rev.*, **30**, 293–331.

Nielsen, S. T., Beninati, L. and Chang, J. (1987). REV 5901 and Ly 171 883 protect rat gastric mucosa against ethanol-induced damage, *Agents Actions*, **21**, 3–4.

Oates, J. and Hakkinen, P. (1988). Studies on the mechanism of ethanol-induced gastric damage in rats, *Gastroenterology*, **94**, 10–21.

Pawlik, W., Konturek, S. J., Gustaw, P. *et al.* (1987). Gastric vasoconstrictive and secretory effects of leukotrienes C_4 and D_4 in canine stomach. In B. Samuelsson, R. Paoletti and P. W. Ramwell (eds) *Advances in Prostaglandin, Thromboxane and Leukotriene Research*, Vol. 17, Raven Press, New York, pp. 357–60.

Peskar, B. M., Lange, K., Hoppe, V. and Peskar, B. A. (1986). Ethanol stimulates formation of leukotriene C_4 in the rat gastric mucosa, *Prostaglandins*, **31**, 283–93.

Pihan, G. and Szabo, S. (1988). Microvascular injury and the role of leukotrienes and prostaglandins in acute mucosal damage and protection. In W. Domschke, H. G. Dammann, B. M. Peskar and K. H. Holtermuller (eds) *Prostaglandins and Leukotrienes in Gastrointestinal Diseases*, Springer-Verlag, Berlin, pp. 23–9.

Price, C. A., Pipkin, G., Currington, A., Davies, L., Darling, L. and Parsons, M. E. (1985). Thromboxanes and gastric mucosal damage, *Gut*, **26**, A1145.

Rachmilewitz, D., Branski, D., Sharon, P. and Karmeli, F. (1984). Possible role of endogenous prostanoids in the pathogenesis of peptic ulcer. In A. Allen, G. Flemström, A. Garner, W. Silen and L. A. Turnberg (eds) *Mechanisms of Mucosal Protection in the Upper Gastrointestinal Tract*, Raven Press, New York, pp. 329–33.

Rainsford, K. D. (1987). The effects of 5-lipoxygenase inhibitors and leukotriene antagonists on the development of gastric lesions induced by nonsteroidal anti-inflammatory drugs in mice, *Agents Actions*, **21**, 3–4.

Robert, A. (1981). Prostaglandins and the gastrointestinal tract. In L. R. Johnson (ed.) *Physiology of the Gastrointestinal Tract*, Raven Press, New York, pp. 1407–34.

Rosam, A. C., Wallace, J. L. and Whittle, B. J. R. (1986). Potent ulcerogenic actions of platelet-activating factor on the stomach, *Nature*, **319**, 54–6.

Samuelsson, B. (1983). Leukotrienes: mediators of immediate hypersensitivity reactions and inflammation, *Science*, **220**, 568–75.

Szabo, S., Trier, J. S., Brown, A. and Schnoor, J. (1985). Early vascular injury and increased vascular permeability in gastric mucosal injury caused by ethanol in the rat, *Gastroenterology*, **88**, 228–36.

Tateson, J. E., Randall, R. W., Reynolds, C. H. *et al.* (1988). Selective inhibition of arachidonate 5-lipoxygenase by novel acetohydroxamic acids: biochemical assessment *in vitro* and *ex vivo*, *Br. J. Pharmacol.*, **94**, 528–39.

Wallace, J. L. (1987). Glucocortoid-induced gastric mucosal damage: inhibition of leukotriene, but not prostaglandin biosynthesis, *Prostaglandins*, **34**, 311–23.

Wallace, J. L. and Whittle, B. J. R. (1985). Role of prostanoids in the protective actions of BW 755C on the gastric mucosa, *Eur. J. Pharmacol.*, **115**, 45–51.

Wallace, J. L. and Whittle, B. J. R. (1986a). Effects of inhibition of arachidonic acid metabolism on PAF-induced gastric mucosal necrosis and haemoconcentration, *Br. J. Pharmacol.*, **89**, 415–22.

Wallace, J. L. and Whittle, B. J. R. (1986b). Prevention of endotoxin-induced gastrointestinal damage by CV-3988, an antagonist of platelet-activating factor, *Eur. J. Pharmacol.*, **124**, 209–10.

Wallace, J. L., Beck, P. L. and Morris, G. P. (1988). Is there a role for leukotrienes as mediators of ethanol-induced gastric mucosal damage?, *Am. J. Physiol.*, **254**, G117–23.

Wallace, J. L., Steel, G., Whittle, B. J. R., Lagente, V. and Vargaftig, B. (1987). Evidence for platelet-activating factor as a mediator of endotoxin-induced gastrointestinal damage in the rat: effects of three platelet-activating factor antagonists, *Gastroenterology*, **93**, 765–73.

Walt, R. P., Kemp, R. T., Filipowicz, B., Davies, J. G., Bhaskar, N. K. and Hawkey, C. J. (1987). Gastric mucosal protection with selective inhibition of thromboxane synthesis, *Gut*, **28**, 541–4.

Walus, K. M., Gustaw, P. and Konturek, S. J. (1980). Differential effects of prostaglandins and arachidonic acid on gastric circulation and oxygen consumption, *Prostaglandins*, **20**, 1089–102.

Whittle, B. J. R. (1984). Cellular mediators in gastric damage: actions of thromboxane A_2 and its inhibitors. In A. Allen, A. Garner, G. Flemström, W. Silen, and L. A. Turnberg (eds) *Mechanisms of Mucosal Protection in the Upper Gastrointestinal Tract*, Raven Press, New York, pp. 295–301.

Whittle, B. J. R. and Boughton-Smith, N. K. (1984). Biosynthesis of endogenous arachidonate products involved in gastric damage and protection. In W. Paton, J. Mitchell and P. Turner (eds) *Proceedings of IUPHAR 9th International Congress of Pharmacology*, MacMillan Press, London, pp. 345–54.

Whittle, B. J. R. and Moncada, S. (1983a). The pharmacological interactions between prostacyclin and thromboxanes, *Br. Med. Bull.*, **39**, 232–8.

Whittle, B. J. R. and Moncada, S. (1983b). Ulceration induced by an endoperoxide analogue and by indomethacin in the canine stomach. In B. Samuelsson, R. Paoletti and P. Ramwell (eds) *Advances in Prostaglandin, Thromboxane and Leukotriene Research*, Raven Press, New York, pp. 373–8.

Whittle, B. J. R. and Vane, J. R. (1987). Prostanoids as regulators of gastrointestinal function. In L. R. Johnson (ed.) *Physiology of the Gastrointestinal Tract*, 2nd edn, Vol. 1, Raven Press, New York, pp. 601–38.

Whittle, B. J. R., Kauffman, G. L. and Moncada, S. (1981). Vasoconstriction with thromboxane A_2 induces ulceration of the gastric mucosa, *Nature*, **292**, 472–4.

Whittle, B. J. R., Kauffman, G. L. and Moncada, S. (1986). Hemostatic mechanisms, independent of platelet aggregation arrest gastric mucosal bleeding, *Proc. Natl. Acad. Sci. USA*, **83**, 5683–7.

Whittle, B. J. R., Kauffman, G. L. and Wallace, J. L. (1987). Gastric vascular and mucosal damaging actions of platelet activating factor in the canine stomach. In B. Samuelsson, R. Paoletti and P. Ramwell (eds) *Advances in Prostaglandin, Thromboxane and Leukotriene Research*, Raven Press, New York, pp. 285–92.

Whittle, B. J. R., Oren-Wolman, N. and Guth, P. H. (1985). Gastric vasoconstrictor actions of leukotriene C_4, $PGF_{2\alpha}$, and thromboxane mimetic U-46619 on rat submucosal microcirculation *in vivo*, *Am. J. Physiol.*, **248**, G580–6.

Whittle, B. J. R., Morishita, T., Ohya, Y., Leung, F. W. and Guth, P. H. (1986). Microvascular actions of platelet-activating factor on the rat gastric mucosa and submucosa, *Am. J. Physiol.*, **251**, G772–8.

Whittle, B. J. R., Boughton-Smith, N. K., Hutcheson, I. R., Esplugues, J. V. and Wallace, J. L. (1987). Increased intestinal formation of PAF in endotoxin-induced damage in the rat, *Br. J. Pharmacol.*, **92**, 3–4.

Whittle, B. J. R., Boughton-Smith, N. K., Hutcheson, I. and Esplugues, J. V. (1988). Intestinal release of eicosanoids and PAF-acether as pathological mediatiors of endotoxin-induced damage. *Gastroenterology*, **94**, A495.

Zamecnik, A. M., Cerskus, J., Stoessl, A. L., Barnett, A. J. and McDonald, J. W. D. (1977). Synthesis of thromboxane B_2 and prostaglandins by bovine gastric mucosal microsomes, *Prostaglandins*, **14**, 819–27.

Advances in Drug Therapy of Gastrointestinal Ulceration
Edited by A. Garner and B. J. R. Whittle
©1989 John Wiley & Sons Ltd

Chapter Fourteen

Pharmacological Interventions in Intestinal Ulcerative Disease

B. M. Peskar

Department of Experimental Clinical Medicine, Ruhr-University of Bochum, D-4630 Bochum, FRG

INTRODUCTION

The chronic inflammatory bowel diseases, ulcerative colitis and Crohn's disease, are among the clinically most important ulcerative disorders of the small and/or large intestine. It has been suggested that interactions between host responses, immunological or genetic influences, and external agents may be involved in the pathogenesis of such inflammatory bowel diseases (Kirsner and Shorter, 1982), but the precise events initiating the mucosal inflammation are still unknown. Since the underlying cause is unknown, the aim of medical treatment is to interrupt the chain of reactions that triggers the amplification of the inflammatory process. Numerous chemically distinct endogenous agents have been found to elicit pathobiological events such as vasodilatation, increased vasopermeability, sensitization of nociceptors, activation of inflammatory cells and local tissue destruction, which finally result in clinical inflammation. These mediators include vasoactive amines such as histamine, peptides like bradykinin, the various fractions of complement, bacterial-derived peptides including formylmethionylleucylphenylalanine (FMLP) and lipid-derived mediators such as arachidonate metabolites and platelet activating factor.

Development of drugs beneficial in the treatment of inflammatory bowel diseases is hampered by the fact that the chemical mediators responsible for the maintenance of the chronic inflammatory process have not been identified so far. Furthermore, a spectrum of different mediators may be generated in response to the initiating event, which may act in concert. Selective inhibition of biosynthesis or antagonism of action of a single type of mediator may, therefore, not necessarily interrupt the inflammatory reaction.

ARACHIDONATE METABOLITES

Biosynthesis of cyclo-oxygenase and lipoxygenase products

In recent years, search for new anti-inflammatory drugs has focused on compounds that modulate biosynthesis and actions of lipid-derived mediators, particularly the prostaglandins (PG), thromboxanes (TX), leukotrienes (LT) and, more recently, platelet activating factor. Arachidonic acid is a normal constituent of cellular phospholipids and is the predominant polyunsaturated 20-carbon fatty acid present in mammalian tissues. Arachidonic acid is liberated from the phospholipid stores by the action of phospholipases as a result of a variety of biological events such as specific receptor activation, antigen–antibody interaction and physical stimuli. Metabolism of the free fatty acid can occur via several different pathways (Figure 14.1).

Arachidonic acid is transformed via the cyclo-oxygenase pathway to the unstable endoperoxide intermediates PGG_2 and PGH_2, which are subsequently metabolized to the prostaglandins PGE_2, $PGF_{2\alpha}$, PGD_2, PGI_2 and TXA_2. While PGE_2, $PGF_{2\alpha}$ and PGD_2 are chemically stable, PGI_2 and TXA_2 are rapidly converted non-enzymatically to the stable, but biologically inactive, compounds 6-keto-$PGF_{1\alpha}$ and TXB_2 respectively. Alternatively, arachidonic

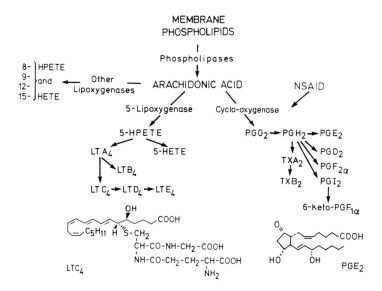

Figure 14.1 Major pathways of arachidonic acid metabolism. The enzyme cyclo-oxygenase catalyses formation of the various prostaglandins and thromboxane and is inhibited by non-steroid anti-inflammatory drugs (NSAIDs). Lipoxygenases transform arachidonic acid to monohydroperoxy- and monohydroxy-acids (HPETEs, HETEs) and the leukotrienes

acid can be metabolized by lipoxygenases leading to formation of various monohydroperoxy acids (HPETEs) and monohydroxy acids (HETEs).

Arachidonic acid is transformed via the 5-lipoxygenase pathway to 5-HPETE, which is either processed to the hydroxy fatty acid 5-HETE or acts as a precursor in the biosynthesis of the leukotrienes. Thus, further conversion of 5-HPETE by the enzyme 5-lipoxygenase results in formation of the unstable intermediary 5,6-epoxide LTA_4. This may undergo enzymatically catalysed hydration yielding the 5-12-di-HETE, LTB_4. An alternative pathway of metabolism of LTA_4 is mediated by addition of glutathione by the enzyme glutathione-S-transferase leading to the formation of LTC_4. Successive shortening of the peptide side-chain results in conversion of LTC_4 to LTD_4 and further to LTE_4. With respect to the related chemical structure and similarity in biologic actions LTC_4, LTD_4 and LTE_4 as a group are termed cysteinyl or sulphidopeptide leukotrienes (for review see Granström, 1983; Hammarström, 1984).

Pro-inflammatory effects of eicosanoids

Both cyclo-oxygenase- and lipoxygenase-derived products of arachidonate metabolism possess pronounced pro-inflammatory properties. E-type prostaglandins and PGI_2 are potent vasodilators in the microcirculation and the generation of these cyclo-oxygenase products in damaged tissues can explain the characteristic erythema of acute inflammation. Prostaglandins have no significant direct effects on blood vessel permeability. Vasodilator prostaglandins, however, potentiate the effect of other inflammatory mediators such as bradykinin, histamine or LTB_4 on plasma exudation. Lipoxygenase products may also increase vascular permeability. Thus, the cysteinyl leukotrienes cause widespread plasma leakage from post-capillary venules in a number of vascular beds. Although LTB_4 does not directly influence vascular permeability, it causes marked plasma leakage when combined with a vasodilator prostaglandin. This effect is proposed to be mediated by polymorphonuclear cells.

Arachidonate metabolites do not cause overt pain. E-type prostaglandins, however, potentiate the pain-producing effects of histamine or bradykinin by a sensitization of nociceptors resulting in hyperalgesia. Furthermore, PGE_2 is a potent pyretic agent which may be involved in the elevated temperature found in patients with inflammatory disorders. While PGE_2 and PGI_2 suppress leukocyte functions such as phagocytosis and motility, the monohydroxy fatty acids 5-HETE and 12-HETE and particularly the dihydroxy fatty acid LTB_4 are chemotactic for polymorphonuclear cells. LTB_4 is one of the most potent endogenous chemotactic factors and in addition induces chemokinesis, aggregation, adherence, margination and lysosomal enzyme release. Generation of LTB_4 by inflamed tissues may be an important factor in the recruitment and activation of inflammatory cells (for a review, see Higgs, Moncada and Vane, 1984).

EICOSANOIDS IN INFLAMMATORY BOWEL DISEASES

Cyclo-oxygenase products

Numerous studies have shown that mucosal tissue obtained from patients with inflammatory bowel diseases synthesizes more cyclo-oxygenase-derived arachidonate metabolites than normal colonic mucosa (for review see Rampton and Hawkey, 1984). Thus, homogenates of inflamed mucosa of these patients converted exogenous arachidonic acid more effectively to the various prostaglandins and TXB_2 than non-inflamed tissue (Harris, Smith and Swan, 1978; Boughton-Smith, Hawkey and Whittle, 1983). Biopsy specimens of inflamed mucosa exhibited an enhanced release of PGE_2, 6-keto-$PGF_{1\alpha}$ and TXB_2 during incubation *in vitro* (Sharon *et al.*, 1978; Ligumsky *et al.*, 1981), while release of cyclo-oxygenase products from non-inflamed mucosa was not different from that in normal mucosa.

Significantly increased accumulation of PGE_2 and TXB_2 was found in the medium of cultured peripheral blood mononuclear cells (Rachmilewitz *et al.*, 1982) and intestinal mononuclear cells (Zifroni *et al.*, 1983) from patients with active Crohn's disease. Increased formation of cyclo-oxygenase products from mononuclear cells did not occur in the absence of mucosal inflammation and seemed to be restricted to Crohn's disease as blood and intestinal mononuclear cells obtained from patients with active ulcerative colitis did not show an increased prostanoid release.

Enhanced formation of cyclo-oxygenase-derived arachidonate metabolites in patients with inflammatory bowel diseases has also been observed *in vivo*. Increased levels of prostaglandin-like activity have been found in the stools and colorectal venous plasma from patients with active ulcerative colitis. Furthermore, urinary excretion of a PGF metabolite was significantly higher in patients with active ulcerative colitis and returned to normal as the disease became quiescent (Gould *et al.*, 1981). Plasma levels of eicosanoids as well as excretion of eicosanoid metabolites in the urine may not represent local production in the gut, however.

The *in vivo* formation of intestinal eicosanoids has been measured more appropriately as the rate of eicosanoids accumulating in dialysis bags placed in the empty rectum, or the equilibrium concentrations of eicosanoids, using the same technique or the original method of *in vivo* dialysis of faeces (for review see Lauritsen *et al.*, 1987). Such studies have demonstrated that the luminal concentrations of PGE_2, $PGF_{2\alpha}$ and TXB_2, but not of 6-keto-$PGF_{1\alpha}$, were significantly elevated in patients with active ulcerative colitis and decreased toward normal levels after successful treatment (Lauritsen *et al.*, 1986a,b).

Lipoxygenase products

More recently, interest has focused on a potential contribution of lipoxygenase-derived arachidonate metabolites in the pathogenesis of inflammatory bowel diseases. Incubation of homogenates of inflammatory bowel disease mucosa with exogenous arachidonic acid resulted in formation of lipoxygenase products such as LTB_4, 5-HETE, 12-HETE and 15-HETE in addition to generation of the cyclo-oxygenase products, PGE_2 and TXB_2 (Boughton-Smith, Hawkey and Whittle, 1983; Sharon and Stenson, 1984). Biopsy specimens obtained from patients with active ulcerative colitis also generate significantly more cysteinyl leukotrienes, consisting of a mixture of LTC_4, LTD_4 and LTE_4, in addition to LTB_4 and PGE_2, during incubation *in vitro* (Figure 14.2). Similarly, colonic mucosal fragments obtained from patients undergoing surgery for active Crohn's disease synthesized more cysteinyl leukotrienes, LTB_4 and PGE_2 than mucosa obtained from patients undergoing surgery for colonic cancer. Increased formation of 5-lipoxygenase and cyclo-oxygenase products by Crohn's mucosa was observed only when the tissue was taken from inflamed regions of the surgical specimens, and not in the absence of mucosal inflammation (Peskar *et al.*, 1986; Dreyling *et al.*, 1987).

Enhanced intestinal production of LTB_4 in patients with active inflammatory bowel diseases could also be demonstrated *in vivo* (Lauritsen *et al.*, 1986b). Luminal concentrations of LTB_4 as measured by rectal equilibrium dialysis were positively correlated with disease activity and significantly decreased in patients responding to anti-inflammatory therapy. Interestingly, in patients with *Clostridium difficile*-associated colitis, luminal concentrations of PGE_2, $PGF_{2\alpha}$ and TXB_2 determined by equilibrium *in vivo* dialysis were abnormally high, but, in contrast to patients with ulcerative colitis, no rise in local concentrations of LTB_4 occurred (Lauritsen *et al.*, 1986a). It remains to be elucidated whether the increased intestinal production of 5-lipoxygenase-derived arachidonate metabolites is related to the specific pathogenesis of chronic inflammatory bowel diseases or is also found with other types of intestinal inflammatory disorders.

Possible pathogenic role of lipoxygenase
products in inflammatory bowel diseases

Histologically, ulcerative colitis and Crohn's disease are characterized by a mixed type of acute and chronic inflammation. Thus, in addition to the presence of mononuclear cells, which are a typical feature of chronic inflammation, the mucosa is heavily infiltrated with neutrophils. Both in Crohn's disease and in ulcerative colitis, movement of large numbers of neutrophils out of the circulation into the inflamed mucosa and then into the intestinal lumen has been demonstrated using ^{111}In-labelled neutrophils (Saverymuttu *et al.*, 1985). Movement of neutrophils to sites of inflammation is triggered by chemotactic

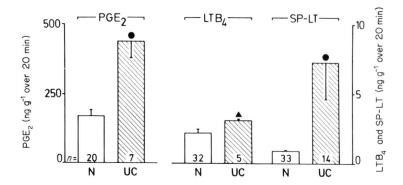

Figure 14.2 Release of PGE_2, LTB_4 and the cysteinyl-containing sulphidopeptide leukotrienes (SP-LT) from rectal mucosa obtained by endoscopy from patients with active ulcerative colitis (UC) or patients without rectal disease (N). Biopsy specimens were incubated in oxygenated Tyrode's solution and release of eicosanoids into the medium was measured using radioimmunoassays. Values represent the mean ± s.e.m. of n experiments. Statistical difference is shown as: ▲, $P < 0.05$; ●, $P < 0.001$, compared to normal mucosa. (Data derived from Peskar *et al.* (1987))

agents present in the tissues. Various soluble mediators have been shown to possess marked chemotactic and/or chemokinetic actions, including the complement fraction C5a, bacterial-derived peptides such as FMLP, lymphocyte-derived chemotactic factors and the 5-lipoxygenase products LTB_4 and 5-HETE (for review see Higgs, Moncada and Vane, 1984). Recent work compared the chemotactic activity of colonic mucosa from patients with inflammatory bowel disease and from normal colonic mucosa by measuring the movement of ^{51}Cr-labelled neutrophils in a Boyden chamber (Lobos, Sharon and Stenson, 1987). Using this method, it was found that the chemotactic response of neutrophils to ulcerative colitis mucosa was more than 20 times that to normal mucosa, and the response to Crohn's colitis mucosa was more than 10 times that to normal mucosa. Further investigations revealed that up to 90% of the chemotactic activity of mucosal homogenates was lipid extractable and co-chromatographed with LTB_4 using high-pressure liquid chromatography separation, suggesting that LTB_4 is the major chemotactic agent in ulcerative colitis mucosa.

Another characteristic feature of inflammatory bowel disease mucosa is severe oedema formation. Swollen and thickened mucosa and blurred vascular patterns are typical endoscopic signs of active disease. The cysteinyl leukotrienes cause widespread plasma leakage in a variety of vascular beds (Dahlen *et al.*, 1981). Enhanced vascular permeability is also found in various organs including the small bowel and the caecum after injection of LTB_4 in rats, and is even more pronounced when LTB_4 is combined with PGE_2 (Stenson, Chang and Williamson, 1986). Furthermore, cysteinyl leukotrienes have been demonstrated to produce small intestinal secretory and anti-absorptive effects in rats (Montzka, Smith and Fondacaro, 1987). Thus, increased formation of 5-lipoxygenase-derived arachidonate metabolites could significantly contribute to the main features of mucosal inflammation, that is cellular infiltration and mucosal oedema, and possibly to the diarrhoea in patients with inflammatory bowel disease.

CYCLO-OXYGENASE INHIBITORS IN INFLAMMATORY BOWEL DISEASES

Cyclo-oxygenase-derived arachidonate metabolites seem to play a crucial role in the pathogenesis of a variety of inflammatory disorders. This is suggested from the increased production of prostaglandins and thromboxane in disease states such as rheumatoid arthritis, osteoarthritis and other chronic inflammatory joint disorders (for review see Higgs, Moncada and Vane, 1984) as well as by the prompt relief of symptoms brought about in these patients by treatment with non-steroid anti-inflammatory drugs. These drugs inhibit the enzyme cyclo-oxygenase and thereby reduce formation of prostaglandins and thromboxanes.

In contrast, in patients with active ulcerative colitis, treatment with indomethacin does not improve clinical symptoms and endoscopic appearance of the mucosa (Gilat et al., 1979; Campieri et al., 1980). In some patients indomethacin even causes a deterioration of the clinical condition. Similarly, in acute attacks of ulcerative colitis, oral flurbiprofen was significantly inferior to conventional treatment with sulphasalazine and corticosteroids in respect of rectal mucosal appearance at sigmoidoscopy, rectal electrical potential difference, rectal mucosal sodium absorption and rectal bleeding, although intraluminal release of PGE_2 fell by 44% (Rampton and Sladen, 1981). In patients in remission, ingestion of non-steroid anti-inflammatory drugs has even been suspected to provoke acute attacks (Rampton, McNeil and Sarner, 1983). From these results it seems likely that, in inflammatory bowel diseases, cyclo-oxygenase products of arachidonate metabolism do not have the same pathogenic relevance in triggering the inflammatory reaction as in other inflammatory disorders, and that other mediators may be of greater importance.

ANTI-INFLAMMATORY DRUGS BENEFICIAL IN INFLAMMATORY BOWEL DISEASES

Corticosteroids

Corticosteroids are the most powerful drugs used to treat acute clinical attacks of ulcerative colitis and Crohn's disease. Glucocorticoids can interfere with the release of arachidonic acid from the phospholipid stores and thus prevent formation of both cyclo-oxygenase and lipoxygenase products. This effect is believed to be mediated by the production of a protein that inhibits phospholipase A_2 activity (for review see Higgs, Moncada and Vane, 1984). Glucocorticoids have been found to reduce release *in vitro* of cyclo-oxygenase-derived arachidonate metabolites from ulcerative colitis mucosa (Ligumsky *et al.*, 1981; Hawkey and Truelove, 1981) and from normal and Crohn's disease monocytes (Maxwell *et al.*, 1985). Corticosteroid-induced inhibition of release of lipoxygenase products from human intestinal tissues *in vitro* has not been demonstrated so far. Topical and systemic administration of prednisolone, however, significantly reduced luminal rectal concentrations of LTB_4 in addition to PGE_2 and $PGF_{2\alpha}$ within less than 72 h in patients with active ulcerative colitis (Lauritsen *et al.*, 1986b, 1987). It remains to be established whether this effect results from reduced arachidonate availability or is secondary to anti-inflammatory actions not primarily mediated by effects on arachidonic acid metabolism.

Sulphasalazine, 5-aminosalicylic acid and related drugs

In patients with ulcerative colitis, sulphasalazine (SASP) has been found to be an effective treatment both in mild to moderate clinical attacks and as maintenance therapy to reduce the risk of relapse. In the colon, SASP is broken down by bacterial enzymes liberating 5-aminosalicylic acid (5-ASA) and sulphapyridine (SP). While SP is rapidly absorbed, most of the 5-ASA remains in the gut lumen. Azad Khan, Piris and Truelove (1977) first reported that topical 5-ASA, but not SP, has therapeutic efficacy comparable to that of SASP in patients with ulcerative colitis. These findings have been confirmed by others and gave rise to the concept that 5-ASA is the active moiety of the SASP molecule, while SP acts as an inert carrier to prevent small intestinal absorption of 5-ASA. As most side-effects of SASP are attributed to the SP moiety, efforts have been made to replace the SP moiety of SASP by a less toxic carrier molecule or to develop slow-release preparations of 5-ASA which ensure delivery of the drug to the colon. During recent years, considerable evidence has accumulated that the new orally active 5-ASA preparations favourably influence the outcome of acute attacks of ulcerative colitis and help to maintain remission. Similar to topical 5-ASA, enemas of 4-ASA, which differs in the position of the amino group, have been reported to be effective in the treatment of mild to moderate distal ulcerative colitis.

Human colonic epithelial cells rapidly acetylate 5-ASA (Ireland, Priddle and Jewell, 1986) and most of the 5-ASA which can be measured in plasma and urine is in the acetylated form. This raises the possibility that at least part of the therapeutic efficacy of 5-ASA is due to the metabolite acetyl-5-ASA. Topical acetyl-5-ASA induced histological and sigmoidoscopic improvement and relief from symptoms in patients with active ulcerative colitis in one study (Willoughby, Piris and Truelove, 1980), but not in other trials. This inconsistent efficacy has been attributed to the fact that, contrary to unmetabolized 5-ASA, acetyl-5-ASA is not readily taken up into intestinal epithelial cells (Ireland, Priddle and Jewell, 1987).

In patients treated with SASP or azodisalicylate, high (millimolar) concentrations of SASP, 5-ASA and acetyl-5-ASA are reached in the gut lumen (Table 14.1), while serum concentrations are considerably lower. Most pharmacological effects of SASP and its metabolites, including the modulatory actions on arachidonate metabolism, are only observed at the high concentrations found in the gut lumen. Thus, SASP inhibits formation of 5-HETE and LTB_4 by human peripheral blood neutrophils with an IC_{50} of 1.5 mmol l^{-1} and 0.9 mmol l^{-1}, respectively (Stenson and Lobos, 1982). 5-ASA inhibited formation of LTB_4 (IC_{50} mmol l^{-1}), but not formation of 5-HETE, by human neutrophils, while SP caused partial inhibition of the synthesis of both compounds, reaching a maximum of 30% inhibition at 4–6 mmol l^{-1}. SASP (1–2.5 mmol l^{-1}) was also found to inhibit conversion of exogenous arachidonic acid to various HETEs and LTB_4 by homogenates of inflammatory bowel diseased colonic mucosa (Sharon and Stenson, 1984; Hawkey, Boughton-Smith and Whittle, 1985). On the other hand, 5-ASA was reported to selectively inhibit the cyclo-oxygenase pathway of arachidonate metabolism without affecting formation of lipoxygenase products in rat colonic mucosa (Sharon and Stenson, 1985) and human colonic mucosal homogenates (Hawkey, Boughton-Smith and Whittle, 1985) in concentrations >5 mmol l^{-1} and up to 1 mmol l^{-1}, respectively.

As discussed, 5-ASA is now considered to be the active moiety of the SASP molecule (although there is substantial evidence that the parent compound,

Table 14.1 Luminal concentrations of sulphasalazine (SASP), 5-aminosalicylic acid (5-ASA) and acetyl-5-ASA in patients treated with SASP or azodisalicylate

Treatment	SASP (mmol l^{-1})	5-ASA (mmol l^{-1})	Ac-5-ASA (mmol $^{-1}$)	Reference
SASP* 3–12 g day^{-1}	2.0–4.2	7.3–12	2.2–7	Peppercorn and Goldmann (1973)
SASP† 2 g day^{-1}	ND	3.9–12	1.0–16	Lauritsen et al. (1984)
ADS† 2 g day^{-1}	ND	4.6–21	1.0–11	Lauritsen et al. (1984)

*Patients with inflammatory bowel disease were treated with SASP for at least 4 weeks. Concentrations of SASP, 5-ASA and acetyl-5-ASA (Ac-5-ASA) were determined in extracts of faeces
†Patients with inactive ulcerative colitis were on maintenance therapy with SASP or azodisalicylate (ADS) for 1 week. Concentrations of SASP, 5-ASA and Ac-5-ASA were determined by in vivo dialysis
ND, not determined

SASP, possesses biological activities distinct from those of 5-ASA). We have therefore compared the effects of SASP, 5-ASA, 4-ASA, the acetylated metabolites of 5-ASA and 4-ASA and indomethacin on the formation of LTB_4, cysteinyl leukotrienes and PGE_2 by fragments of human colonic mucosa during incubation *in vitro*. This *in vitro* technique should allow differentiation between direct effects on arachidonate metabolism and secondary effects resulting from anti-inflammatory actions not primarily related to the eicosanoid system.

As shown in Figure 14.3, formation of LTB_4 and cysteinyl leukotrienes by normal human colonic mucosa was dose-dependently reduced in the presence of 5-ASA in concentrations greater than 1 mmol l^{-1}. At 7.5 mmol l^{-1}, 5-ASA practically abolished leukotriene synthesis. The parent compound, SASP, was found to be about 20 times more active in inhibiting human colonic mucosal leukotriene formation than its metabolite 5-ASA, while 4-ASA and acetyl-5-ASA had comparable inhibitory actions to that of 5-ASA. The acetylated metabolite of 4-ASA did not achieve a significant inhibitory action up to a concentration of 15 mmol l^{-1}. The IC_{50} values for inhibition of human colonic mucosal cysteinyl leukotriene formation are given in Table 14.2. Formation of LTB_4 was affected in a similar way. Experiments with colonic mucosa obtained from patients operated on for active Crohn's disease showed that SASP and 5-ASA

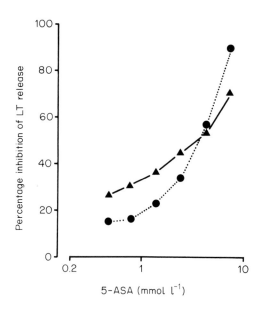

Figure 14.3 Effect of 5-ASA on formation of LTB_4 (▲) and cysteinyl leukotrienes (●) *in vitro* by human colonic mucosa obtained from patients undergoing surgery for colonic cancer. Formation of leukotrienes was stimulated by ionophore A23187 (5 μg ml^{-1}). Dose–response curves were calculated from 5–8 incubations for each concentration. (Data derived from Peskar *et al.* (1987))

Table 14.2   Inhibition of release of cysteinyl leukotrienes and PGE_2 from human colonic mucosa by various anti-inflammatory drugs

Compound	Cysteinyl leukotrienes (IC_{50}, mmol l^{-1})	PGE_2
SASP	0.2	No inhibition
5-ASA	3.7	1.7
4-ASA	5.2	15
Ac-5-ASA	5.6	>15
Ac-4-ASA	>15	>15
SP	1.4	>15
Indomethacin	No inhibition	0.001

Mucosal fragments obtained from patients undergoing surgery for colonic cancer were incubated in the absence or presence of various concentrations of drugs *in vitro*. Effects of drugs on PGE_2 release and their effects on ionophore A23187-stimulated release of cysteinyl leukotrienes were evaluated during a 20 min incubation period. IC_{50} (concentration causing 50% inhibition) values of SASP (sulphasalazine), SP (sulphapyridine), 5-ASA (5-aminosalicylic acid) and the other salicylates were calculated from 5–8 dose–response curves each. Methods used have been described previously (Dreyling *et al.*, 1987)

also inhibited the increased release of LTB_4 and cysteinyl leukotrienes from inflamed mucosal tissues (Dreyling *et al.*, 1987), the IC_{50} values being of the same order of magnitude as that found in non-inflamed mucosa.

In contrast to the results of Stenson and Lobos (1982), who found no significant inhibitory action of SP on formation of 5-HETE and LTB_4 by human peripheral blood neutrophils, SP dose-dependently inhibited formation of leukotrienes from human colonic mucosal fragments *in vitro*. The inhibitory action was at least as marked as that of 5-ASA, a concentration of 7.5 mmol l^{-1} causing nearly complete inhibition of cysteinyl leukotriene release. It remains to be elucidated whether the different clinical efficacy of SP and 5-ASA, despite comparable inhibitory actions on colonic mucosal leukotriene formation *in vitro*, is evidence against a relevant contribution of these mediators in inflammatory bowel diseases. Alternatively, the therapeutic activity of 5-ASA may be due to the drug being retained in the gut lumen and reaching high local concentrations, while SP is rapidly absorbed. In this context, it may be of interest that, recently, SASP has been reintroduced as a second line agent in the treatment of patients with rheumatoid arthritis. In these patients, the disease-modifying activity of SASP can be attributed to the SP moiety of the molecule, while 5-ASA was found to be ineffective (Pullar, Hunter and Capell, 1985). Similar to colonic mucosa, SP inhibits synthesis of cysteinyl leukotrienes by human synovial tissue *in vitro* (Wittenberg *et al.*, 1987). The concentrations of SP necessary to affect synovial cysteinyl leukotriene formation are higher than the plasma levels reached in rheumatoid patients treated with SASP. Nevertheless, it is tempting to speculate that the clinical efficacy of SASP in both rheumatoid arthritis and inflammatory bowel diseases is related to effects of its constituents on formation of 5-lipoxygenase products and that differences in the pharmacokinetic properties determine which is the active component in the treatment of arthritic conditions and intestinal inflammation, respectively.

Contrary to the uniform inhibitory action of SASP and the various salicylates studied on human colonic leukotriene formation, the compounds have divergent effects on colonic release of PGE_2 (Table 14.2). In the concentrations used, 5-ASA and 4-ASA dose-dependently reduce PGE_2 formation, whereas their acetylated metabolites have only minor or no effects, and SASP actually increases release of PGE_2. SASP has complex actions on the various enzymes of prostaglandin synthesis and degradation. Thus, the drug has been found to both inhibit (for review see Rampton and Hawkey, 1984) and stimulate (Schlenker and Peskar, 1981) human colonic prostaglandin synthesis depending on the amount of fatty acid substrate present. Furthermore, SASP inhibits the prostaglandin-degrading enzymes 15-hydroxyprostaglandin dehydrogenase and $^{13}\Delta$-prostaglandin reductase (Hoult and Moore, 1980; Peskar, Schlenker and Weiler, 1982). These complex actions may explain the divergent results observed with SASP on prostaglandin formation using different experimental models. In contrast to SASP and the various salicylates, indomethacin, which is of no benefit in the treatment of intestinal inflammation, selectively inhibits human colonic formation of PGE_2, while release of LTB_4 and cysteinyl leukotrienes even tends to be increased (Table 14.2).

LIPOXYGENASE INHIBITORS IN ANIMAL MODELS OF INFLAMMATORY BOWEL DISEASE

The correlation between the clinical efficacy of the drugs studied and their inhibitory action on human colonic leukotriene formation may suggest that leukotrienes are of pathobiological relevance in inflammatory bowel diseases. Recently, the effect of lipoxygenase inhibitors has been studied in an experimental colitis in rats induced by intracolonic instillation of trinitrobenzene sulphonic acid (TNB). Similar to human inflammatory bowel disease, TNB-induced colitis is accompanied by increased formation of cyclo-oxygenase- and 5-lipoxygenase-derived arachidonate metabolites. Treatment with selective 5-lipoxygenase inhibitors significantly reduced the ulceration, inflammation and diarrhoea in TNB-treated rats (MacNaughton, Morris and Wallace, 1988; Allgayer and Stenson, 1988). In another study, however, treatment with the dual inhibitor of cyclo-oxygenase and lipoxygenase BW755C in doses that significantly reduced colonic LTB_4 and 6-keto-$PGF_{1\alpha}$ synthesis did not affect TNB-induced colonic damage (Boughton-Smith et al., 1988).

CONCLUSIONS

While inhibition of formation of cyclo-oxygenase products of arachidonate metabolism has been shown unequivocally to be of no benefit in the treatment of inflammatory bowel diseases, the therapeutic effect of blockade of the lipoxygenase pathway is still unclear. A number of compounds are currently under development, which are considerably more potent as inhibitors of leukotriene formation than SASP and the salicylates. Clinical trials with such drugs in patients with inflammatory bowel disease should clarify whether leukotrienes are indeed relevant mediators of such inflammation. SASP and the salicylates have a wide spectrum of biological effects, including modulation of lymphocyte functions (for review see Hoult, 1986) and radical scavenging activity (Ahnfelt-Ronne and Haagen Nielsen, 1987). The pluripotency of glucocorticoids, SASP and salicylates may be an important contribution to their beneficial actions in inflammatory bowel disease patients. It remains to be established whether compounds which selectively inhibit biosynthesis or actions of single inflammatory mediators have the same, or even superior, therapeutic potential.

ACKNOWLEDGEMENTS

This work was supported by the Deutsche Forschungsgemeinschaft grant Pe-215/6. I thank Ms I. Schönewolff for excellent secretarial work.

REFERENCES

Ahnfelt-Ronne, I. and Haagen Nielsen, O. (1987). The anti-inflammatory moiety of sulfasalazine, 5-aminosalicylic acid, is a radical scavenger, *Agents Actions*, **21**, 191–4.
Allgayer, H. and Stenson, W. F. (1988). Role of lipoxygenase pathway products in an animal model of colitis: effect of pretreatment with 5-lipoxygenase inhibitors, *Gastroenterology*, **94**, A6.
Azad-Khan, A. H., Piris, J. and Truelove, S. C. (1977). An experiment to determine the active therapeutic moiety of sulphasalazine, *Lancet*, **ii**, 892–5.
Boughton-Smith, N. K., Hawkey, C. J. and Whittle, B. J. R. (1983). Biosynthesis of lipoxygenase and cyclo-oxygenase products from (^{14}C)-arachidonic acid by human colonic mucosa, *Gut*, **24**, 1176–82.
Boughton-Smith, N. K., Wallace, J. L., Morris, G. P. and Whittle, B. J. R. (1988). The effect of anti-inflammatory drugs on eicosanoid formation in a chronic model of inflammatory bowel disease in the rat, *Br. J. Pharmacol.*, **94**, 65–72.
Campieri, M., Lanfranchi, G. A., Bazzochi, G. *et al.* (1980). Prostaglandins, indomethacin, and ulcerative colitis, *Gastroenterology*, **78**, 193.
Dahlen, S. E., Björk, J., Hedqvist, P. *et al.* (1981). Leukotrienes promote plasma leakage and leukocyte adhesion in postcapillary venules: *in vivo* effects with relevance to the acute inflammatory response, *Proc. Natl. Acad. Sci., USA*, **78**, 3887–91.
Dreyling, K. W., Hoppe, U., Peskar, B. A., Schaarschmidt, K. and Peskar, B. M. (1987). Leukotrienes in Crohn's disease: effect of sulfasalazine and 5-aminosalicylic acid. In B. Samuelsson, R. Paoletti and P. W. Ramwell (eds) *Advances in Prostaglandin, Thromboxane, and Leukotriene Research*, Vol. 17, Raven Press, New York, pp. 339–43.

Gilat, T., Ratan, J., Rosen, P. and Peled, J. (1979). Prostaglandins and ulcerative colitis, *Gastroenterology*, **77**, 1083.

Gould, S. R., Brash, A. R., Conolly, M. E. and Lennard-Jones, J. E. (1981). Studies of prostaglandins and sulphasalazine in ulceration colitis, *Prostaglandins Med.*, **6**, 165–82.

Granström, E. (1983). Biochemistry of the prostaglandins, thromboxanes, and leukotrienes. In J. J. Bonica, N. Lindblom and A. 'Jggo (eds) *Advances in Pain Research and Therapy*, Vol. 5, Raven Press, New York, pp. 605–15.

Hammarström, S. (1984). The leukotrienes. In G. Litwack (ed.) *Biochemical Actions of Hormones*, Vol. 11, Academic Press, New York, pp. 1–23.

Harris, D. W., Smith, P. R. and Swan, C. H. J. (1978). Determination of prostaglandin synthetase activity in rectal biopsy material and its significance in colonic disease, *Gut*, **19**, 875–7.

Hawkey, C. J., Boughton-Smith, N. K. and Whittle, B. J. R. (1985). Modulation of human colonic arachidonic acid metabolism by sulfasalazine, *Dig. Dis. Sci.*, **30**, 1161–5.

Hawkey, C. J. and Truelove, S. C. (1981). Effect of prednisolone on prostaglandin synthesis by rectal mucosa in ulcerative colitis: investigation by laminar flow bioassay and radioimmunoassay, *Gut*, **22**, 190–3.

Higgs, G. A., Moncada, S. and Vane, J. R. (1984). Eicosanoids in inflammation, *Ann. Clin. Res.*, **16**, 287–99.

Hoult, J. R. S. (1986). Pharmacological and biochemical actions of sulphasalazine, *Drugs*, **32** (Suppl. 1), 18–26.

Hoult, J. R. S. and Moore, P. K. (1980). Effects of sulphasalazine and its metabolites on prostaglandin synthesis, inactivation and actions on smooth muscle, *Br. J. Pharmacol.*, **68**, 719–30.

Ireland, A., Priddle, J. D. and Jewell, D. P. (1986). Acetylation of 5-aminosalicylic acid by human colonic epithelial cells, *Gastroenterology*, **90**, 1471.

Ireland, A., Priddle, J. D. and Jewell, D. P. (1987). A comparison of the uptake of 5-aminosalicylic acid (5-ASA) and *N*-acetylaminosalicylic acid (Ac-ASA) into the isolated colonic epithelial cell, *Gastroenterology*, **92**, 1447.

Kirsner, J. B. and Shorter, R. G. (1982). Recent developments in nonspecific inflammatory bowel disease, *New Engl. J. Med.*, **306**, 775–85, 837–48.

Lauritsen, K., Hansen, J., Ryde, M. and Rask-Madsen, J. (1984). Colonic azodisalicylate metabolism determined by *in vivo* dialysis in healthy volunteers and patients with ulcerative colitis, *Gastroenterology*, **86**, 1496–500.

Lauritsen, K., Laursen, L. S., Bukhave, K. and Rask-Madsen, J. (1986a). Profiles of arachidonic acid metabolites determined by equilibrium *in vivo* dialysis of rectum in active ulcerative colitis, Crohn's colitis, and *C. difficile*-associated colitis, *Gastroenterology*, **90**, 1514.

Lauritsen, K., Laursen, L. S., Bukhave, K. and Rask-Madsen, J. (1986b). Effects of topical 5-aminosalicylic acid and prednisolone on prostaglandin E_2 and leukotriene B_4 levels determined by equilibrium *in vivo* dialysis of rectum in relapsing ulcerative colitis, *Gastroenterology*, **91**, 837–44.

Lauritsen, K., Laursen, L. S., Bukhave, K. and Rask-Madsen, J. (1987). Role of eicosanoids in inflammatory bowel disease. In G. Jarnerot (ed.) *Inflammatory Bowel Disease*, Raven Press, New York, pp. 83–94.

Ligumsky, M., Karmeli, F., Sharon, P., Zor, U., Cohen, F. and Rachmilewitz, D. (1981). Enhanced thromboxane A_2 and prostacyclin production by cultured rectal mucosa in ulcerative colitis and its inhibition by steroids and sulphasalazine, *Gastroenterology*, **81**, 444–9.

Lobos, E. A., Sharon, P. and Stenson, W. F. (1987). Chemotactic activity in inflammatory bowel disease: role of leukotriene B_4, *Dig. Dis. Sci.*, **32**, 1380–8.

MacNaughton, W. K., Morris, G. P. and Wallace, J. L. (1988). Inhibition of leukotriene synthesis markedly enhances healing in a rat model of inflammatory bowel disease, *Gastroenterology*, **94**, A618.

Maxwell, W. J., Bloomfield, F. J., Hogan, F. P., Kelleher, J. P. and Keeling, P. W. N. (1985). Inhibition of PGE_2 secretion by salazopyrin and prednisolone in normal and Crohn's disease monocytes, *Gut*, **26**, P74.

Montzka, D. M., Smith, P. L. and Fondacaro, J. D. (1987). Action of peptidoleukotrienes (PLTs) on electrolyte transport in rat small intestine, *Gastroenterology*, **92**, 1803.

Peppercorn, M. A. and Goldmann, P. (1973). Distribution studies of salicylazo-sulfapyridine and its metabolites, *Gastroenterology*, **64**, 240–5.

Peskar, B. M., Schlenker, T. and Weiler, H. (1982). Effect of sulphasalazine (SASP) and 5-aminosalicylic acid (5-ASA) on the human colonic prostaglandin system, *Gut*, **23**, A444.

Peskar, B. M., Dreyling, K. W., Peskar, B. A., May, B. and Goebell, H. (1986). Enhanced formation of sulfidopeptide-leukotrienes in ulcerative colitis and Crohn's disease: inhibition by sulfasalazine and 5-aminosalicylic acid, *Agent Actions*, **18**, 381–3.

Peskar, B. M., Dreyling, K. W., May, B., Schaarschmidt, K. and Goebell, H. (1987). Possible mode of action of 5-aminosalicylic acid, *Dig. Dis. Sci.*, **32**, 51S–6S.

Pullar, T., Hunter, J. A. and Capell, H. A. (1985). Which component of sulphasalazine is active in rheumatoid arthritis?, *Br. Med. J.*, **290**, 1535–9.

Rachmilewitz, D., Ligumsky, M., Haimowitz, A. and Trewes, A. J. (1982). Prostanoid synthesis by cultured peripheral blood mononuclear cells in inflammatory diseases of the bowel, *Gastroenterology*, **82**, 673–9.

Rampton, D. S. and Hawkey, C. J. (1984). Prostaglandins and ulcerative colitis, *Gut*, **25**, 1399–413.

Rampton, D. S., McNeil, N. I. and Sarner, M. (1983). Analgesic ingestion and other factors preceding relapse in ulcerative colitis, *Gut*, **24**, 187–9.

Rampton, D. S. and Sladen, G. E. (1981). Prostaglandin synthesis inhibitors in ulcerative colitis: flurbiprofen compared with conventional treatment, *Prostaglandins*, **21**, 417–25.

Saverymuttu, S. H., Peters, A. M., Lavender, J. P., Chadwick, V. S. and Hodgson, H. J. (1985). *In vivo* assessment of granulocytic migration to diseased bowel in Crohn's disease, *Gut*, **26**, 378–83.

Schlenker, T. and Peskar, B. M. (1981). Dual effect of sulphasalazine on colonic prostaglandin synthetase, *Lancet*, **ii**, 815.

Sharon, P. and Stenson, W. F. (1984). Enhanced synthesis of leukotriene B_4 by colonic mucosa in inflammatory bowel disease, *Gastroenterology*, **86**, 453–60.

Sharon, P. and Stenson, W. F. (1985). Metabolism of arachidonic acid in acetic colitis in rats: similarity to human inflammatory bowel disease, *Gastroenterology*, **88**, 55–62.

Sharon, P., Ligumsky, M., Rachmilewitz, D. and Zor, U. (1978). Role of prostaglandins in ulcerative colitis: enhanced production during active disease and inhibition by sulphasalazine, *Gastroenterology*, **75**, 638–40.

Stenson, W. F. and Lobos, E. (1982). Sulfasalazine inhibits the synthesis of chemotactic lipids by neutrophils, *J. Clin. Invest.*, **69**, 494–7.

Stenson, W. F., Chang, K. and Williamson, J. R. (1986). Tissue differences in vascular permeability induced by leukotriene B_4 in the rat, *Prostaglandins*, **32**, 5–19.

Willoughby, C. P., Piris, J. and Truelove, S. C. (1980). The effect of topical *N*-acetyl-5-aminosalicylic acid in ulcerative colitis, *Scand. J. Gastroenterol.*, **15**, 715–19.

Wittenberg, H. R., Kleemeyer, K., Hoppe, U., Peskar, B. M. and Peskar, B. A. (1987). Release of eicosanoids from human synovial tissue and the effect of anti-inflammatory drugs. In H. Sinzinger and K. Schrör (eds) *Prostaglandins in Clinical Research*, Alan R. Liss, New York, pp. 277–82.

Zifroni, A., Treves, A. J., Sachar, D. B. and Rachmilewitz, D. (1983). Prostanoid synthesis by cultured intestinal epithelial and mononuclear cells in inflammatory bowel disease, *Gut*, **24**, 659–64.

Advances in Drug Therapy of Gastrointestinal Ulceration
Edited by A. Garner and B. J. R. Whittle
© 1989 John Wiley & Sons Ltd

Chapter Fifteen

Pharmacological Modulation of Cellular, Vascular and Motility Factors

Sandor Szabo
Departments of Pathology, Brigham & Women's Hospital, Harvard Medical School, Boston, Massachusetts 02115, USA

Pharmacological modulation of cellular and vascular factors in the stomach and duodenum provides a potential approach in the medical treatment or prevention of erosions and ulcers in these two organs. Until recently, such a comprehensive approach to ulcer disease was unthinkable since ulcer therapy has historically been equated with neutralization of gastric acid. Reduction of acidity has dominated the relief of ulcer pain, practically from prehistoric times until the 1970s when, in addition to the potent antacids, novel antisecretory agents with minimal side-effects became available (Figure 15.1). Gastric acid thus could not only be neutralized once it had been released into the lumen, but its secretion could be reduced at the parietal cell responsible for secretion of hydrochloric acid by blocking one of the rate-limiting receptors, e.g. the histamine H_2-receptor on the basolateral plasma membrane of these cells. The revolutionary first drug was burimamide, followed by metiamide, but the first representative compound to be tested in worldwide clinical studies and which became a top selling drug was actually cimetidine (Durant, 1987). New derivatives and clones of its structure have been tested and released every few years since.

The other surprising new development in ulcer pharmacology was the revolutionary recognition in the late 1970s and early 1980s that gastric and duodenal ulcers may be prevented and their healing accelerated by drugs such

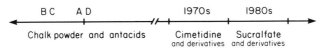

Figure 15.1 Schematic presentation of the history of ulcer pharmacology

as sucralfate which are virtually ineffective toward gastric acid (Marks and Samloff, 1985). The discovery of this drug was independent of but parallel with the emergence of the concept of gastric 'cytoprotection' (Robert, 1979). This phenomenon, initially recognized with prostaglandins (PG), refers to prevention of chemically induced acute haemorrhagic erosions by very low doses of PG which do not inhibit gastric acid secretion in the rat (Robert, 1979). The stage has thus been set both from clinical observations (Marks and Samloff, 1985) and from laboratory experience with experimental animals to suggest that there might be cells other than parietal cells and functions other than acid neutralization or inhibition of secretion which may play a crucial role in both ulcer development and prevention.

This chapter provides a cellular pharmacological overview of ulcer disease in the stomach and duodenum, and emphasizes 'new' cell types whose pharmacological modulation may provide a promising novel lead for ulcer prevention and treatment. Both positive and important negative results will be reviewed in order to obtain a balanced and realistic cellular approach to ulcer pharmacology.

GASTRIC CELL TYPES AND THEIR
POSSIBLE PHARMACOLOGICAL MODULATION

The gastrointestinal tract contains numerous cell types and the complexity of this tissue resembles that of the neuroendocrine system (Table 15.1). This is reinforced by the fact that the gut, unlike most other tissues and organs, possesses a semi-independent enteric nervous system responsible for endogenous regulation in addition to being influenced by the central nervous system. The gastrointestinal tissue with its complex regulation and different cell types thus represents a unique challenge for pharmacological modulation (Table 15.1). It is not surprising, either, that ulcer diseases of the stomach and duodenum are complex, multifactorial or pluricausal diseases, with poorly understood aetiology

Table 15.1 Pharmacological modulation of cellular and vascular factors

Cell types	Function/product	Modulation
Surface mucous	Mucus, bicarbonate	+
Parietal	Hydrochloric acid	+ + +
Chief	Pepsin	±
Neuroendocrine	Gastrin, somatostatin	±
Fibroblasts	Ulcer healing	+
Endothelium	Vascular permeability, blood flow	+ +
Nerve fibres	Secretion, vascular permeability and blood flow, motility	+
Smooth muscle	Motility, blood flow	±

and pathogenesis (Szabo, 1986; Szabo and Bynum, 1988). The heterogeneity of ulcer disease also adds to the complexity and challenge to drug design and the *new* pharmacology of ulcer disease (Szabo and Bynum, 1988).

Parietal cells have, historically, received the most attention and hence drugs are available in abundance for their pharmacological modulation at two (H_2 and acetylcholine) of their surface receptors, although neither gastrin nor somatostatin receptor antagonists are widely available yet (Table 15.1). One significant achievement in ulcer research over the last decade is the demonstration that surface mucous cells of stomach and duodenum secrete measurable quantities of bicarbonate (Flemström and Garner, 1982). The bicarbonate secretion, in addition to the previously recognized mucus secretion (Allen and Garner, 1980), represents one of the first lines of defence against luminal acid and pepsin, and has been called the 'mucus–bicarbonate barrier'.

Chief cells and their secretory product, pepsinogen, cannot yet be specifically modulated by drugs. This might not be such a great disadvantage, since, if we derive the pharmacology from our knowledge of pathogenesis, it is apparent that the role of pepsin in the mechanism of gastric and duodenal ulceration is not at all clear (Brooks, 1985). Hence the unfortunate misnomer 'peptic ulcer' needs no further comment (Szabo, 1984; Szabo and Bynum, 1988).

Fibroblasts are essential for wound healing because of their participation in formation of granulation tissue which fills up the gap when a necrotic specialized tissue such as smooth muscle cannot regenerate. Thus, epithelialization, which assures the surface continuity of gastric and duodenal mucosa, can take place only if a connective tissue scaffolding such as the granulation tissue is present to provide a ground framework. Specific growth factors, such as the fibroblast growth factor, have been isolated during the last few years but they have not yet been used in ulcer research.

Neuroendocrine cells produce important regulatory factors such as gastrin and somatostatin, but their pharmacological potential has either not been explored (for example, due to lack of specific antagonists such as for gastrin) or else the early results have not been conclusive (as with, for example, somatostatin) (Kayasseh and Gyr, 1987; Szabo and Usadel, 1982).

Roles exist for the vascular endothelium and smooth muscle in the pathogenesis of both acute and chronic ulcers. Because of the complexity of their actions, as well as the multiplicity of pharmacological control, vascular and motility elements will be discussed separately. Vascular, or blood flow, and motility factors are closely related in every organ where muscle tissue is preponderant, for example skeletal muscle, heart and gut. It is not surprising that in the stomach, with its relatively thick muscle layer and unusual disposition of blood vessels traversing the muscle not only perpendicularly but obliquely (Piasecki and Wyatt, 1986), motility factors markedly influence blood flow and the development of mucosal lesions (Mersereau and Hinchey, 1980; Takeuchi and Nobuhara, 1985; Janicek *et al.*, 1988). Furthermore, both vascular and motility factors have been somewhat neglected in elucidating the pathogenesis of gastric and duodenal ulcers, and their pharmacological modulation.

VASCULAR ENDOTHELIUM AND MICROCIRCULATION

Blood flow *per se* and its relationship to gastric acid secretion and ulcer localization in the duodenum have been widely investigated. However, systematic studies of vascular factors, especially the emphasis of structural (e.g. endothelial cells and smooth muscle) and functional (e.g. blood flow and vascular permeability) elements in both gastric mucosal injury *and* protection are relatively recent developments (Table 15.2). Thus, the vascular tree is not only passively compressed by outside forces (by muscle) or obstructed internally (e.g. by thrombus) but it actively participates in the development and prevention of mucosal lesions.

The reasons for this relatively recent recognition of the key role of vascular factors are complex, and are both conceptual and methodological (Table 15.2). Essentially, the causes are related to obsession with epithelial and secretory components in gastric pathophysiology, and lack of specialized methods and of a conceptual framework integrating epithelial and endothelial alteration in gastric mucosal injury and protection. With the recognition that vascular injury is a very early event in the pathogenesis of chemically induced gastric erosions (Szabo and Trier, 1984; Szabo *et al.*, 1985), and with the availability of collodial

Table 15.2   Vascular factors in gastric and mucosal injury and protection

---

History
Obsession with epithelial, especially parietal and chief cells
Lack of adequate methods
Importance of blood flow *per se*
Ischaemia: external narrowing (e.g. compression, spasms)
             internal obstruction (e.g. thrombosis, embolism)

Present
Ethanol: rapidly developing and early vascular injury
Endothelial damage is non-specific: HCl, NaOH, aspirin, indomethacin
Vascular injury: associated with functional impairment of microcirculation
Gastroprotective agents decrease vascular damage and maintain blood flow
Maintenance of blood flow: essential for restitution and regeneration

Future
Mechanism of vascular injury: direct and indirect aetiological factors
Endogenous mediators of vascular damage: monoamines, leukotrienes, TX, PAF, etc.
Endogenous vasoprotectors: prostacyclin, glucocorticoids, etc.
Role in both mucosal injury and protection
Pharmacological target

---

carbon or monastral blue to visualize vascular lesions macroscopically or at the light and electron microscopy levels, increasing attention is being devoted to vascular factors in gastric protection. Furthermore, other new techniques such as *in vivo* microscopy of gastric blood flow as well as laser Doppler velocimetry and hydrogen clearance methods helped to demonstrate that the *structural* endothelial lesions are accompanied by rapid *functional* impairment of microcirculation (Leung, Robert and Guth, 1985; Pihan *et al.*, 1986; Szabo, Pihan and Trier, 1986).

Gastric protective PG and sulphydryl (SH) groups not only prevent the microvascular injury demonstrable by vascular tracers (Szabo *et al.*, 1985; Szabo, Pihan and Trier, 1986) but they also *maintain* blood flow in subepithelial capillaries after topical application of damaging agents (Leung, Robert and Guth, 1985; Pihan *et al.*, 1986). This is an important new development since initially increased blood flow was thought to be involved in gastric mucosal protection. New and independent results from two laboratories demonstrate that in healthy control rats prostaglandins alone (i.e. without ethanol) decreases while thiosulphate increases mucosal blood flow (Leung, Robert and Guth, 1985; Pihan *et al.*, 1986). Both agents nevertheless maintain blood flow at control level after administration of ethanol (Figure 15.2). The functional microcirculation ensures that a well oxygenated environment is maintained in the superficial mucosa where epithelial restitution will repair superficial damage.

Epithelial restitution is a relatively recently recognized phenomenon (Lacy and Ito, 1984), but regeneration has been investigated for a long time. Unfortunately, these terms are often used interchangeably, although the distinction should be clear: rapid restitution is cell migration while regeneration involves cell division (proliferation) to replace the defective mucosa. Both are

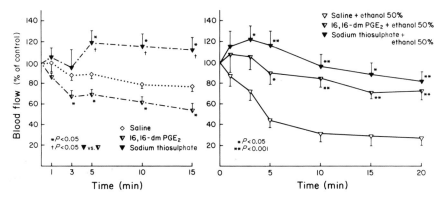

Figure 15.2 Changes in rat gastric mucosal blood flow measured by laser Doppler velocimetry after luminal application of saline, 16,16-dimethyl PGE$_2$ or sodium thiosulphate in the absence and presence of 50% ethanol. (Reprinted with permission from Pihan *et al.*, 1986)

inherent properties which are energy-dependent processes in the gut though more data are available on the direct pharmacological stimulation of cell proliferation than on cell migration.

It is not usually appreciated that epithelial restitution is a truly efficient process only in the case of superficial mucosal injury. Lacy and Ito (1984) ensured such a condition by mechanically removing ethanol from the rat stomach after 30–45 s exposure. Pharmacologically, gastric protective PG and SH achieve this by creating a 'histodilutional' barrier (Dupuy et al., 1988; Pihan and Szabo, 1988) and 'mucoid cap' (Wallace, 1988) by diluting the damaging agent in the perivascular space and limiting its penetration. This minimizes or prevents endothelial injury, maintains blood flow in subepithelial capillaries and ensures an energy-rich environment for rapid epithelial restitution to repair the superficial epithelial defect (Lacy and Ito, 1984; Leung, Robert and Guth, 1985; Tarnawski et al., 1985; Pihan et al., 1986). If the damage is deep (i.e. deep erosion or ulcer), cell proliferation or regeneration (e.g. epithelial cells, fibroblasts, angiogenesis) is also required to repair the mucosal defect. Epithelial restitution and regeneration thus extensively depend on vascular factors.

Studies of vascular factors have greatly contributed to our present advanced understanding of gastric mucosal injury and protection by drugs which do not affect gastric secretion (e.g. low doses of PG and SH). The present developments concerning vascular factors (Table 15.2) had such a widespread influence that now even investigators who earlier assigned little significance to vascular factors in gastric protection now consider maintenance of blood flow as a key event in mucosal protection (Robert, 1987; Silen, 1988). The Japanese school (e.g. Kitajima, Nagashima, Oda, Tsuchiya, Yabana) recognized the importance of microcirculatory changes in gastric ulcerogenesis some years ago (Tsuchiya et al., 1987).

The molecular and biochemical mechanisms of vascular injury and protection are nevertheless poorly understood. Blood vessels, especially capillaries and venules, can be damaged and protected by direct or indirect factors. Direct effects are produced by the chemicals and their metabolites. Indirect actions are induced when compounds or their metabolites cause the modification or liberation of vasoactive products. Sulphydryl compounds may then directly influence membrane permeability or enzymes in the endothelium, smooth muscle or deep epithelial cells, indirectly prevent the release of vasoactive substances (e.g. from mucosal and submucosal mast cells or macrophages), or hinder the access of exogenous damaging agents (e.g. epithelial and endothelial basement membrane). Mast cell degranulation accompanies ethanol-induced haemorrhagic erosions in the stomach (Bose, Brown and Szabo, 1985), thus supporting the idea that liberation of vasoactive products leads to gastric mucosal injury. Preventing the release (by cromolyn or doxantrazole) or action (by diphenylhydramine) of vasoactive substances from mast cells decreased the ethanol-induced mucosal lesions (Bose, Brown and Szabo, 1985). In addition, these erosions were significantly decreased in a mouse strain genetically deficient in mast cells (Galli, Bose and Szabo, 1985). One should recall that many receptors are SH-sensitive (e.g. cholinergic, adrenergic, dopaminergic) and the state of these membrane SH groups influences secretion, membrane permeability and enzyme activation.

Leukotrienes (e.g. LTC_4 or LTD_4) are much more potent at increasing vascular permeability when compared to biogenic amines (e.g. histamine, serotonin) and both are released when mast cells degranulate. Glutathione (GSH) is a precursor for leukotriene synthesis. The reaction involves the combination of LTA_4 and GSH by the enzyme glutathione-S-transferase. GSH levels have been shown to affect the synthesis of slow reacting substance, a crude form of leukotrienes. It is tempting to postulate that the gastric protective effect of GSH depletors such as DEM may be due, at least in part, to decreased production of certain leukotrienes because of the unavailability of GSH.

Proteases from the damaged epithelium and other cells as well as those released into the extracellular matrix by inflammatory cells have been shown to be SH sensitive (Khar, 1986). Inhibition of these proteases or their specific endogenous inhibitors could lead to protection or damage to the extracellular matrix respectively. One could envision a balance of protease activation with inhibition being offset in acute gastric mucosal injury. Thus, if the inhibitors were inactivated, the proteases could not be prevented from digesting the extracellular matrix, leading to tissue injury (Figure 15.3). On the other hand, if proteases themselves are inactivated, digestion of the extracellular matrix will not occur.

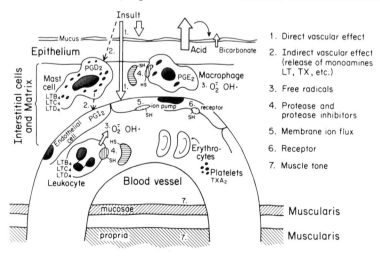

Figure 15.3 Interactions in gastric mucosal injury and protection, with special reference to the role of blood vessel and microcirculation. (The details of blood vessel are derived from a summary slide provided by Professor M. Tsuchiya, Tokyo, Japan)

This system of proteases and their inhibitors has been shown to be involved in lung injury (Campbell, Senior and Welgus, 1987) and, as our preliminary data indicate, in gastric mucosal damage as well.

Last, but not least, the smooth muscle in vessel walls, muscularis mucosae and muscularis propria (Figure 15.3) might have an important function in regulating blood flow to the mucosa. The end-artery models of gastric mucosal blood supply indicate a very important role for the muscularis mucosae since blood vessels cross it not only perpendicularly but also obliquely (Piasecki and Wyatt, 1986). The thin-walled veins seem to be especially sensitive to external compression. Indeed, after intragastric administration of damaging agents (e.g. concentrated ethanol, HCl, NaOH) mild to severe venoconstriction has been described in several studies (Pihan *et al.*, 1986; Oates and Hakkinen, 1988). In addition to endothelial injury caused by damaging chemicals and the released mediators (e.g. monoamines, leukotrienes) smooth muscle contraction at the outflow seems to also contribute to severe mucosal congestion seen early after administration of gastrotoxic agents. Blood flow and motility thus seem to be closely connected.

MOTILITY FACTORS

Motility changes seem to contribute to the pathogenesis of both gastric and duodenal ulceration. Historically, only gastric motility as it relates to emptying of acid had been considered. New data, however, implicate motility alterations leading to congestive hypoxia in the gastric mucosa. The area of congestion actually seems to determine the localization of haemorrhagic injury; for example 10 ml of 100% ethanol, 0.6 mol l^{-1} HCl or 0.2 mol l^{-1} NaOH put in the rabbit stomach causes virtually no grossly visible lesions. Partial narrowing of intramural veins, on the other hand, produces haemorrhagic injury similar to that which these chemicals cause if administered in 1 ml into the rat stomach (Janicek *et al.*, 1988). Relieving the apparent muscular spasm by papaverine or related drugs prevents the acute haemorrhagic mucosal injury. Prostaglandin derivatives might also exert at least part of their gastric protective effects by this muscle relaxing action (Mersereau and Hinchey, 1980).

Duodenal ulceration is associated with motility alteration both in human studies and in animal models (Szabo, 1984; Szabo *et al.*, 1984; Pihan *et al.*, 1985; Takeuchi, Nishiwaki and Okabe, 1987). Motility controls fluid transfer in the proximal duodenum and it is thus not surprising that motility may have a role in duodenal ulceration. Furthermore, in patients with duodenal ulcer, abnormal peristaltic waves and intraluminal pressure have been recorded (Szabo, 1984; Pihan, Gallagher and Szabo, 1985).

At least two motility factors are of potential pathogenic value: gastric emptying and duodenal motility. The available studies indicate that gastric emptying of both solids and liquids is delayed by the duodenal ulcerogen cysteamine (Lichtenberger, Szabo and Reynolds, 1977). This seems to be due to decreased fundic motility and increased antral activity (Pihan *et al.*, 1985). The results from animal models, however, seem in contradiction with those obtained in duodenal ulcer patients in whom gastric emptying is either normal or accelerated (Malagelada and Larach, 1980). The human studies, however, have been performed in patients with well developed ulcers and not during ulceration. In fact, in rats with chronic duodenal ulcers induced by cysteamine, gastric emptying of liquids was either normal or accelerated. Thus, both in animal models and in humans, the acute changes in gastric emptying during ulceration might prevent further damage. The chronic motility alterations, on the other hand, are probably a response to the formation of the ulcer.

The duodenal motility changes are specific and caused only by cysteamine and propionitrile and not by the non-ulcerogen structural analogue ethanolamine (Pihan *et al.*, 1985). The changes consist of a dose-dependent disruption of the fasting migrating myoelectric complex, a marked and prolonged increase in the spiking activity which indicates a state of sustained hypermotility, and a decrease in the frequency of slow myoelectric waves (Pihan *et al.*, 1985). These motility alterations are suppressed by dopamine (Szabo *et al.*, 1984) (Figure 15.4) and

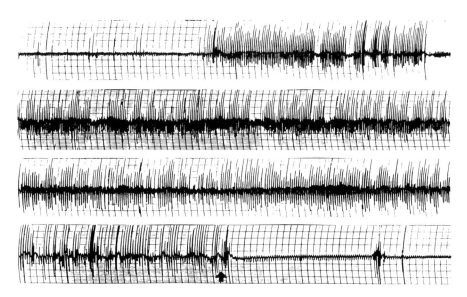

Figure 15.4 Recordings of myoelectric activity of proximal duodenum in fasted rat. Top row: slow waves of phase I (left) and spiking activity in phase III of control rat. Second and third rows: virtually continuous spiking activity after injection of cysteamine or propionitrile, respectively. Bottom row: sudden blockade of increased myoelectric activity in cysteamine-treated rat by start of dopamine infusion. (Reproduced with permission from Szabo *et al.* 1984)

this may be related to the relatively high number of dopamine binding sites in gastric and duodenal muscle, especially in comparison with the mucosa (Szabo *et al.*, 1982). These are important findings because the anti-ulcer effect of dopamine agonists is not dependent on their effects on gastric acid secretion (Gallagher, Brown and Szabo, 1987).

Further studies have revealed that, during the phase of hypermotility, the proximal to distal duodenal transit is faster and consequently the distal to proximal is slower which leads to a decrease in amount of pancreatic and biliary bicarbonate in the proximal duodenum (Szabo *et al.*, 1984; Pihan *et al.*, 1985). That delivery of pancreatic and biliary secretions can influence duodenal ulcerogenesis has been clearly demonstrated by experiments in which the pancreatic and/or biliary secretions have been re-routed to the proximal duodenum or distally into the jejunum, resulting in amelioration or aggravation of cysteamine-induced duodenal ulcers (Pihan *et al.*, 1985). The contribution of pancreatobiliary secretions to acid neutralization in the proximal duodenum is also demonstrated by the fact that more acid is recovered through an open proximal duodenal fistula (implanted at the sites where ulcers develop) when pancreatic secretions are drained, compared with when they are not (Gallagher and Szabo, 1984).

Duodenal dysmotility thus seems to play as important if not a more crucial role in the pathogenesis of duodenal ulceration than acid secretion since motility affects not only acid but bicarbonate secretion as well. Under normal conditions, the 'proper mix' of acid and base products is located near the pylorus, but either increased or decreased contractions of duodenal muscle seems to impair the delivery of pancreatic and biliary bicarbonate from the distal to the proximal duodenum, resulting in a 'misplaced mix' of neutralization (Figure 15.5) (Szabo, 1984; Szabo *et al.*, 1984; Takeuchi, Nishiwaki and Okabe, 1987). Taking into consideration motility factors thus helps to explore the acid-sensitivity of duodenal ulcers even in patients in whom gastric secretion is normal or below the usual amount. As studies with animal models revealed, 5–10 times higher activity can be demonstrated at the site of duodenal ulceration if delivery of bicarbonate from the distal duodenum is impaired (Gallagher and Szabo, 1984). The pharmacological sensitivity of this duodenal dysmotility for example to dopamine-like drugs (Szabo *et al.*, 1984; Takeuchi, Nishiwaki and Okabe, 1987), offers a new therapeutic or preventive approach to ulcer disease.

COMPARATIVE PHARMACOLOGY OF CELL-SPECIFIC AND TISSUE-SPECIFIC APPROACH TO ULCER DISEASE

The basic principle of any pharmacological (medical as opposed to surgical) treatment or prevention is to achieve a high degree of specificity with minimal or no side-effects. This criterion has been largely satisfied by the new

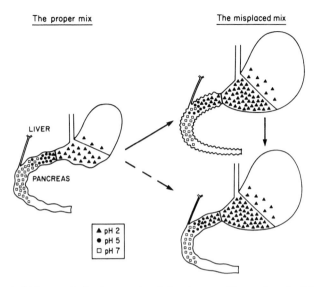

The proper mix   The misplaced mix

LIVER

PANCREAS

▲ pH 2
● pH 5
□ pH 7

Figure 15.5 Acid-base mix in the proximal duodenum. (Reproduced with permission from Szabo, 1984)

antisecretory agents introduced during the last 10 years. Thus, receptor antagonism (e.g. histamine H_2-receptors) and enzyme inhibition (e.g. $^+H,^+K$-ATPase) usually ensure a high degree of specificity (Table 15.3). Modulation of membrane transports or potential is less specific, although it may be enhanced by making it tissue-specific (e.g. affecting only certain nerve terminals or smooth muscle). Chemical scavenging (e.g. by SH and non-SH antioxidants) and chemical neutralization (e.g. of gastric acid) are the least specific, though useful, approaches. For centuries, neutralization of secreted gastric acid had been the only therapeutic option to relieve ulcer pain. Furthermore, scavenging of the multiple and chemically toxic free radicals (e.g. superoxide, hydroxyl, singlet

Table 15.3 Mechanisms of action of anti-ulcer agents

Mechanism	Example	Specificity
Receptor antagonism	Cimetidine, ranitidine	+ + +
Enzyme inhibition	Omeprazole	+ + +
Membrane transport (e.g. secretion, absorption)	Prostaglandins, metals, fatty acids, phospholipids	+ +
Membrane potential (e.g. nerve, muscle)	Domperidone, metoclopramide	+ +
Chemical scavenging	Sulphydryls, non-SH anti-oxidants	+
Chemical neutralization	Antacids	+

oxygen) may be a very beneficial approach when dealing with the type of gastric mucosal injury where such a pathogenic pathway is operational and substantial (e.g. 'stress ulceration').

An alternative analysis of cellular-oriented pharmacology of ulcer disease is based on single or multiple mechanisms of action (Table 15.4). Most of the anti-ulcer drugs used until now act through a single mechanism by affecting only one cell type and only one function in the stomach. The emerging new 'cytoprotective' or 'gastroprotective' drugs, on the other hand, exert multiple mechanisms of action (Table 15.4) and among these only prostaglandins and dopamine might inhibit gastric acid secretion under certain conditions. The accumulating clinical evidence with CBS (colloidal bismuth subcitrate) (De-Nol) and sucralfate indicates that, without modifying gastric acid, these drugs achieve healing rates of gastric and duodenal ulcers comparable to the efficacy of H_2-antagonists or antacids (Bianchi Porro, 1985; Brooks, 1985; Marks and Samloff, 1985). Furthermore, CBS and sucralfate exert gastroprotection which cannot be proved with cimetidine and ranitidine. These facts alone underscore the validity of an alternative approach (Szabo and Bynum, 1988) to ulcer disease despite our lack of understanding as to which, if any, of the known mechanisms contributes most to their mechanism of action. The frequent objection that drugs with multiple mechanisms are not significantly better in treating this multifactorial ulcer disease compared with single-action drugs is not valid on ethical grounds and because of restrictions in study design. Hence, in all the comparative studies the dosage of all the drugs is chosen to achieve maximal or submaximal healing or pain-relief rates (e.g. 85–95%), which cannot be enhanced in a statistically significant manner without enlisting a huge number of patients. If the dose and thus healing rates of single mechanism of action drugs were adjusted to around 50%, a statistically significant superiority of multiple-action drugs should be demonstrable.

Table 15.4 Single versus multiple effects of mediators and modulators of gastroduodenal ulcers

	Actions
Single	
Antacids*	HCl neutralization
H_2-receptor antagonists	HCl secretion
ATPase inhibitors	HCl secretion
Polyamines	Cell proliferation
Growth factors*	Cell growth and proliferation
Multiple	
CBS, sucralfate	Pepsin, mucus secretion, blood flow
Prostaglandins	HCl, HCO_3^-, mucus secretion, blood flow
Sulphydryls	Free radical scavenging, mucus secretion, blood flow
Dopamine	HCl, pepsin, HCO_3^- secretion, blood flow, motility

*New data indicate additional actions

The experimental drugs, e.g. prostaglandins, SH compounds and dopamine-derivatives, with their multiplicity of gastroprotection and anti-ulcer effects, deserve special attention (Table 15.4). In addition to further mechanistic pharmacological studies, clinical studies are needed with these new agents. In the meantime, we propose to use a mechanistic classification of anti-ulcer drugs (Szabo and Bynum, 1988) (Table 15.5). If the mechanism of action can be defined biochemically, chemical categories may be established, while if the mode of action is unknown descriptive morphologic terms such as 'cytoprotection' or 'organoprotection' may be used.

SUMMARY

Among the many cell types in the gastric mucosa, historically only the parietal cell was the subject of intensive pharmacological research. Consequently, drugs that neutralize luminal acid and inhibit its secretion have been developed. These drugs, however, have not solved the problem of ulcer disease, since although the healing rates are very high (e.g. 85–95%), recurrence rates are also substantial (30–50% during the first year after stopping treatment with H_2-antagonists). New cellular pharmacological targets include the mucous cells which secrete mucus and bicarbonate and the vascular endothelium which is crucial in regulating permeability and blood flow. Smooth muscle and motility also affect mucosal blood flow, thus recent studies indicate that muscular compression of venules seems to contribute, in addition to endothelial injury, to the vascular congestion after intragastric administration of gastrotoxic chemicals. In the future, motility factors should include not only gastric but duodenal emptying as well, since the site of acid–base mix and neutralization is also affected by duodenal motility. Drugs of the future for such a multifactorial or pluricausal

Table 15.5 Mechanistic classification of anti-ulcer agents

Mechanism of action clarified or suspected (defined by biochemical process or target)	Unknown mechanism(s) of action (defined in morphologic terms by structural target)
Antisecretory agents (e.g. HCl, pepsin)	Cytoprotection
Prosecretory agents (e.g. HCO_3^-, mucus)	Histoprotection (e.g. vasoprotection)
Neutralizing drugs (e.g. antacids)	Organoprotection (e.g. gastroprotection, enteroprotection)
Antioxidants (e.g. free radical scavengers)	
Oxidizing agents (e.g. mild stimulants, metals)	

Modified from Szabo and Bynum (1988)

disorder as ulcer disease should include compounds with multiple actions and high-specificity local effects, acting on the basis of aetiology and pathogenic elements.

REFERENCES

Allen, A. and Garner, A. (1980). Mucus and bicarbonate secretion in the stomach and their possible role in mucosal protection, *Gut*, **21**, 249–62.

Bianchi Porro, G. (ed.) (1985). DeNol: a new concept in cytoprotection, *Scand. J. Gastroenterol.*, **21** (Suppl. 122), 1–54.

Bose, R., Brown, A. and Szabo, S. (1985). Histochemical and pharmacological studies related to mast cells with ethanol- or aspirin-induced gastric erosions, *Fed. Proc.*, **44**, 733.

Brooks, F. P. (1985). The pathophysiology of peptic ulcer: an overview. In F. P. Brooks, S. Cohen and R. D. Soloway (eds) *Peptic Ulcer Disease*, Churchill Livingstone, New York, pp. 45–149.

Campbell, E. J., Senior, R. M. and Welgus, H. G. (1987). Extracellular matrix injury during lung inflammation, *Chest*, **92**, 161–9.

Dupuy, D., Kronague, J. F., Jones, A. G. and Szabo, S. (1988). Gastric mucosal protection may be mediated through increases in vascular permeability which create a histodilutional barrier, *Gastroenterology*, **94**, A615.

Durant, G. J. (1987). Histamine H_2 receptor antagonists as gastric acid secretion inhibitors. In S. Szabo and G. Mozsik (eds) *New Pharmacology of Ulcer Disease*, Elsevier, New York, pp. 264–77.

Flemström, G. and Garner, A. (1982). Gastroduodenal HCO_3-transport: characteristics and proposed role in acidity regulation and mucosal protection, *Am. J. Physiol.*, **242**, G183–93.

Gallagher, G. T. and Szabo, S. (1984). Direct measurement of duodenal acid–pepsin exposure at the site of ulceration in rats, *Am. J. Physiol.*, **246**, G5660–5.

Gallagher, G. T., Brown, A. and Szabo, S. (1987). Effect of dopamine-related drugs on duodenal ulcer induced by cysteamine or propionitrile: prevention and aggravation may not be mediated by gastrointestinal secretory changes in the rat, *J. Pharmacol. Exp. Ther.*, **240**, 883–9.

Galli, S. J., Bose, R. and Szabo, S. (1985). Mast cell-dependent augmentation of ethanol-induced acute gastric damage in mice, *Dig. Dis. Sci.*, **30**, 375.

Janicek, M., Hollenberg, M. K., Lin, Y. S. and Szabo, S. (1988). Area of congestion in angiography and rise of intravenous pressure determine the localization and extent of chemically-induced gastric mucosal injury, *Gastroenterology*, **94**, A206.

Kayasseh, L. and Gyr, K. (1987). Clinical aspects of somatostatin in ulcer disease. In S. Szabo and G. Mozsik (eds) *New Pharmacology of Ulcer Disease*, Elsevier, New York, pp. 360–8.

Khar, A. (1986). Activation of collagenase production in a rat macrophage-like cell line, *Biochem. Int.*, **13**, 565–70.

Lacy, E. R. and Ito, S. (1984). Rapid epithelial restitution in the rat gastric mucosa after ethanol injury, *Lab. Invest.*, **51**, 573–83.

Leung, F. W., Robert, A. and Guth, P. H. (1985). Gastric mucosal blood flow in rats after administration of 16,16-dimethyl prostaglandin E_2 at a cytoprotective dose, *Gastroenterology*, **88**, 1948–53.

Lichtenberger, L. M., Szabo, S. and Reynolds, E. S. (1977). Gastric emptying in the rat is inhibited by the duodenal ulcerogens, cysteamine and propionitrile, *Gastroenterology*, **73**, 1072–6.

Malagelada, J. R. and Larach, J. R. (1980). Gastric emptying in duodenal ulcer, *Scand. J. Gastroenterol.*, **15**, 115–30.

Marks, I. N. and Samloff, I. M. (eds) (1985). Sucralfate in peptic ulcer and gastritis: a worldwide view, *Am. J. Med.*, **79**(2C), 1–64.

Mersereau, W. A. and Hinchey, E. J. (1980). Prevention of indomethacin-induced gastric hypercontractility: a mucosal protective mechanism of prostaglandin E_2, *Gastroenterology*, **78**, 1221.

Oates, P. J. and Hakkinen, J. P. (1988). Studies on the mechanism of ethanol-induced gastric damage in rats, *Gastroenterology*, **94**, 10–21.

Piasecki, C. and Wyatt, C. (1986). Patterns of blood supply to the gastric mucosa: a comparative study revealing an end-artery model, *J. Anat.*, **149**, 21–39.

Pihan, G. and Szabo, S. (1988). 16,16-DMPGE$_2$ and thiosulfate decrease gastric mucosal penetration in hypertonic NaCl and increase net transmucosal water flux, *Gastroenterology*, **94**, A354.

Pihan, G., Gallagher, G. T. and Szabo, S. (1985). Biliary and pancreatic secretions influence experimental duodenal ulcer without affecting gastric secretion in the rat, *Dig. Dis. Sci.*, **30**, 240–6.

Pihan, G., Kline, T. J., Hollenberg, N. K. and Szabo, S. (1985). Duodenal ulcerogens cysteamine and propionitrile induce gastroduodenal motility alterations in the rat, *Gastroenterology*, **88**, 989–97.

Pihan, G., Majzoubi, D., Haudenschild, C., Trier, J. S. and Szabo, S. (1986). Early microcirculatory stasis in acute gastric mucosal injury in the rat and prevention by 16,16-dimethyl prostaglandin E_2 or sodium thiosulfate, *Gastroenterology*, **91**, 1415–26.

Robert, A. (1979). Cytoprotection by prostaglandins, *Gastroenterology*, **77**, 761–7.

Robert, A. (1987). Gastric antisecretory, antiulcer, and cytoprotective properties of prostaglandins. In S. Szabo and G. Mozsik (eds) *New Pharmacology of Ulcer Disease*, Elsevier, New York, pp. 322–8.

Silen, W. (1988). What is cytoprotection of the gastric mucosa?, *Gastroenterology*, **94**, 232–5.

Szabo, S. (1984). Biology of disease—pathogenesis of duodenal ulcer disease, *Lab. Invest.*, **51**, 121–47.

Szabo, S. (1986). Mechanisms of mucosal injury in the stomach and duodenum: time-sequence analysis of morphologic functional, biochemical and histochemical studies, *Scand. J. Gastroenterol.*, **22** (Suppl. 127), 21–8.

Szabo, S. and Bynum, T. E. (1988). Alternatives to the acid-oriented approach to ulcer disease: does 'cytoprotection' exist in man? A new classification of antiulcer agents, *Scand. J. Gastroenterol.*, **23**, 1–6.

Szabo, S. and Trier, J. S. (1984). Pathogenesis of acute gastric mucosal injury: sulfhydryls as a protector, andrenal cortex as a modulator, and vascular endothelium as a target. In A. Allen, G. Flemström, A. Garner, W. Silen and L. A. Turnberg (eds) *Mechanisms of Mucosal Protection in the Upper Gastrointestinal Tract*, Raven Press, New York, pp. 287–93.

Szabo, S. and Usadel, K. H. (1982). Cytoprotection–organoprotection by somatostatin: gastric and hepatic lesions, *Experientia*, **38**, 254–5.

Szabo, S., Pihan, G. and Trier, J. S. (1986). Alterations in blood vessels during gastric injury and protection, *Scand. J. Gastroenterol.*, **21** (Suppl. 125), 92–6.

Szabo, S., Sandrock, A. W., Nafradi, J., Maull, E. A., Gallagher, G. T. and Blyzniuk, A. (1982). Dopamine and dopamine receptors in the gut—their possible role in duodenal ulceration. In M. Kohsaka, T. Shohmori, Y. Tsukada and G. N. Woodruff (eds) *Advances in Dopamine Research*, Pergamon Press, New York, pp. 165–70.

Szabo, S., Pihan, G., Gallagher, G. T. and Brown, A. (1984). Role of local secretory and motility changes in the pathogenesis of experimental duodenal ulceration, *Scand. J. Gastroenterol.*, **19** (Suppl. 92), 106–11.

Szabo, S., Trier, J. S., Brown, A. and Schnoor, J. Jr (195). Early vascular injury and increased permeability in gastric mucosal injury caused by ethanol in the rat, *Gastroenterology*, **88**, 228–36.

Takeuchi, K., Nishiwaki, H. and Okabe, S. (1987). Role of local motility changes in the pathogenesis of duodenal ulcers induced by cysteamine in rats, *Dig. Dis. Sci.*, **32**, 295–304.

Takeuchi, K. and Nobuhara, Y. (1985). Inhibition of gastric motor activity by 16,16-dimethyl prostaglandin E_2, *Dig. Dis. Sci.*, **30**, 1181–8.

Tarnawski, A., Hollander, D., Stachura, J., Krause, W. J. and Gergely, H. (1985). Prostaglandin protection of the gastric mucosa against alcohol injury — a dynamic time-related process, *Gastroenterology*, **88**, 334–52.

Tsuchiya, M., Ansano, M., Mishima, Y. and Oda, M. (eds) (1987). *Microcirculation: An Update*, Elsevier, Amsterdam.

Wallace, J. L. (1988). Increased resistance of the rat gastric mucosa to hemorrhagic damage after exposure to an irritant: role of the 'mucoid cap' and prostaglandin synthesis, *Gastroenterology*, **94**, 22–32.

Advances in Drug Therapy of Gastrointestinal Ulceration
Edited by A. Garner and B. J. R. Whittle
©1989 John Wiley & Sons Ltd

Chapter Sixteen

Stress Ulceration and Mucosal Acid–Base Balance

Rudolf Schiessel

1st Clinic of Surgery, University Hospital, A-1090 Vienna, Austria

STRESS ULCER: THE CLINICAL SITUATION

Stress ulceration of the stomach and duodenum are epithelial defects of the mucosa that penetrate as far as the submucosa or the lamina propria. The mucosal defects can appear either as multiple small erosions or as single large ulcerations. The development of such lesions occurs usually within a few hours after burns, polytrauma, big operations, apoplexia and sepsis. We know from prospective studies with routine endoscopy that the incidence of stress ulcers ranged between 80 and 100% in burns, polytrauma and sepsis before the era of routine prophylaxis (Table 16.1).

Acute stress lesions are still a serious threat to a severely ill patient, because complications such as bleeding and perforation are common. For this reason, several clinical trials have been undertaken to study different forms of

Table 16.1 Incidence of stress lesions: prospective studies with routine endoscopy

Nature of stress	Number of patients (*n*)	Incidence of Mucosal lesion (%)	Incidence of Bleeding (%)	Reference
Burns	32	86	22	Czaja, McAlhany and Pruitt (1974)
Polytrauma	38	97	42	Schiessel *et al.* (1978)
Sepsis	14	100	68	Le Gall *et al.* (1976)
Apoplexia	177	52	19	Kitamura and Ho (1976)
Renal transplant	28	28	7	Schiessel *et al.* (1981)

prophylactic therapy to reduce especially the risk of bleeding. The first series of trials compared the effect of antacids versus placebo (Table 16.2). McAlhany, Czaja and Pruitt (1976) and Hastings *et al.* (1978) showed a significant reduction in the frequency of stress ulcer bleeding in burn patients and intensive-care patients, respectively. In other series of trials, cimetidine has been evaluated against placebo (Table 16.3). Thus, McDougall, Bailey and Williams (1977) showed a significant reduction in the bleeding frequency in patients with liver failure; Halloran *et al.* (1980) showed a significant reduction of the bleeding frequency in brain trauma; while Lorenz *et al.* (1980) demonstrated a similar effect in polytrauma. However, a trial from our group (Schiessel *et al.*, 1981) showed no effect in patients after renal transplantation.

A further series of trials has compared the effects of cimetidine with those of antacids (Table 16.4). Three groups showed no difference between cimetidine

Table 16.2 Treatment of stress bleeding: antacids versus placebo

Nature of stress	Treatment	Number of patients (*n*)	Number of cases of bleeding	Reference
Burns	Antacid	24	1*	McAlhany, Czaja and
	Placebo	24	6	Pruitt (1976)
ICU	Antacid	51	2*	Hastings *et al.* (1978)
	Placebo	49	12	

*$P<0.05$

Table 16.3 Treatment of stress bleeding: cimetidine versus placebo

Nature of stress	Treatment	Dose (g)	Number of patients *n*	Number of cases of Bleeding	Blood loss (ml)	Reference
Liver failure	Cimetidine	2.4	26	1	—	McDougall,
	Placebo		24	13*		Bailey and
						Williams
						(1977)
Brain injury	Cimetidine	1.8	26	5	18	Halloran *et al.*
	Placebo		24	18*	21	(1980)
Brain injury	Cimetidine	1.0	10	0	0	Silvestri *et al.*
	Placebo		10	0	70*	(1980)
Polytrauma	Cimetidine	1.2	14	0	—	Lorenz *et al.*
	Placebo		14	5*	—	(1980)
Renal transplant	Cimetidine	1.6	27	3	27	Schiessel *et al.*
	Placebo		28	2	28	(1981)

*$P<0.05$

Table 16.4 Treatment of stress bleeding: cimetidine versus antacids

	Treatment	Dose	Number of patients (n)	Number of cases of Bleeding	Blood loss (ml)	Reference
Burns	Cimetidine	1.6 g	13	0	30	McElwee,
	Antacid	15 ml h^{-1}	14	0	79*	Sirinek and Levine (1979)
ICU	Cimetidine	1.2 g	65	1	—	Stothert *et al.*
	Antacid	30–60 ml h^{-1}	58	0	—	(1980)
ICU	Cimetidine	1.8 g	40	3	—	Martin, Max
	Antacid	60 ml h^{-1}	37	2	—	and Polk (1980)
ICU	Cimetidine	1.2–2.4 g	38	7	—	Priebe *et al.*
	Antacid	30–120 ml h^{-1}	37	0*	—	(1980)

*$P < 0.05$

and antacid treatment on the frequency of bleeding (McElwee, Sirinek and Levine, 1979; Stothert *et al.*, 1980; Martin, Max and Polk, 1980). Only the study by Priebe *et al.* (1980) has shown a significantly lower bleeding frequency in the antacid group. A trial by Zinner *et al.* (1981) with intensive-care patients also showed a better result with antacids than with cimetidine or placebo. In a similar trial by Basso *et al.* (1981), cimetidine and antacids were equally active in reducing the bleeding frequency and more effective than placebo.

From these studies, we have learned that antacids, as well as cimetidine and ranitidine, can reduce the incidence of stress ulcer bleeding in comparison to placebo. In a recent review of 16 clinical trials (Shuman, Schuster and Zuckerman, 1987), 2133 patients were evaluated. The frequency of bleeding was 15% with placebo, whereas in patients receiving antacids this frequency was 3.3%, and in those given cimetidine it was 2.8%. There have, however, been several problems associated with increasing the pH of the gastric contents. It has been shown that the reduction of the H$^+$ ion concentration in gastric juice leads to bacterial contamination, which is linearly correlated with the pH (Moulin *et al.*, 1982). Thus, the higher the pH in the stomach, the higher is the bacterial count. In addition, it has been shown that the same type of bacteria found in the stomach can also be cultivated from the tracheobronchial tree. From this finding, it has been proposed that gastrobronchial reflux in intensive-care patients may lead to severe pulmonary infections. To overcome this problem, several trials have been conducted with substances that do not influence gastric pH. Skillman *et al.* (1984) published a study on intensive-care patients comparing (15R)-15-methyl-PGE$_2$ with antacid. The results were disappointing, however, since antacid was more effective than the prostaglandin. Furthermore, van Essen *et al.* (1985) showed no difference between PGE$_2$ and placebo.

Levine, Sirinek and Gaskill (1985) used prostaglandins in a study on gastric bleeding resulting from erosions, but no difference between placebo and 15-methyl-PGE$_2$ could be demonstrated. Thus, no clinical study has yet shown that PGE is effective in stress ulcer prophylaxis.

Recently, trials have been conducted with sucralfate, a substance that can stimulate endogenous prostaglandin biosynthesis. Borrero et al. (1985) published a study comparing antacid with sucralfate which showed no difference between these agents. Tryba et al. (1985) compared sucralfate, antacid and cimetidine and showed no difference between the three groups. Recently, a study published by Driks et al. (1987) has shown that the incidence of nosocomial pneumonia was much lower in intubated patients given sucralfate as compared with antacids or H$_2$-blockers. In that study of a total of 130 patients given mechanical ventilation in an intensive-care unit, the incidence of stress ulcer bleeding was nearly equal in the sucralfate group and the antacid, H$_2$-blocker group. Although the rate of nosocomial pneumonia was reduced, the results did not reach statistical significance with the same being found in respect of mortality.

In our institution, the incidence of stress ulceration has decreased from about 20 cases per year to just two cases in 1986. These data are derived from an intensive care unit with 250 patients per year. The composition of the patients has not changed over the years. Two factors may have contributed to this decrease: firstly, routine prophylaxis with H$_2$-blockers and antacids; secondly, better understanding of the pathophysiology of this syndrome.

PATHOPHYSIOLOGY OF STRESS ULCER

For many years it was assumed that an overproduction of acid was the main reason for the development of stress ulceration. More recently, the mechanisms allowing the mucosa to withstand the enormous H$^+$ ion concentration gradient between the lumen and the cells on the surface have been identified. It is now assumed that an imbalance between the aggressive factors, hydrochloric acid and pepsin, and the protective mechanisms of the stomach and the duodenum causes acute ulceration. The most important factors in the stomach are:

(1) the impermeability of the mucosa to H$^+$ ions,
(2) mucus,
(3) alkaline secretion,
(4) blood flow,
(5) secretory state,
(6) intracellular pH regulation,
(7) rapid epithelial restitution.

In the duodenum, the most important factors are:

(1) mucus,
(2) alkaline secretion,
(3) blood flow,
(4) intraluminal buffering,
(5) intracellular pH regulation,
(6) rapid epithelial restitution.

Role of mucosal blood flow and bicarbonate

The following section focuses on the two main factors influencing mucosal acid–base balance, namely blood flow and the role of bicarbonate. The role of blood flow is not only to transport oxygen and substrates to the mucosa, but also to remove H^+ ions and to bring bicarbonate to the mucosa. The importance of blood flow for acid–base balance was clearly demonstrated in experiments in which the pH of the lamina propria was measured with a microelectrode in the anaesthetized rabbit. At the same time, mucosal blood flow was measured with microspheres (Starlinger et al., 1981a,b). When the gastric lumen was perfused with acid, the intramural pH dropped for a short time, but then returned to baseline. However, during this period, mucosal blood flow had substantially increased. When this mechanism was blocked with vasopressin, gross ulceration of the stomach became visible. The increase in mucosal blood flow correlated well with the luminal acid concentration. From these results, we assumed that H^+ back-diffusion stimulated an autoregulatory mechanism causing an increase in mucosal blood flow. A similar mechanism was found to operate in the duodenum (Starlinger et al., 1987).

In another series of experiments, we investigated the effects of shock on the gastric mucosa. When the rat stomach is filled with acid and the rat is subjected to shock, ulceration occurs over 100% of the mucosal surface. Treatment of the rats with prostacyclin resulted in recovery of gastric mucosal blood flow to control levels but, despite normal blood flow, the stomachs still ulcerated. When the shocked rats were treated with parenteral bicarbonate, the stomachs did not ulcerate, despite a very low mucosal blood flow. With TRIS buffer, ulceration could also be avoided. In addition, when a carbonic anhydrase inhibitor was used, parenteral bicarbonate was no longer effective in preventing damage (Starlinger et al. 1981b).

These results clearly indicated that it is the availability of bicarbonate that is the critical factor in the development of lesions under conditions of reduced blood flow, rather than the limited supply of oxygen or substrates per se. There are no data available about the dependence of gastric bicarbonate secretion in the lumen on mucosal blood flow. However, experiments in our laboratory have clearly demonstrated that changes in blood flow are directly related to changes in alkaline secretion from the duodenal mucosa (Schiessel et al., 1984). When the bicarbonate delivery, expressed as bicarbonate ion concentration × blood flow, was plotted against alkaline secretion, the curve demonstrated a saturable process. Thus alkaline secretion is to some degree dependent on bicarbonate delivery to the mucosa. Continuation of these experiments showed that the mucosal tolerance of the duodenum to luminal acid is dependent on the amount of alkaline secretion. Thus, inhibition of alkaline secretion with metabolic acidosis caused severe damage, whereas stimulation of alkaline secretion with glucagon or bicarbonate infusions caused minimal damage to the mucosa (Wenzl *et al.*, 1987). From these experiments, we obtained a linear correlation between the amount of alkaline secretion and the amount of damage caused by luminal acid.

In the stomach, bicarbonate comes from two sources: plasma bicarbonate and bicarbonate from the oxyntic cells ('alkaline tide') resulting from acid production by parietal cells (Figure 16.1). O'Brien and Silen (1976) first discovered that the acid tolerance of an inhibited gastric mucosa was much lower than that of a histamine-stimulated mucosa. In further experiments, we demonstrated that the reason for the lower acid tolerance is bicarbonate deficiency. The reduced acid tolerance *in vitro*, shown by a decrease in potential difference and short-circuit current could be overcome by a high bicarbonate concentration in the nutrient bathing solution (Schiessel *et al.*, 1980). On the other hand, removal of bicarbonate did not affect histamine-stimulated tissues, whereas inhibited tissues showed a drastic fall in potential difference. Interestingly, Gannon *et al.* (1984) have demonstrated that there are small vessels coming from the gastric glands which go up to the surface, and which seem to be the pathway for bicarbonate delivery from parietal to surface cells.

Bicarbonate is not only important for protection of the mucosa, but also for the repair process. In recent experiments on the duodenal mucosa, we have found that, after mucosal damage with luminal acid, alkaline secretion is increased

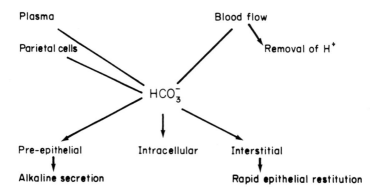

Figure 16.1 Determinants of gastric mucosal acid–base balance. HCO_3^- has a central role for the protection of the gastric mucosa

(Vattay *et al.*, 1988), as shown in Figure 16.2. The repair process after damage requires about 5 h (Feil *et al.* 1987). The mucosal defects are bridged by migration of the remaining, viable cells. This process operates even at a luminal pH of 3. When we removed the necrotic layer of cells and mucus after damage, we found that the process of epithelial restitution was inhibited. However, when we substituted bicarbonate with HEPES in the nutrient solution, alkaline secretion after damage and the repair process were almost completely inhibited (Figures 16.3 and 16.4). This study therefore demonstrates that the availability of bicarbonate is also important for the repair process in the mucosa, which occur in response to damage.

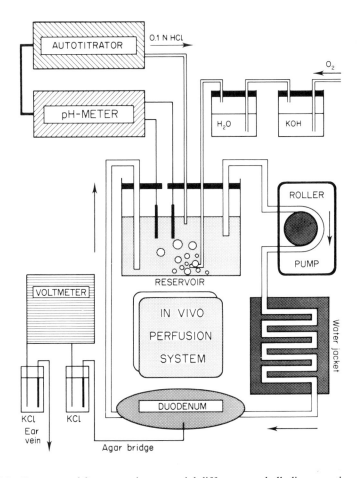

Figure 16.2 System used for measuring potential difference and alkaline secretion during damage and repair of duodenal mucosa *in vitro*

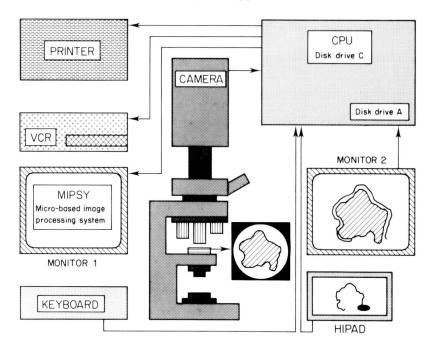

Figure 16.3 Computer-based morphometry to quantitate damage and repair of the duodenum

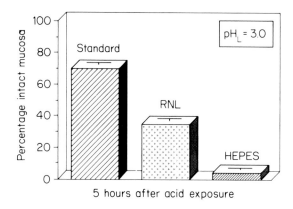

5 hours after acid exposure

Figure 16.4 Epithelial restitution in the rabbit duodenum *in vitro* following a 5 h exposure to acid (luminal pH 3). Removal of the necrotic layer (RNL) or of HCO_3^- from nutrient solution in exchange for HEPES results in inhibition of epithelial restitution. Results are expressed as mean ± s.e.m.

REFERENCES

Basso, N., Bagarani, M., Materia, A., Fiorani, S., Lunardi, P. and Speranza, V. (1981). Cimetidine and antacid prophylaxis of acute upper gastrointestinal bleeding in high risk patients, *Am. J. Surg.*, **141**, 339–41.

Borrero, E., Bank, S., Margolis, I., Schulman, N. D. and Chardavoyne, R. (1985). Comparison of antacid and sucralfate in the prevention of gastrointestinal bleeding in patients who are critically ill, *Am. J. Med.*, **7** (Suppl. 2C), 62–4.

Czaja, A. J., McAlhany, J. C., Pruitt, B. A. (1974). Acute gastroduodenal disease after thermal injury: an endoscopic evaluation of incidence and natural history, *New Engl. J. Med.*, **291**, 925–9.

Driks, M. R., Craven, D. E., Colli, B. R. *et al.* (1987). Nosocomial pneumonia in intubated patients given sucralfate as compared with antacids or histamine type 2 blockers: the role of gastric colonization, *New Engl. J. Med.*, **317**, 1376–82.

Feil, W., Wenzl, E., Vattay, P., Starlinger, M., Sogukoglu, T. and Schiessel, R. (1987). Repair of rabbit duodenal mucosa after acid injury *in vivo* and *in vitro*, *Gastroenterology*, **92**, 1973–86.

Gannon, B., Browning, J., O'Brien, P. and Rogers, P. (1984). Mucosal microvascular architecture of the fundus and body of human stomach, *Gastroenterology*, **86**, 866–75.

Halloran, L.G., Zfass, A. M., Gayle, W. E., Wheeler, C. B. and Miller, J. D. (1980). Prevention of acute gastrointestinal complications after severe head injury: a controlled trial of cimetidine prophylaxis, *Am. J. Surg.*, **139**, 44–8.

Hastings, P. R., Skillmann, J. J., Bushnell, L. S. and Silen, W. (1978). Antacid titration in the prevention of acute gastrointestinal bleeding: a controlled randomized trial in 100 critically ill patients, *New Engl. J. Med.*, **298**, 1041–5.

Kitamura, T. and Ho, K. (1976). Acute gastric changes in patients with acute stroke. Part 1: With reference to gastroendoscopic findings, *Stroke*, **7**, 460–3.

Le Gall, J. R., Mignon, F. C., Rapin, M. *et al.* (1976). Acute gastroduodenal lesion related to severe sepsis, *Surg. Gynecol. Obstet.*, **142**, 377–80.

Levine, B. A., Sirinek, K. R. and Gaskill, H. V. (1985). Topical prostaglandin E_2 in the treatment of acute upper gastrointestinal tract hemorrhage: a prospective, randomized, double-blind study, *Arch. Surg.*, **120**, 600–4.

Lorenz, W., Fischer, M., Rhode, H., Troidl, H., Reimann, H. J. and Obmann, C. (1980). Histamine and stress ulcer: new components in organizing a sequential trial of cimetidine prophylaxis in seriously ill patients and definition of a special group at risk (severe polytrauma), *Klin. Wochenschr.*, **58**, 653–65.

McAlhany, J. C. Jr, Czaja, A. J. and Pruitt, B. A. (1976). Antacid control of complications from acute gastroduodenal disease after burns, *J. Trauma*, **16**, 645–9.

McDougall, B. R. D., Bailey, R. J. and Williams, R. (1977). H_2-receptor antagonists and antacids in the prevention of acute gastrointestinal hemorrhage in fulminant hepatic failure: two controlled trials, *Lancet*, **i**, 617–19.

McElwee, H. P., Sirinek, K. R. and Levine, B. A. (1979). Cimetidine affords protection equal to antacids in prevention of stress ulceration following thermal injury, *Surgery*, **86**, 620–5.

Martin, L. F., Max, M. H. and Polk, H. C. Jr. (1980). Failure of gastric pH control by antacids or cimetidine in the critically ill: a valid sign of sepsis, *Surgery*, **88**, 59–66.

Moulin, G. C. du, Patenson, D. G., Hedley-White, J. and Lisbon, A. (1982). Aspiration of gastric bacteria in antacid-treated patients: a frequent cause of postoperative colonisation of the airway, *Lancet*, **i**, 242–5.

O'Brien, P. and Silen, W. (1986). Influence of acid secretory state on the gastric mucosal tolerance to back diffusion of H^+, *Gastroenterology*, **92**, 1973–86.

Priebe, H. J., Skillmann, J. J., Bushnell, L. S., Lang, P. C. and Silen, W. (1980). Antacid versus cimetidine in preventing acute gastrointestinal bleeding: a randomized trial in 75 critically ill patients, *New Engl. J. Med.*, **302**, 426–30.

Schiessel, R., Deisenhammer, N., Opitz, A. *et al.* (1978). Stressveränderungen des Magens und Duodenums bei Mehrfachverletzten: Ergebnis einer prospektiven Studie. In E. Wayland and P. Brücke (eds) *Kongressbericht der Österr.Ges.f.Chirurgie*, Egermann Verlag, Vienna, pp. 53–6.

Schiessel, R., Merhav, A., Matthews, J. B., Fleischer, L., Barzilai, A. and Silen, W. (1980). Role of nutrient HCO_3^- in protection of amphibian gastric mucosa, *Am. J. Physiol.*, **239**, G536–42.

Schiessel, R., Starlinger, M., Wolf, A. *et al.* (1981). Failure of cimetidine to prevent gastroduodenal ulceration and bleeding after renal transplantation, *Surgery*, **90**, 456–8.

Schiessel, R., Starlinger, M., Kovats, E., Appel, W., Feil, W. and Simon, A. (1984). Alkaline secretion of rabbit duodenum *in vivo*: its dependence on acid base balance and mucosal blood flow. In A. Allen *et al.* (eds) *Mechanisms of Mucosal Protection in the Upper Gastrointestinal Tract*, Raven Press, New York, pp. 267–71.

Shuman, R. B., Schuster, D. P. and Zuckerman, G. R. (1987). Prophylactic therapy for stress ulcer bleeding: a reappraisal, *Ann. Int. Med.*, **104**, 562–7.

Silvestri, N., Curzio, M., Motta, M., Pletrio, P. de, Bonanzina, F. and Minoja, G. (1980). Cimetidine to prevent stress ulcers, *Lancet*, **i**, 885.

Skillmann, J. J., Lisbon, A., Long, P. C. and Silen, W. (1984). 15(R)-15-Methyl-prostaglandin E_2 does not prevent gastrointestinal bleeding in seriously ill patients, *Am. J. Surg.*, **147**, 451–5.

Starlinger, M., Schiessel, R., Hung, C. K. and Silen, W. (1981a). H^+ back diffusion stimulating gastric mucosal blood flow in the rabbit fundus, *Surgery*, **89**, 232–6.

Starlinger, M., Jakesz, R., Matthews, J. B., Yoon, C. and Schiessel, R. (1981b). The relative importance of HCO_3^- and blood flow in the protection of rat gastric mucosa during shock, *Gastroenterology*, **81**, 732–5.

Starlinger, M., Matthews, J. B., Yoon, C., Wenzl, E., Feil, W. and Schiessel, R. (1987). The effect of acid perfusion on mucosal blood flow and intramural pH of rabbit duodenum, *Surgery*, **101**, 433–8.

Stothert, J. C., Simonowitz, D. A., Dellinger, E. P. *et al.* (1980). Randomized prospective evaluation of cimetidine and antacid control of gastric pH in the critically ill, *Ann. Surg.*, **192**, 169–74.

Tryba, M., Zervounov, F., Torok, M. and Zenz, M. (1985). Prevention of acute stress bleeding with sucralfate, antacids or cimetidine, *Am. J. Med.*, **79** (Suppl. 26), 55–61.

van Essen, H. A., van Blankenstein, M., Wilson, J. H. P., van den Berg, B. and Bruining, H. A. (1985). Intragastric prostaglandin E_2 and the prevention of gastrointestinal hemorrhage in ICU patients, *Crit. Care Med.*, **13**, 957–60.

Vattay, P., Feil, W., Klimesch, S., Wenzl, E., Starlinger, M. and Schiessel, R. (1988). Acid stimulated alkaline secretion in the rabbit duodenum is passive and correlates with mucosal damage, *Gut*, **29**, 284–90.

Wenzl, E., Feil, W., Starlinger, M. and Schiessel, R. (1987). Alkaline secretion: a protective mechanism against acid injury in rabbit duodenum, *Gastroenterology*, **92**, 709–15.

Zinner, M. J., Zuidema, G. D., Smith, P. L. and Mignosa, M. (1981). The prevention of upper gastrointestinal tract bleeding in patients in an intensive care unit, *Surg. Gynecol. Obstet.*, **153**, 214–20.

Advances in Drug Therapy of Gastrointestinal Ulceration
Edited by A. Garner and B. J. R. Whittle
©1989 John Wiley & Sons Ltd

Chapter Seventeen

Peptide Control Systems of the Gut as Therapeutic Targets

G. J. Dockray

MRC Secretory Control Research Group, Department of Physiology, University of Liverpool, Liverpool L69 3BX, UK

INTRODUCTION

Until about 15 years ago, hormonal mechanisms were thought to be the only way that peptides regulated digestion, that is to say they were delivered to their targets in the blood stream. The well known actions of gastrin, secretin and cholecystokinin on gastric and pancreatic secretion, and on gall bladder contraction, were considered to be models of this type of control system. There have been several important developments since that time in our ideas of how peptides regulate gut function. For example, it is now clearly recognized that peptides released from gut endocrine cells can also act on neighbouring cells in local or paracrine control systems, and that gut neurones can make and release a wide variety of peptides that have neurotransmitter-like actions. The same or closely related groups of peptides can function in each type of control system. Moreover, it is now clear beyond any reasonable doubt that a single peptide does not have exclusive control over any particular aspect of gastrointestinal function (for reviews see Dockray, 1987; Walsh, 1987). Instead it is apparent that interactions between regulatory peptides and other transmitters, e.g. paracrine agents such as histamine and the prostaglandins, and neurotransmitters like acetylcholine and noradrenaline are of primary importance in the control of the gut. The widespread involvement of peptides in the regulation of digestion would appear at first sight to justify the idea that manipulation of these systems might provide scope for treating disorders of the gut; set against this, however, are obvious problems in developing drugs of the appropriate specificity.

The development of drugs that can be used to manipulate regulatory peptide systems has, until recently, been slow. In part, this is attributable to the fact that peptides are relatively complex molecules and the chemistry needed to produce analogues is elaborate. In addition, most peptides are relatively rapidly degraded in the body and are not readily absorbed intact by the gut mucosa. In recent years, however, good progress has been made with the elucidation of structure–activity relationships, and several novel drugs, including non-peptides, that act on regulatory peptide systems have been developed. The present account will focus on general aspects of organization of peptide-producing systems, and potential sites at which drugs might influence these systems; the role that peptides play in upper gastrointestinal function, and therefore the scope for applications of novel pharmacologically active compounds; and, finally, recent progress in the development of antagonists for peptides of the gastrin-cholecystokinin group.

ORGANIZATION OF PEPTIDERGIC SYSTEMS

By analogy with other systems, it is possible to conceive of potentially useful drugs that influence peptide synthesis, degradation or action. These mechanisms are essentially similar for peptides working through the endocrine, paracrine and neurotransmitter modes; the differences between these systems are largely limited to the time and distance over which a particular peptide acts.

Biosynthesis

Regulatory peptides are synthesized initially as large precursor molecules, which are converted, usually within their cells of origin, to smaller forms. The genes encoding most of the major gut peptides have now been cloned and the nucleotide base sequences of the precursor peptides have been determined. In principle, this should make it possible to bring molecular biological methods to experimental, diagnostic and therapeutic problems of regulatory peptides in gut disease. For the most part, these possibilities have not yet been exploited.

The pyloric antral hormone, gastrin, has been intensively studied and offers a convenient illustration of biosynthetic mechanisms (see Dockray and Gregory, 1989, for review). The initial precursor is a molecule of 101 (man) or 104 (pig) residues; there is a signal sequence of 21 amino acid residues which is rapidly cleaved leaving (in man) progastrin or preprogastrin 22–101 (Figure 17.1). The major steps leading to the production of biologically active material take place in the Golgi and in immature secretory granules. They include cleavage of the chain, and amidation of the C-terminus of the major active form, G17. Other post-translational modifications include tyrosine sulphation (which also occurs in cholecystokinin (CCK) where it is essential for biological activity) and serine phosphorylation. The phosphorylation site is immediately adjacent to the cleavage point that subsequently yields the biologically important C-terminus

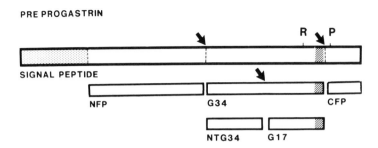

Figure 17.1 Schematic representation of the gastrin precursor showing cleavage points (arrows), sulphation (R) and phosphorylation (P) sites. Major biologically active products are G17 and G34. The signal sequence is removed rapidly. In antral mucosa, post-translational processing generates G17 as the predominant product; in human duodenal gastrin cells G34 is the main product. In some gastrinomas there are large quantities of unprocessed progastrin. Both sulphated and unsulphated gastrins occur naturally

of G17 (Figure 17.2); phosphorylation sites are also found in similar positions in the precursors of several other peptides (Dockray *et al.*, 1987).

Within individual cells expressing the gastrin gene, there are differences in processing so that the final products are distributed in cell-specific patterns. In antral gastrin cells the major products are G17, C- and N-terminal flanking peptides, and the N-terminal tryptic peptide of G34; in human duodenal gastrin cells G34 occurs as a major product, but in some gastrinomas there is little or no cleavage of the precursor and intact progastrin predominates (Pauwels *et al.*, 1986). In these gastrinoma cells, therefore, the primary product does not even possess the normal biological activity of the hormone. This is not an isolated instance associated with neoplastic cells; there are other examples where the primary product of a particular cell is apparently inactive. In the case of the opioid peptides, many central neurones expressing the proenkephalin A gene process the precursor to yield active opioid peptides (Leu and Met-enkephalin and C-terminally extended variants, Met-enkephalin $Arg^6Gly^7Leu^8$ and Met-enkephalin Arg^6Phe^7). However, in bovine adrenal chromaffin cells, larger inactive forms predominate. We have recently found a number of similarities in enkephalin biosynthesis between bovine adrenal chromaffin cells and opiate-producing neurons and endocrine cells of the pig antrum and duodenum, where inactive peptides including N-terminally extended forms of Met-enkephalin $Arg^6Gly^7Leu^8$ and Met-enkephalin Arg^6Phe^7 appear to predominate (Watkinson and Dockray, unpublished observations). The importance of these differences for present purposes is that they indicate that biosynthetic processing events are likely to be regulated and consequently that pharmacological intervention in the regulatory pathway is a possibility, albeit a presently remote one. The factors that determine the selection of different processing pathways are still largely unknown. One possibility is that serine phosphorylation might have a

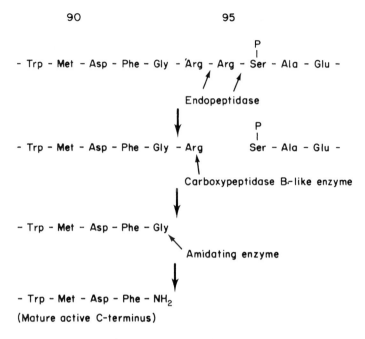

Figure 17.2   Important steps leading to the production of the biologically active C-terminal end of G17 and G34. There is an initial endopeptidase cleavage between Arg residues or between Arg and the phosphorylation site. Carboxypeptidase B-like cleavage generates a Gly-extended intermediate which is the substrate for an amidating enzyme which produces the active amidated peptide

regulatory role in determining processing, but direct evidence is still needed for this. Characterization of the enzymes involved in cleavage of the chain, amidation and phosphorylation ought to be a practical first step in exploiting the biosynthetic pathway as a target for therapeutic control of hormone production.

Metabolism

The idea that there might be specific degrading enzymes for different peptides has fallen from favour in recent years. Instead, there is now considerable evidence to suggest that a common group of proteolytic enzymes might degrade a wide variety of regulatory peptides. Two enzymes that appear to degrade many small active peptides and that have been relatively well studied are peptidyl dipeptidase (angiotensin converting enzyme) and neutral endopeptidase 24.11 (also known as enkephalinase). These are widely distributed and act on many different substrates, and in both instances inhibitors are available. Endopeptidase 24.11 cleaves peptide bonds to the N-terminus of hydrophobic aminoacid residues. Recent studies suggest that in pig it is involved in the cleavage of G17, at or soon after secretion; thus administration of an inhibitor (phosphoramidon) resulted in the appearance of material in the antral venous outflow that had the chromatographic and immunochemical properties of intact G17, whereas in control animals the major products were a complex mixture of C-terminal immunoreactive G17 fragments (Power *et al.*, 1987). Moreover, in man, the main products of G17 metabolism found in the circulation during infusion of G17 were the same as those produced by *in vitro* incubation of the synthetic peptide with purified endopeptidase 24.11 as shown in Figure 17.3 (Deschodt-Lanckman *et al.*, 1988). Bado *et al.* (1987) have reported that an inhibitor of this enzyme, acetorphan, increased acid secretion from Heidenhain pouches in cat, which would be compatible with preservation of circulating G17. The mechanisms are complex, however, because acetorphan also depressed the acid secretory response of the Heidenhain pouch and gastric fistula to pentagastrin. In the case of the gastric fistula response this effect was reversed by naloxone, suggesting an opioid-mediated inhibition of acid secretion (Bado *et al.*, 1987). It is evident from these results that inhibition of endopeptidase 24.11 could depress acid secretion by blocking degradation of peptide inhibitors of acid secretion, or might increase secretion by prolonging the effects of gastric acid stimulants. Studies of the proteases for gut peptides are plainly still at an early

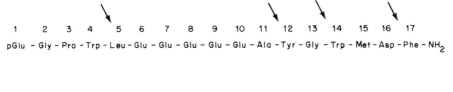

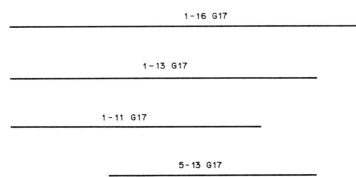

Figure 17.3 Major metabolic cleavage sites in G17. Neutral endopeptidase 24.11 cleaves G17 to the N-terminal side of hydrophobic residues, i.e. Trp⁴Leu⁵, Ala¹¹Tyr¹², Gly¹³Trp¹⁴, and Asp¹⁶Phe¹⁷. Some of the major intermediates and products are found in plasma during infusion of G17 in man, namely 1–11 G17, 1–13 G17, 1–16 G17 and 5–13 G17. In experimental animals there is evidence that inhibitors of endopeptidase 24.11 delay G17 metabolism

stage, but in trying to assess whether or not these enzymes are a potentially useful therapeutic target the central question is whether they show the appropriate selectivity. The presently available evidence is not encouraging on this point.

In a number of instances it has been possible to obtain degradation-resistant analogues of active peptides. Amongst the peptides with gastrointestinal actions, particularly good illustrations of this approach are provided by somatostatin analogues (Figure 17.4). One of these, SMS 201-995 (Bauer *et al.*, 1982), has been used by a number of centres for clinical studies (Long, 1987). There are potential applications of these and similar somatostatin analogues in the control of gastro-intestinal bleeding, and in the management of carcinoid patients and patients with endocrine tumours of the pancreas. Hormone secretion is inhibited in the latter patients with amelioration of symptoms, and in some cases with tumour regression.

Receptors

Early studies of the structure–activity relationships of gut peptides, particularly gastrin, seemed to indicate that it might be difficult to obtain antagonists.

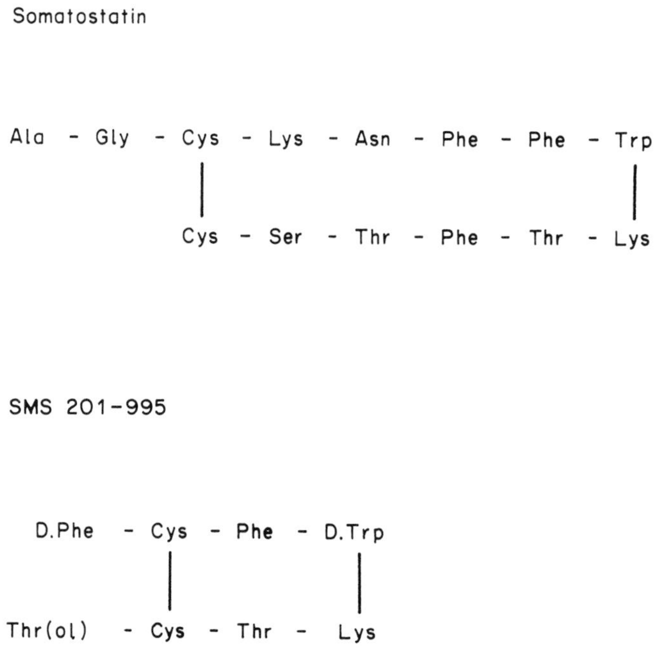

Somatostatin

```
Ala  - Gly  - Cys  - Lys  - Asn  - Phe  - Phe  - Trp
               |                                  |
             Cys  - Ser  - Thr  - Phe  - Thr  - Lys
```

SMS 201-995

```
D.Phe   - Cys  - Phe  - D.Trp
             |             |
Thr(ol)  - Cys  - Thr  - Lys
```

Figure 17.4 The structure of somatostatin and an analogue SMS 201-995, which is a long-acting agonist and has been used in the treatment of patients with endocrine tumours of the pancreas and carcinoid tumours

There is now abundant evidence, however, that peptide antagonists can be obtained for any of a variety of different peptides, although in the case of the gut peptides only a few of these have so far proved to be useful (Table 17.1). Substituted analogues, particularly with D-residues, have yielded antagonists of vasoactive intestinal peptide, substance P and gastrin-releasing peptide (GRP) (Waelbroeck *et al.*, 1985; Pandol *et al.*, 1986; Heinz-Erian *et al.*, 1987). For the most part, the application of these antagonists has been limited to *in vitro* experimental studies or local administration *in vivo*. Most of these compounds have relatively low affinity and it is unlikely that they will be of clinical value.

Recently there has been good progress with the development of CCK antagonists; in particular, antagonists for the peripheral CCK type of receptor suitable for *in vivo* applications are now available. The development and application of these drugs is covered in more detail below.

PEPTIDES AND THE CONTROL OF GASTRIC FUNCTION

A detailed review of the role of regulatory peptides in the control of gastric function is beyond the scope of this account. It will, however, be useful to summarize the role of peptides in gastric function as it relates to ulcer disease with the object of identifying potential targets for novel compounds acting on regulatory peptide control systems.

Table 17.1 Peptide analogues of gut peptides with potentially useful pharmacological properties

Peptide	Analogue	Properties
CCK	(des-Phe) CCK8 amide*	Antagonist on stomach, brain and pancreatic acinar cells
GRP	D-Phe^{12} bombesin analogues	Antagonist on pancreatic acinar cells
VIP	(N-Ac Tyr^1, D-Phe^2) GRF 1–29 amide, (4 Cl-D-Phe^{6}Leu^{17}) VIP	Antagonists on pancreatic acinar cells
Somatostatin	SMS 201-995	Long-acting agonist
Opioid peptides	D-Ala^2, MePhe^4, Gly-ol^6 enkephalin	μ-selective agonist
	D-Pen^2, D-Pen^5 enkephalin	δ-selective agonist
Substance P	D-Arg^1, D-Pro^2, D-Trp^{7,9} Leu^{11}, SP	Antagonist (also interacts with GRP receptors on pancreatic acinar cells)

*See also Table 17.2

Acid-secreting mucosa

Many of the known gut peptides either increase or decrease acid secretion, but most of these actions are not physiological. On present evidence, the stimulation of acid secretion by gastrin is one of the three primary drives to the parietal cell, the others being acetylcholine and histamine (Figure 17.5). In the dog, a species which has been intensively studied, all three are able to stimulate parietal cells directly, and there is a potentiating interaction between them. In other species, e.g. the rabbit, gastrin may act through the release of histamine (Soll, 1987). The role of somatostatin in the inhibition of acid secretion is a good example of paracrine control. Plainly gastrin antagonists or somatostatin agonists might have a potential application in the control of gastric acid secretion. Both might have special advantages in the treatment of patients with increased acid secretion due to hyper-gastrinaemia, either from gastrinomas or from G-cell hyperfunction (Dockray and Calam, 1989). Beyond this, however, it is not immediately clear whether control of acid secretion by manipulation of gastrin or somatostatin offers advantages over the presently available approaches, including for example histamine H_2-receptor antagonist therapy. There may, however, be special advantages in the use of gastrin antagonists as antitrophic factors (see below).

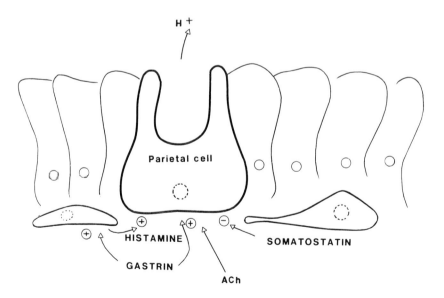

Figure 17.5 Interaction of peptides and other factors in the control of parietal cell function. Gastrin, together with histamine and acetylcholine, stimulates acid secretion; gastrin may also release histamine. Somatostatin inhibits acid secretion

Pyloric antral mucosa

The control of gastrin release in the pyloric antral part of the stomach reflects the interplay of luminal, nervous and paracrine control mechanisms (Figure 17.6). Polypeptides and amino acids in the lumen release gastrin; acid in the lumen inhibits gastrin release (Dockray and Gregory, 1989). The cellular and molecular mechanisms involved in mediating these effects are still poorly understood. Several observations support the idea that somatostatin acts locally in the antral mucosa to depress gastrin release. Thus, somatostatin is released by acid and is known to inhibit secretion of gastrin as well as other hormones. Moreover, neutralizing antibodies to somatostatin enhance gastrin release. It is reasonable to suppose that somatostatin plays a part in paracrine inhibition of gastrin release in response to luminal acid. Nervous control mechanisms play an important part in gastrin release both early in digesting a meal (cephalic phase) and later in the gastric phase; there is evidence for local cholinergic muscarinic control mechanisms, but there are also important non-cholinergic neurotransmitters that release gastrin. The best candidate for the latter is GRP, which is the mammalian counterpart of bombesin. GRP occurs in gastric mucosal nerve fibres, is released by nerve stimulation, and stimulates gastrin release.

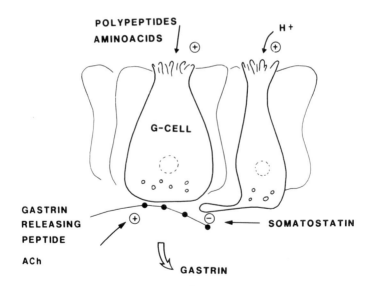

Figure 17.6 Interaction of peptides and other factors in the control of gastrin cell function. Gastrin is released by luminal chemicals (polypeptides, amino acids), and the peptide neurotransmitter GRP; somatostatin is released by luminal acid and suppresses gastrin secretion. Long-term inhibition of acid secretion leads to an increased number of gastrin cells, and to increased activity

Trophic effects

Inhibition of gastric secretion is a primary therapeutic objective in most treatments of peptic ulcer. Because acid inhibits gastrin release, it is not surprising to find enhanced plasma gastrin following treatment with inhibitors of acid secretion. A prolonged decrease in gastric acid secretion, e.g. by drugs that inhibit the parietal cell or by surgical manipulation (vagotomy, fundusectomy, etc.), is also associated with an increase in G-cell numbers. The consequences are also strikingly apparent in patients with achlorhydria who after several years develop a marked G-cell hyperplasia and increased basal and stimulated gastrin release. In these conditions antral acidification can partially, but not completely, reverse the elevated plasma gastrin. The mechanisms involved are uncertain. One possibility is that normal G-cell function reflects a balance between the stimulatory actions of GRP and the inhibitory actions of somatostatin, and that in the absence of acid-evoked release of somatostatin the drive on the G-cell by GRP is enhanced. It is known that GRP is mitogenic to several cell types, so that this mechanism could account both for increased G-cell numbers and gastrin release. The mechanisms are important because gastrin is trophic to the body of the stomach. In conditions associated with hypergastrinaemia, there is a tendency to develop enterochromaffin-like (ECL) hyperplasia (Hakanson, Ekelund and Sundler, 1984; Larsson *et al.*, 1986). There has been some debate about the possible mechanisms involved, but given the well established trophic effect of gastrin it is reasonable to postulate that gastrin is responsible for the ECL cell hyperplasia. However, the precise site and mechanism of action of gastrin and the specificity of the receptor are still unknown. The development of an antagonist for this action of gastrin is of obvious importance.

Motility

The rate of gastric emptying determines the delivery of acid to the duodenum. Mechanisms activated from the duodenum regulate gastric emptying of liquids by control of the pylorus and of the pressure gradient between the body of the stomach and the duodenum. In some species, opioid peptides control the sphincter and opiate antagonists enhance gastric emptying (Dockray, 1987). CCK released by fat and protein inhibits gastric emptying and CCK antagonists increase gastric emptying. These effects could be mediated either by direct actions on the pylorus or by indirect effects producing relaxation of the body of the stomach. Although there is evidence of increased emptying rates in duodenal ulcer, the evidence does not suggest that this is due to a failure of the CCK mechanism.

Mucosal protection

Detailed accounts of mucosal protection mechanisms appear elsewhere in this volume. Two facets are of relevance here. First, a number of peptides are able to either increase (glucagon, CCK) or decrease (GRP) bicarbonate secretion from gastric mucosa *in vitro* and so have potential regulatory roles in protective mechanisms (Flemström, Heylings and Garner, 1982). For the present, however, prostaglandins would appear to offer more profitable opportunities for controlling this system. Second, there is now evidence that the extrinsic afferent innervation of the gut helps protect against ulcerogenic stimuli. Thus, rats pretreated soon after birth with capsaicin (which selectively lesions small-diameter primary afferents) are more prone to develop haemorrhagic lesions of the gastric mucosa in response to any of a variety of ulcerogenic stimuli (Holzer and Sametz, 1986). It seems possible that the peripheral terminals of afferent nerve fibres exert a protective role in the mucosa. These fibres contain substance P and calcitonin gene-related peptide (Green and Dockray, 1988), both of which are potent vasodilators. One possibility is that peripheral release of these peptides increases local mucosal blood flow which has a protective effect. For the present, however, the therapeutic potential in manipulating this mechanism remains remote.

ANTAGONISTS OF CCK–GASTRIN-RELATED PEPTIDES

The progress made with the development of antagonists to the CCK–gastrin group of peptides has been impressive. The lessons may also be valuable in comparable studies with other peptides. It is still only quite recently that orally active antagonists have been available, and the impact of these compounds in experimental studies has so far been greater than that in the clinic.

Gastrin–CCK receptors

Radioligand binding studies and structure–activity studies suggest the occurrence of several different receptors for the gastrin–CCK group of peptides. On pancreatic acinar cells CCK interacts with receptors that show high affinity for molecules with a sulphated tyrosine at position 7 from the C-terminus; gastrin (sulphated or unsulphated) and desulphated CCK have 1000 times lower affinity than CCK at this target. Essentially similar specificity is found for CCK-stimulated gall bladder contraction, guinea-pig ileum contraction, and relaxation of the rat stomach. These effects are mediated by the so-called peripheral CCK receptor. The central CCK receptor shows an affinity for gastrin, or desulphated CCK, only 10–100 fold lower than that for sulphated CCK. This receptor is thought to mediate most CNS effects of CCK, although in the nucleus tractus solitarius and interpeduncular nucleus there are peripheral-type receptors. The so-called gastrin receptor found on dog parietal cell shows little or no discrimination between gastrin and CCK. Within this broad classification there is evidence of different subclasses of receptors. Of the presently available drugs, some are antagonists at all three receptor subtypes, and others show marked preference for the peripheral CCK receptor.

Discovery of CCK antagonists

The discovery of non-peptide CCK antagonists originated with the finding by Peikin, Costenbader and Gardner (1979) that dibutyryl cyclic guanosine monophosphate (Bt_2cGMP) acted as a competitive antagonist of CCK effects on the pancreas. The concentrations required for inhibition of CCK-stimulated pancreatic secretion were relatively high and perhaps not surprisingly Bt_2cGMP has not been useful for *in vivo* work. The same group subsequently discovered several other types of CCK antagonist, e.g. proglumide (Figure 17.7) and benzotript (Hahne *et al.*, 1981). Proglumide, in particular, has been quite widely used in experimental studies. This is a glutaramic acid derivative; it has a relatively low potency and needs to be used in the low millimolar range. Proglumide also has poor selectivity, and appears not to discriminate between peripheral and central CCK receptors or gastrin receptors (Table 17.2). More recently developed proglumide-related peptides include CR 1409 which has greatly increased potency and shows selectivity for peripheral CCK receptors (Makovec *et al.*, 1986). In addition, other recently developed proglumide-related compounds show some selectivity between pancreas and gall bladder CCK receptors, suggesting subclasses of the peripheral CCK receptor (Jensen *et al.*,

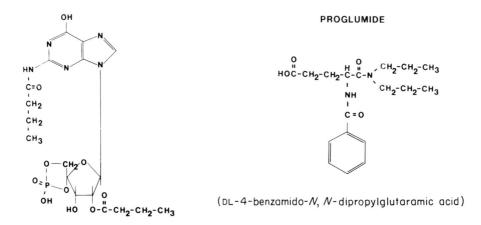

Figure 17.7 Structures of the CCK antagonists dibutyryl cyclic guanosine monophosphate (Bt_2cGMP) and proglumide

Table 17.2 Properties of antagonists of the CCK–gastrin group

Compound	Identity	Concentration for 50% inhibition*		
		Pancreas	Brain	Stomach
Proglumide	Glutaramic acid derivative	0.2–6 mmol l^{-1}	0.8–10 mmol l^{-1}	1 mmol l^{-1}
Bt$_2$cGMP	Cyclic nucleotide	30–90 μmol l^{-1}	1.6–2.3 mmol l^{-1}	1–2 mmol l^{-1}
(des Phe) CCK8 amide	Peptide	2–3.5 μmol l^{-1}	3–80 μmol l^{-1}	—
CR 1409	Proglumide derivative	18–130 nmol l^{-1}	0.2–2.2 μmol l^{-1}	2 μmol l^{-1}
Asperlicin	Mold metabolite	0.18–1.4 μmol l^{-1}	>100 μmol l^{-1}	>100 μmol l^{-1}
L-364 718	Benzodiazepine-related	80 pmol l^{-1}	245 nmol l^{-1}	300 nmol l^{-1}

*Compiled from Vigna, Szecowka and Williams (1985), Makovec *et al.* (1986), Chang *et al.* (1985), Chang and Lotti (1986). Based on competition with ^{125}I-labelled CCK8 or CCK33 for binding to guinea-pig or rat pancreas acinar cells, guinea-pig or mouse brain membrane and ^{125}I-labelled gastrin binding to guinea-pig gastric glands

1986). These compounds have already proved useful in a variety of ways, not least in defining more precisely different subclasses of receptor for the gastrin and CCK family of peptides.

Peptide antagonists

Following the characterization of proglumide and benzotript as CCK antagonists, Spanarkel *et al.* (1983) reasoned that it might be possible to develop other peptide-based antagonists. They found that many derivatives of tryptophan acted as weak antagonists of the action of CCK on the exocrine pancreas. Particularly striking, however, was the finding that removal of the C-terminal Phe residue of CCK to give des-Phe CCK8 amide produced a relatively good antagonist. A range of shorter des-Phe analogues has also now been made. Some, including phenethyl ester derivatives of the C-terminal tetrapeptide, inhibit gastrin-stimulated acid secretion (Martinez and Bali, 1984; Martinez *et al.*, 1986). Most have not yet been fully characterized, but they would appear to have low selectivity (Vigna, Szecowka and Williams, 1985).

Asperlicin and 1,4-benzodiazepine-like antagonists

During a screen of microbial broths, Chang *et al.* (1985) discovered a mold metabolite, asperlicin, which was an antagonist of CCK action on pancreatic acinar cells. This compound had somewhat higher affinity than proglumide, but more importantly it proved to be the starting point for the development of CCK antagonists with improved selectivity. There is a similarity in structure between asperlicin and the benzodiazepines and, on this basis, Evans *et al.* (1986) screened a number of benzodiazepine analogues for CCK antagonist activity.

They discovered several antagonists, including L-364 718 which is active in the sub-micromolar range and shows selectivity for peripheral rather than central CCK receptors (Figure 17.8). It appears that L-364 718 does not interact with central benzodiazepine binding sites or for that matter with other well characterized neuronal receptors (Chang and Lotti, 1986).

L-364 718: pharmacology and importance for physiology

Binding studies suggest that L-364 718 is selective for peripheral type CCK receptors; at least 1000 times higher concentrations are needed for displacement of label at gastrin receptors or at central CCK receptors. It should be noted that L-364 718 is nevertheless active in brain and gastric mucosa at concentrations similar to those of the unselective antagonist proglumide. The selectivity of L-364 718 has made it particularly valuable for studies of CCK physiology. In recent years there has been controversy over the physiological significance of the classical actions of CCK in the stimulation of gall bladder contraction and in pancreatic enzyme secretion. At the same time other actions, notably inhibition

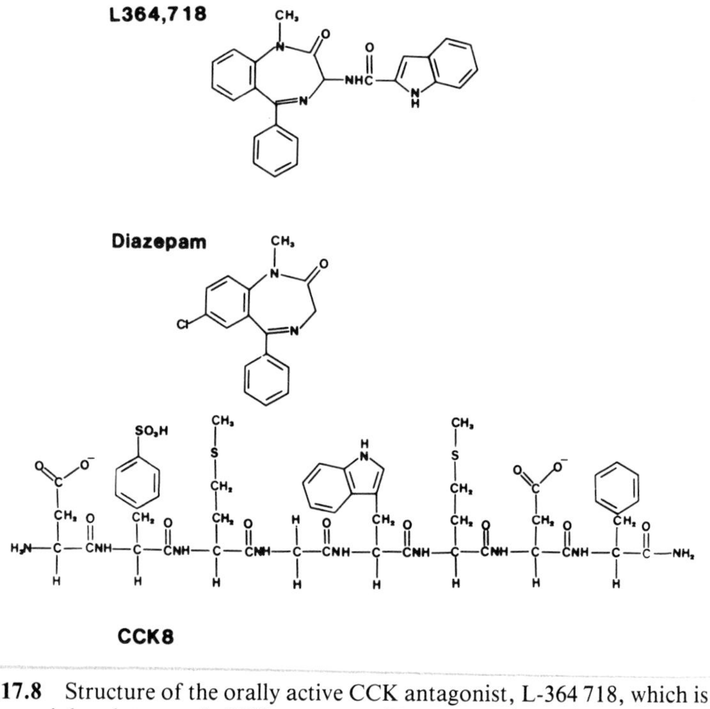

Figure 17.8 Structure of the orally active CCK antagonist, L-364 718, which is selective for the peripheral type of CCK receptor. For comparison the chemically related benzodiazepine, diazepam, and CCK8 are shown. L364 718 does not act at central benzodiazepine binding sites

of gastric emptying and inhibition of food intake, have attracted attention as potentially of physiological importance. The availability of good *in vivo* antagonists has now opened the way for critical studies of some of these problems.

Pendleton *et al.* (1987) showed that L-364 718 inhibited the action of exogenous CCK on gall bladder contraction, pancreatic enzyme secretion and gastric emptying in the dog. They also showed that it inhibited gall bladder contraction in response to a meal, suggesting a physiological role for endogenous CCK in mediating this effect. Surprisingly, however, pancreatic enzyme responses and the delay in gastric emptying produced by a test meal were not suppressed by L-364 718, suggesting that these responses were not CCK-mediated. In conscious gastric fistula rats, however, we have found that L-364 718 reverses the inhibition of gastric emptying of liquid meals containing peptone or a protease inhibitor, FOY-305, which releases CCK from the intestine by depressing the inhibitory action of proteases on CCK secretion (Dimaline, Dockray and Green, 1988). The specificity of the response was established by showing that hyperosmolal solutions and acid also depressed gastric emptying but these effects were not influenced by L-364 718 (Figure 17.9). In this preparation, then, it would appear that protein-rich meals delay gastric emptying by releasing CCK. It is not yet clear whether the different results in dog and rat are attributable to species differences in the physiological roles of CCK or to different experimental protocols. The target for CCK in producing inhibition of gastric emptying in the rat appears to be the vagal afferent innervation of the stomach. This is supported by recent findings that, in rats pretreated soon after birth with the sensory neurotoxin capsaicin, the action of protein, protease inhibitors and exogenous CCK on gastric emptying is impaired (Green and Dockray, unpublished observations). It would appear that CCK might act directly on the vagal afferents that mediate gastric mechanoreceptor discharge to produce a vagovagal relaxation of the body of the stomach.

OVERVIEW

Some progress has now been made with the development of long-acting, metabolism-resistant peptide analogues; for example, somatostatin analogues that have clinical applications. There are further possibilities for the development of novel drugs along these lines. In addition, the way forward in the development of antagonists to gut peptides is already clear from studies with CCK. In the immediate future, CCK antagonists are likely to have considerable impact on our view of the physiology of this and related peptides. It would also seem reasonable to explore the possible development of antagonists selective for gastrin receptors using the presently available compounds as a lead. Control of acid secretion is an obvious application of gastrin antagonists, but regulation

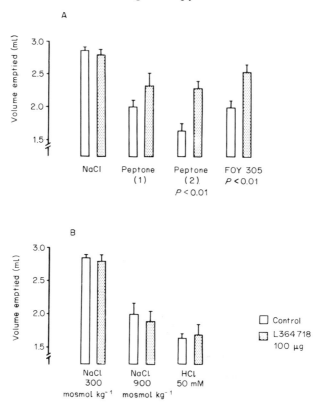

Figure 17.9 Inhibition of the action of two CCK-releasing liquid test meals on gastric emptying in the conscious gastric fistula rat by L-364 718. (A) Gastric emptying of peptone and the protease inhibitor FOY-305 is delayed compared with saline; peptone was studied both alone (1) and following a preload with peptone (2); for details see Dimaline, Dockray and Green (1988). (B) Hyperosmolal saline and acid also delay emptying. Prior administration of L-364 718 into the gastric fistula suppresses the action of peptone and FOY-305 but not hyperosmolal saline and acid

of the trophic effects of this hormone is also likely to be particularly rewarding. In view of the evidence associating present acid-inhibitory therapies with hypergastrinaemia and ECL cell hyperplasia, the scope for application of antitrophic gastrin antagonists needs no emphasis.

REFERENCES

Bado, A., Chicau-Chovet, M., Appia, F., Dubrasquet, M., Lecomte, J. M. and Roze, C. (1987). Acetorphan, an enkephalinase inhibitor, decreases gastric secretion in cats, *Peptides*, **8**, 89–93.

Bauer, W., Briner, U., Doepfner, W. *et al.* (1982). SMS 201-995: a very potent and selective octapeptide analogue of somatostatin with prolonged action, *Life Sci.*, **31**, 1133–40.

Chang, R. S. L. and Lotti, V. J. (1986). Biochemical and pharmacological characterization of an extremely potent and selective nonpeptide cholecystokinin antagonist, *Proc. Natl. Acad. Sci. USA*, **83**, 4923–6.

Chang, R. S. L., Lotti, V. J., Monaghan, R. L. *et al.* (1985). A potent nonpeptide cholecystokinin antagonist selective for peripheral tissues isolated from *Aspergillus alliaceus*, *Science*, **230**, 177–9.

Deschodt-Lanckman, M., Pauwels, S., Najdvoski, T., Dimaline, R. and Dockray, G. J. (1988). Degradation of heptadecapeptide gastrin by endopeptidase 24.11 *in vitro*, and identification of the products *in vivo*, *Gastroenterology*, **94**, 712–21.

Dimaline, R., Dockray, G. J. and Green, T. (1988). The action of the cholecystokinin antagonist L364,718 on gastric emptying in the rat, *J. Physiol.*, **396**, 17P.

Dockray, G. J. (1987). Physiology of enteric neuropeptides. In L. R. Johnson (ed.) *Physiology of the Gastrointestinal Tract*, 2nd edn, Raven Press, New York, pp. 41–66.

Dockray, G. J. and Calam, J. (1988). Peptic ulcer. In R. D. Cohen, K. G. M. M. Alberti, B. Lewis and A. M. Denman (eds) *The Metabolic and Molecular Basis of Acquired Disease*, Ballière Tindall. (In press)

Dockray, G. J. and Gregory, R. A. (1988). Gastrin. In G. M. Makhlouf (ed.) *Handbook of Physiology*, American Physiological Society. (In press)

Dockray, G. J., Varro, A., Desmond, H., Young, J., Gregory, H. and Gregory, R. A. (1987). Post-translational processing of the porcine gastrin precursor by phosphorylation of the COOH-terminal fragment, *J. Biol. Chem.*, **262**, 8643–7.

Evans, B. E., Bock, M. G., Rittle, K. E. *et al.* (1986). Design of potent, orally effective, nonpeptidal antagonists of the peptide hormone cholecystokinin, *Proc. Natl. Acad. Sci. USA*, **83**, 4918–22.

Flemström, G., Heylings, J. R. and Garner, A. (1982). Gastric and duodenal HCO_3^- transport *in vitro*: effects of hormones and local transmitters, *Am. J. Physiol.*, **242**, G100–10.

Green, T. and Dockray, G. J. (1988). Characterization of peptidergic afferent innervation of the stomach in rat, mouse and guinea pig, *Neuroscience*, **25**, 181–93.

Hakanson, R., Ekelund, M. and Sundler, F. (1984). Activation and proliferation of gastric endocrine cells. In S. Falkmer, R. Hakanson and F. Sundler (eds) *Evolution and Tumour Pathology of the Neuroendocrine System*, Elsevier, Amsterdam, pp. 371–98.

Hahne, W. F., Jensen, R. T., Lemp, G. F. and Gardner, J. D. (1981). Proglumide and benzotript: members of a different class of cholecystokinin receptor antagonists, *Proc. Natl. Acad. Sci. USA*, **78**, 6304–8.

Heinz-Erian, P., Coy, D. H., Tamura, M., Jones, S. W., Gardner, J. D. and Jensen, R. T. (1987). [D-Phe^{12}]bombesin analogues: a new class of bombesin receptor antagonists, *Am. J. Physiol.*, **252**, G439–42.

Holzer, P. and Sametz, W. (1986). Gastric mucosal protection against ulcerogenic factors in the rat mediated by capsaicin-sensitive afferent neurons, *Gastroenterology*, **91**, 975–81.

Jensen, R. T., Zhou, Z-C., Murphy, R. B. *et al.* (1986). Structural features of various proglumide-related cholecystokinin receptor antagonists, *Am. J. Physiol.*, **251**, G839–46.

Larsson, H., Carlsson, E., Mattson, H. *et al.* (1986). Plasma gastrin and gastric enterochromaffin-like activation and proliferation: studies with omeprazole and ranitidine in intact and antrectomized rats, *Gastroenterology*, **90**, 391–9.

Long, R. G. (1987). Review: long-acting somatostatin analogues, *Aliment. Pharmacol. Ther.*, **1**, 191–200.

Makovec, F., Bani, M., Chiste, R., Revel, L., Rovati, L. C. and Rovati, L. A. (1986). Differentiation of central and peripheral cholecystokinin receptors by new glutaramic acid derivatives with cholecystokinin-antagonist activity, *Arzneim. Forsch.*, **36**, 98–102.

Martinez, J. and Bali, J.-P. (1984). A new class of potent gastrin antagonists, *Reg. Peptides*, **9**, 259–62.

Martinez, J., Rodriguez, M., Bali, J.-P. and Laur, J. (1986). Phenethyl ester derivative analogues of the C-terminal tetrapeptide of gastrin as potent gastrin antagonists, *J. Med. Chem.*, **29**, 2201–6.

Pandol, S. J., Dharmsathaphorn, K., Schoeffield, M. S., Vale, W. and Rivier, J. (1986). Vasoactive intestinal peptide receptor antagonist [4Cl-D-Phe^6,Leu^{17}] VIP, *Am. J. Physiol.*, **250**, G553–7.

Pauwels, S., Desmond, H., Dimaline, R. and Dockray, G. J. (1986). Identification of progastrin in gastrinomas, antrum, and duodenum by a novel radioimmunoassay, *J. Clin. Invest.*, **77**, 376–81.

Peikin, S. R., Costenbader, C. L. and Gardner, J. D. (1979). Actions of derivatives of cyclic nucleotides on dispersed acini from guinea pig pancreas, *J. Biol. Chem.*, **254**, 5321–7.

Pendleton, R. G., Bendesky, R. J., Schaffer, L., Nolan, T. E., Gould, R. J. and Clinischmidt, B. V. (1987). Roles of endogenous cholecystokinin in biliary, pancreatic and gastric function: studies with L-364 718, a specific cholecystokinin receptor antagonist, *J. Pharmacol. Exp. Ther.*, **241**, 110–16.

Power, D. M., Bunnett, N., Turner, A. J. and Dimaline, R. (1987). Degradation of endogenous heptadecapeptide gastrin by endopeptidase 24.11 in the pig, *Am. J. Physiol.*, **253**, G33–9.

Soll, A. H. (1987). Review: antisecretory drugs — cellular mechanisms of action, *Aliment. Pharmacol. Ther.*, **1**, 77–89.

Spanarkel, M., Martinez, J., Briet, C., Jensen, R. T. and Gardner, J. D. (1983). Cholecystokinin 27–32 amide: a member of a new class of cholecystokinin receptor antagonists, *J. Biol. Chem.*, **258**, 6746–9.

Vigna, S. R., Szecowka, J. and Williams, J. A. (1985). Do antagonists of pancreatic cholecystokinin receptors interact with central nervous system cholecystokinin receptors?, *Brain Res.*, **343**, 394–7.

Waelbroeck, M., Robberecht, P., Coy, D. H., Camus, J-C., Neef, P. de and Christophe, J. (1985). Interaction of growth hormone-releasing factor (GRF) and 14 GRF analogs with vasoactive intestinal peptide (VIP) receptors of rat pancreas: discovery of (*N*-Ac-Tyr^1,D-Phe^2)-GRF (1–29)-NH$_2$ as a VIP antagonist, *Endocrinology*, **116**, 2643–9.

Walsh, J. H. (1987). Gastrointestinal hormones. In L. R. Johnson (ed.) *Physiology of the Gastrointestinal Tract*, 2nd edn, Raven Press, New York, pp. 181–253.

Advances in Drug Therapy of Gastrointestinal Ulceration
Edited by A. Garner and B. J. R. Whittle
©1989 John Wiley & Sons Ltd

Chapter Eighteen

Modulation of Cell Turnover and Mucosal Growth

Robert A. Goodlad and Nicholas A. Wright
Imperial Cancer Research Fund Histopathology Unit, Lincoln's Inn Fields, London, and Department of Histopathology, Royal Postgraduate Medical School, Hammersmith Hospital, London W12 0HS, UK

INTRODUCTION

The gastrointestinal epithelium is renewed by a process of continuous cell division and has the fastest turnover of all the body tissues. The study of gastrointestinal epithelial cell proliferation is of great interest in its own right, and also has important implications for the study of gastrointestinal carcinogenesis and pathophysiology. The intestinal mucosa is in many ways an ideal model system for the study of epithelial renewal in general, because of its high rate of cell division and the restriction of proliferation to anatomically discrete zones.

THE CELL CYCLE

There are four phases of cell division which together constitute the cell renewal cycle (see Figure 18.1). The chromosomes separate in mitosis which is thus termed the M phase. Dividing cells then enter the first portion of interphase, the postmitotic, presynthetic gap, called G_1. Cells can remain in G_1 or they may eventually pass some crucial control point and become committed to the next phase of the cell cycle, the DNA synthesis (S) phase, which is followed by another, but much shorter, gap G_2 (see Figure 18.1). There is intense biochemical activity in the G_2 phase as cells prepare for mitosis and assemble the spindle proteins. If differentiation is to occur after mitosis, the cells eventually pass a critical stage and are incapable of re-entering the cell cycle (Aherne, Camplejohn and Wright, 1977; Wright and Alison, 1984a).

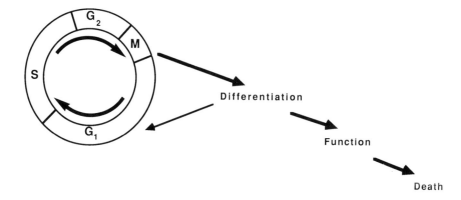

Figure 18.1 The cell cycle. The chromosomes separate by mitosis in the M phase, enter the G_1 gap phase and can then duplicate their DNA in the S phase before entering the G_2 gap and mitosis again. After mitosis the cells may either go round the cycle again or they may start to differentiate and eventually become incapable of rejoining the cell cycle

Mitotic cells can readily be identified by microscopy; however, a much larger sample of dividing cells can be obtained by visualizing S-phase cells (as the duration of the S phase is several times longer than that of the M phase). S-phase cells can be labelled with [^{3}H]thymidine and visualized by auto-radiography. The distribution of labelled and mitotic cells delineates the reproductive compartment, and the change in distribution of labelled cells with time can be utilized for the study of cell migration and transit. Birth rates can be estimated by the ratio of mitotic or labelled cells to other cells. However, such 'state' measures are vulnerable to changes in the duration of their respective phases and it is preferable to measure the rate of entry of cells into the M or the S phase using metaphase arrest or double labelling. While this chapter is not the forum for discussing in detail the methodology involved in the study of intestinal epithelial cell proliferation studies, the vital importance of utilizing appropriate and robust methods cannot be overemphasized (Al-Mukhtar *et al.*, 1982; Goodlad and Wright, 1982; Wright and Alison, 1984b).

INTESTINAL EPITHELIAL CELL RENEWAL

Cells at the base of the intestinal proliferative hierarchy give rise to all the other epithelial cells (Cheng and Leblond, 1974), and can thus be regarded as the functional 'stem' cells (Potten and Loeffler, 1987). These stem cells do not migrate, whereas their daughter cells are transitory, with a limited life expectancy and division capacity. Proliferation in the small intestine is confined to the crypts of Lieberkühn. There is little proliferative activity in the basal cell positions, due to the non-dividing Paneth cells, and the long cell cycle times of the omnipotent, functional, basal stem cells (Al-Dewachi *et al.*, 1979). The daughter cells then divide rapidly in the lower and middle regions of the crypt and leave the cell division cycle and differentiate, so that the top of the crypt is a non-proliferative, maturation compartment, which feeds cells to the villus. The kinetic organization of the small intestinal crypt can thus be portrayed as in Figure 18.2.

The situation in the gastric epithelium is somewhat different in that most proliferation occurs in the neck and isthmus region, and the majority of cells migrate upwards towards the gastric lumen with only a few cells migrating downwards. The common precursor cell in the stomach is probably the

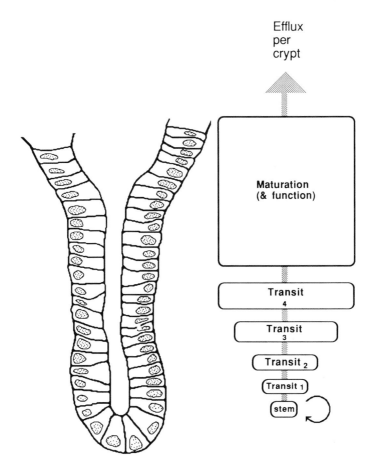

Figure 18.2 The kinetic organization of the small intestinal crypt. A few basal self-renewing stem cells divide and their daughters pass through 3–4 transit divisions after which they decycle and differentiate. Several crypts feed one villus, so that the net villus influx is determined by the product of the crypt efflux and the crypt/villus ratio

undifferentiated neck cell, which may in turn be fed from the mucous neck cell, which may be the gastric 'stem' cell (Goodlad and Wright, 1987a). The general kinetic organization of the colon is broadly similar to that of the small intestine.

MECHANISMS INVOLVED IN THE CONTROL OF INTESTINAL EPITHELIAL CELL PROLIFERATION

The intestinal epithelium can rapidly adapt to a wide variety of altered circumstances, but the main determinant would appear to be increased food intake (Goodlad et al., 1987) or increased nutrient flow to specific areas of the gastrointestinal tract (Williamson, 1978a). Intestinal growth or atrophy can be achieved by altering the production rate of cells per crypt, increasing the lifespan of the functional cells, increasing the absolute number of proliferative units or changing the crypt/villus ratio. Of these, changes in the crypt cell production rate (CCPR) are by far the most important mechanism (Wright and Alison, 1984a). The CCPR is the product of crypt size, growth fraction and cell cycle time and, although all of these factors are known to change, most intestinal adaptation appears to be moderated by alteration in crypt size.

There are probably several mechanisms involved in the control of gastrointestinal epithelial cell renewal (Wright and Alison, 1984b), but the most important of these are generally considered to be:

(1) local negative feedback,
(2) 'luminal nutrition',
(3) humoral factors.

There may also be a small role for the effects of pancreaticobiliary secretions, mucosal blood flow and neuroendocrine factors.

Negative feedback

Negative feedback from the functional to the reproductive compartments has been implicated in several adaptive responses. It is usually a local phenomenon in response to chemical or radiation-induced mucosal damage, and may even involve those exceptionally elusive tissue specific inhibitors known as the chalones. Some of the best evidence for negative feedback mechanisms can be seen in the response of the crypts and villi after chemotoxic ablation of crypt cells. Thus, while there is an immediate reduction in crypt cell population, cell production does not increase until the villus population has become depleted (Wright and Al-Nafussi, 1982). These data can be accommodated by a mathematical model which includes feedback from both the proliferative and the functional compartments (Britton, Wright and Murray, 1982). An exhaustive review of the subject has been presented previously (Wright and Alison, 1984b).

Luminal nutrition

The presence of food in the intestinal lumen is one of the most potent stimuli of intestinal proliferation (Goodlad *et al.*, 1987) and can be considered to be the consequence of the direct and indirect effects of 'luminal nutrition' and/or mucosal workload (Dowling, 1982; Wright and Alison, 1984b). The importance of luminal nutrition is demonstrated in animals subjected to small bowel resection, where there is a massive adaptive response, which is nonetheless almost totally abolished if the same animals are fed intravenously (Al-Mukhtar *et al.*, 1982). Several attempts have been made to distinguish between the effects of extraction of absorbed nutrients by the functional cells (luminal nutrition) and the effects of mucosal workload or functional demand. Although this question has not been fully resolved, the response to sugars which are absorbed and metabolized seems to be similar to that to sugars which are absorbed but not metabolized. This finding would tend to favour the mucosal workload hypothesis (Clarke, 1977). It must not be forgotten that luminal nutrients can also stimulate the release of locally and/or systemically active gut peptides.

Another effect of luminal nutrition may be seen in the colon where feeding rats a fibre-free 'elemental' diet leads to disuse atrophy of the distal ileum and of the colon. Addition of fibre restores proliferation, whereas inert bulk does not (Goodlad and Wright, 1983). The stimulatory effect of fibre is most probably the result of the breakdown of fibre into short-chain fatty acids (SCFA) by the microbial flora (Goodlad *et al.*, 1987b), which may have both a direct effect and an indirect systemic effect (Sakata and Yajima, 1984).

Hormonal factors

There is also a large body of evidence for the involvement of humoral factors in the control of mucosal renewal. Parabiotic and cross-circulation studies have shown that a blood-borne stimulant of intestinal epithelial cell proliferation exists (Williamson, 1978b) and studies in isolated loops confirm this (Hanson, 1982).

Gastrin stimulates proliferation in the stomach, but claims for its role in the rest of the gut (Johnson, 1981) can most probably be attributed to poor methodology (Goodlad and Wright, 1987b).

Several other peptides and hormones may also stimulate gastrointestinal renewal and may act either systemically or locally. One of the most likely candidate hormones is enteroglucagon, but most of the evidence for this has had to be circumstantial due to the lack of purified or synthesized enteroglucagon. Nevertheless, the evidence for a trophic role for enteroglucagon has been steadily building up ever since an enteroglucagon secreting tumour was found to be associated with massive villus enlargement (Bloom, 1972). Plasma enteroglucagon levels increase in a wide variety of hyperproliferative models and in several pathological conditions associated with intestinal hyperplasia and

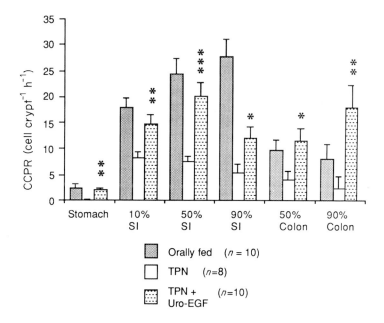

Figure 18.3 The effects of intravenous administration of urogastrone/EGF on intestinal crypt cell production in rats maintained by total parenteral nutrition (TPN). The first group of rats were fed orally *ad lib*. The second were maintained by intravenous feeding (TPN) and the third were on TPN + 60 μg of urogastrone–EGF rat^{-1} day^{-1}. CCPR was determined by the accumulation of vincristine-arrested metaphases in microdissected crypts. Significance levels of *t*-test of TPN + urogastrone versus TPN rats: significantly different, *(P < 0.05); **(P < 0.01); ***(P < 0.001)

correlate well with CCPR in a wide range of experimental models of intestinal adaptation (Goodlad and Wright, 1987b). Enteroglucagon cells are located throughout the gut, but most are localized in the distal regions, which would appear to be the strategic position for monitoring the efficiency of the digestive process.

Another peptide which appears to be co-localized with enteroglucagon is peptide tyrosine–tyrosine (PYY), and like enteroglucagon it can also inhibit gastric acid secretion and emptying. PYY levels also correlate well with enteroglucagon and with intestinal proliferation (Goodlad *et al.*, 1987b).

The polypeptide growth factor, epidermal growth factor (EGF), is intimately associated with the gastrointestinal tract, being present in large amounts in the salivary glands and in the Brunner's glands, and in milk (Goodlad and Wright, 1987b). While its growth promoting effects *in vitro* are well documented its role *in vivo* is uncertain. EGF inhibits gastric acid secretion (Konturek *et al.*, 1984) and may also have a 'cytoprotective' role (Konturek *et al.*, 1981; Olsen *et al.*, 1984). Since the administration of exogenous EGF to animals has produced

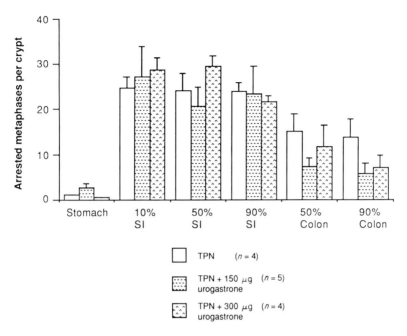

Figure 18.4 Intestinal cell proliferation (as assessed by the collection of vincristine-arrested metaphases over a 2 h period) after intragastric administration of urogastrone–EGF (150 and 300 μg rat^{-1} day^{-1})

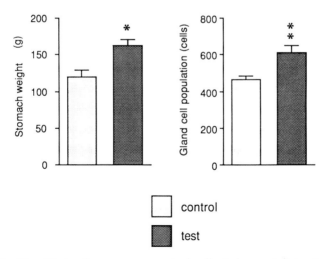

Figure 18.5 The effects of exogenous prostaglandin (misoprostol) treatment on the stomach wet weight and gastric gland cell population (measured from the neck/base junction to the surface), after 77 days of 300 μg kg^{-1} oral misoprostol administration. Significantly different, *($P < 0.05$), **($P < 0.01$)

conflicting results, we decided to infuse recombinant human EGF (urogastrone) into rats where the intrinsic rates of intestinal cell proliferation had been reduced to basal levels by feeding the animals intravenously.

EGF significantly increased crypt cell production rates throughout the entire gastrointestinal tract, in a dose-dependent manner, with the most marked effects occurring in the stomach and colon (Goodlad et al., 1987a). EGF was effective if infused continuously (see Figure 18.3) or if the gut was allowed to atrophy before EGF administration. A similar proliferative effect of intravenous EGF administration has also been seen in a human infant infused with EGF (Walker-Smith et al., 1985). Administration of high doses of EGF intragastrically was without effect (see Figure 18.4).

Intestinal hypertrophy is also seen after the administration of exogenous prostaglandins and their long-lived analogues (Dembinski and Konturek, 1985), and while some workers have found that mucosal DNA synthesis was increased others have not found any effect on proliferative indices (Uribe, Tribukait and Johansson, 1987). A recent study utilizing rigorous cell kinetic methods has, however, shown that while prostaglandin administration may not alter some state parameters, such as the labelling index, if the same data are expressed as number of labelled cells per gland, a significant effect is indeed observed, which is the result of the size of the gastric glands being significantly greater in the treated group (Goodlad et al., 1988). (See Figures 18.5 and 18.6.) The dangers of relying on a static measure when the denominator is also changing are shown diagrammatically in Figure 18.7.

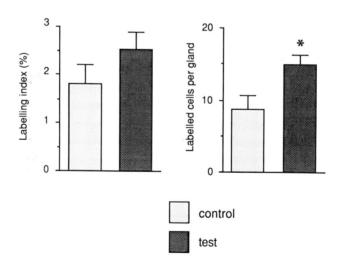

Figure 18.6 The effects of prostaglandin administration on the labelling index (labelled cells ÷ total cells) and on the number of labelled cells per gastric gland. See legend of Figure 18.4 for experimental details. Significantly different *($P < 0.05$)

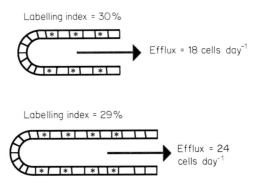

Figure 18.7 Diagram of two intestinal crypts (or glands) showing that, although they may have the same labelling index, they can have vastly different cell outputs due to the difference in size of the two crypts by virtue of differences in gland size (and cell population)

CONCLUSION

The gastrointestinal epithelium is a system well suited for the study of epithelial organization and growth control but, unless appropriate and robust methods are applied, meaningless results may be generated. While the control of gastrointestinal epithelial cell proliferation is undoubtedly a multi-factorial system, most models will have to take negative feedback, 'luminal nutrition' and the effects of systemic agents into account.

Growth control is of vital importance to multicellular organisms and probably involves a complex cascade-like system. It may well prove to be of importance to be able to differentiate between the effects of major control mechanisms and of the consequent secondary messenger signals.

REFERENCES

Aherne, W. A., Camplejohn, R. S. and Wright, N. A. (1977). *An Introduction to Cell Population Kinetics*, Edward Arnold, London.

Al-Dewachi, H. S., Appleton, D. R., Watson, A. J. and Wright, N. A. (1979). Variations in the cell cycle time in the crypts of Lieberkühn of the mouse, *Virchows Arch.*, **31**, 37–44.

Al-Mukhtar, M. Y. T., Polak, J. M., Bloom, S. R. and Wright, N. A. (1982). The search for appropriate measurements of proliferative and morphological status. In J. W. L. Robinson, H. Dowling and E. O. Reicken (eds) *Mechanisms of Intestinal Adaptation*, MTP Press, Lancaster, pp. 3–30.

Al-Mukhtar, M. Y. T., Sagor, G. R., Ghatei, M. A. *et al.* (1982). The relationship between endogenous gastrointestinal hormones and cell proliferation in models of intestinal adaptation. In J. W. L. Robinson, R. H. Dowling and E. O. Reicken (eds) *Mechanisms of Intestinal Adaptation*, MTP Press, Lancaster, pp. 243–53.

Bloom, S. R. (1972). An enteroglucagon tumour in man, *Gut*, **13**, 520–3.

Britton, N. F., Wright, N. A. and Murray, J. D. (1982). A mathematical model for cell population kinetics in the small intestine, *J. Theoret. Biol.*, **98**, 531–42.

Cheng, H. and Leblond, C. P. (1974). Origin, differentiation and renewal of the four main epithelial cell types of the mouse small intestine. V. Unitarian theory of the origin of the four epithelial cell types, *Am. J. Anat.*, **144**, 537–62.

Clarke, R. M. (1977). Luminal nutrition versus functional work load as controllers of mucosal morphology and epithelial replacement in the rat small intestine, *Digestion*, **15**, 411–29.

Dembinski, A. and Konturek, S. (1985). Effects of E, F and I series prostaglandins and analogues on growth of gastroduodenal mucosa and pancreas, *Am. J. Physiol.*, **248**, G170–5.

Dowling, R. H. (1982). Small bowel adaptation and its regulation, *Scand. J. Gastroenterol.*, **17** (Suppl. 74), 54–74.

Goodlad, R. A. and Wright, N. A. (1982). Quantitative studies on epithelial replacement in the gut. In D. A. Titchen (ed.) *Techniques in the Life Sciences. Digestive Physiology*, Vol. P2, Elsevier Biomedical Press, Ireland, pp. P212/2–23.

Goodlad, R. A. and Wright, N. A. (1983). Effects of addition of kaolin or cellulose to an elemental diet on intestinal cell proliferation in the mouse, *Br. J. Nutr.*, **50**, 91–8.

Goodlad, R. A. and Wright, N. A. (1987a). The gastric epithelium, *GI Futures*, **1**, 16–19.

Goodlad, R. A. and Wright, N. A. (1987b). Peptides and epithelial growth regulation, *Experientia*, **43**, 780–4.

Goodlad, R. A., Plumb, J. A. and Wright, N. A. (1987). The relationship between intestinal crypt cell production and intestinal water absorption measured *in vitro* in the rat, *Clin. Sci.*, **72**, 297–304.

Goodlad, R. A., Wilson, T. G. J., Lenton, W., Gregory, H., McCullagh, K. G. and Wright, N. A. (1987a). Proliferative effects of urogastrone-EGF on the intestinal epithelium, *Gut*, **28** (Suppl. 1), 37–43.

Goodlad, R. A., Lenton, W., Ghatei, M. A., Adrian, T. E., Bloom, S. R. and Wright, N. A. (1987b). Proliferative effects of fibre on the intestinal epithelium: relationship to gastric, enteroglucagon and PYY, *Gut*, **28** (Suppl. 1), 221–6.

Goodlad, R. A., Moffat, M. R., Madgwick, A. J., Levin, S., Allen, J. L. and Wright, N. A. (1988). Misoprostol and the gastric epithelium. I. Effects of misoprostol on gastric epithelial cell proliferation, *Gut* (in press).

Hanson, W. R. (1982). Proliferative and morphological adaptation of the intestine to experimental resection. *Scand. J. Gastroenterol.*, **17** (Suppl. 74), 11–20.

Johnson, L. R. (1981). Regulation of gastrointestinal growth. In *Physiology of the Digestive Tract*, Raven Press, New York, pp. 169–96.

Konturek, S. J., Radecki, T., Brzozowski, T. *et al.* (1981). Gastric cytoprotection by epidermal growth factor: role of endogenous prostaglandins and DNA synthesis, *Gastroenterology*, **81**, 438–43.

Konturek, S. J., Cieszkowski, M., Jaworek, J., Konturek, J., Brzozowski, T. and Gregory, H. (1984). Effects of epidermal growth factor on gastrointestinal secretions, *Am. J. Physiol.*, **246**, G580–6.

Olsen, P. S., Poulsen, S. S., Kirkegaard, P. and Nexo, E. (1984). Role of submandibular saliva and epidermal growth factor in gastric cytoprotection, *Gastroenterology*, **87**, 103–8.

Potten, C. S. and Loeffler, M. (1987). A comprehensive model of the crypts of the small intestine of the mouse provides insight into the mechanisms of cell migration and the proliferative hierarchy, *J. Theor. Biol.*, **127**, 381–91.

Sakata, T. and Yajima, T. (1984). Influence of short chain fatty acids on the epithelial cell division of digestive tract, *Q. J. Exp. Physiol.*, **69**, 639–48.

Uribe, A., Tribukait, B. and Johansson, C. (1987). Cell cycle distribution of proliferative and functional cells of the rat jejunum after treatment with oral E_2 prostaglandins, *Scand. J. Gastroenterol.*, **22**, 177–84.

Walker-Smith, J. A., Phillips, A. D., Walford, N. *et al.* (1985). Intravenous epidermal growth factor/urogastrone increases small intestinal cell proliferation in congenital microvillus atrophy, *Lancet*, **ii**, 1239–40.

Williamson, R. C. N. (1978a). Intestinal adaptation. 1. Structural, functional and cytokinetic changes, *New Engl. J. Med.*, **298**, 1393–402.

Williamson, R. C. N. (1978b). Intestinal adaptation. 2. Mechanisms of control, *New Engl. J. Med.*, **298**, 1444–50.

Wright, N. A. and Alison, M. R. (1984a). *The Biology of Epithelial Cell Populations*, Vol. 1, Clarendon Press, Oxford.

Wright, N. A. and Alison, M. R. (1984b). *The Biology of Epithelial Cell Populations*, Vol. 2, Clarendon Press, Oxford.

Wright, N. A. and Al-Nafussi, A. (1982). Kinetics of villus cell populations in the mouse small intestine. II. Negative feedback after death of proliferating cells, *Cell Tissue Kinetics*, **15**, 610–22.

Advances in Drug Therapy of Gastrointestinal Ulceration
Edited by A. Garner and B. J. R. Whittle
©1989 John Wiley & Sons Ltd

Chapter Nineteen

Gastric Protective and Ulcer-Healing Action of Epidermal Growth Factor

S. J. Konturek, T. Brzozowski,
A. Dembinski, Z. Warzecha and J. Yamazaki
*Institute of Physiology, Academy of Medicine, 31-531 Krakow,
Poland and Hitachi Chemical Company, Ibaraki, Japan*

INTRODUCTION

Epidermal growth factor (EGF) is a single-chain polypeptide which is secreted mainly by submandibular glands and duodenal mucosa (Byyny, Orth and Cohen, 1972; Heitz *et al.*, 1978; Gresik, Van der Noen and Barka, 1979). It is a powerful mitogen and an inhibitor of gastric acid secretion (Gregory, 1975; Dembinski *et al.*, 1982; Konturek *et al.*, 1984).

Recent studies have demonstrated that EGF is also capable of protecting the gastric mucosa against the damage caused by various irritants such as aspirin (Konturek *et al.*, 1981b), ethanol (Konturek *et al.*, 1983b) and cysteamine (Olsen *et al.*, 1984). EGF was also reported to promote healing of chronic gastric and duodenal ulceration in rats (Olsen *et al.*, 1986a,b; Konturek *et al.*, 1988). Furthermore, the extirpation of salivary glands (to remove endogenous source of EGF) was accompanied by an increase in the susceptibility of gastric mucosa to damage by ulcerogens (Skinner, Soper and Tepperman, 1984) and by a delay in healing of chronic peptic ulcerations (Olsen *et al.*, 1986a,b; Konturek *et al.*, 1988). The mechanisms of these gastric protective and ulcer-healing effects of EGF are unknown, but they have been attributed, at least in part, to the trophic influence of this peptide on the lining of the gastrointestinal tract (Konturek *et al.*, 1981a; Skinner, Soper and Tepperman, 1984).

In the current study, we have examined the protective effect of EGF against gastric mucosal damage induced by various ulcerogens and the healing action of EGF on chronic acetic acid-induced gastroduodenal ulcerations. Furthermore, the effects of EGF on biochemical indicators of mucosal growth have been determined in an attempt to correlate the protective, ulcer-healing and growth-promoting properties of this peptide.

EFFECTS OF EGF ON EXPERIMENTAL GASTRODUODENAL DAMAGE

Acute gastric mucosal lesions

Male Wistar rats, weighing 150–200 g, were used for the studies on acute gastric mucosal damage, gastric and duodenal ulcerations and mucosal growth. Four types of acute gastric mucosal lesions were developed in 24 h fasted rats using absolute ethanol, acidified aspirin (ASA), acidified taurocholate (TC) and water immersion and immobilization stress (stress) as described previously (Takagi, Kasuya and Watanabe, 1964; Konturek *et al.*, 1983a,b, 1986). Briefly, in tests with ethanol and TC, 1 ml of 100% ethanol or 1 ml of 100 mmol l^{-1} taurocholate in 0.15 mol l^{-1} HCl was introduced intragastrically (i.g.) through a metal orogastric tube. The animals were killed 1 h later and the stomach was removed. The number of gastric necrotic lesions was recorded and their total area was measured by planimetry (Morphomat, Carl Zeiss, Berlin). In tests with aspirin, ASA was dissolved in 0.15 mol l^{-1} HCl and instilled i.g. in a bolus dose of 60 mg kg^{-1} followed by a dose of 42 mg $kg^{-1} h^{-1}$ for a 3 h period. Animals were then killed and the area and number of ulcers were measured planimetrically. Stress ulcers were induced by placing the rats in special restraining cages immersed in a water bath at 23 °C for 7 h. The animals were then killed, the stomach removed and examined grossly for the number and area of gastric ulcerations.

Several groups of 8–20 rats were used in studies with absolute ethanol:

(1) Ethanol alone,
(2) EGF (recombinant human EGF, Chiron Co., USA, and Hitachi Chemical Co., Japan) (25–100 μg $kg^{-1} h^{-1}$ s.c.) followed 30 min later by ethanol in rats with and without submandibular salivary glands,
(3) EGF (100 μg kg^{-1} p.o.) followed 30 min later by ethanol,
(4) difluoromethyl ornithine (DFMO; MDL 71 782) (200 mg kg^{-1} i.p.) followed 2 h later by EGF (100 μg $kg^{-1} h^{-1}$ s.c.) and then 30 min later by ethanol,
(5) DFMO (200 mg kg^{-1} i.p.) followed 2 h later by ethanol,
(6) 16,16-dimethyl PGE$_2$ (10–40 μg kg^{-1} p.o.) followed 30 min later by ethanol in rats with and without submandibular glands.

In experiments with acidified ASA, acidified TC and stress, the following groups were investigated:

(1) ASA, TC or stress alone,
(2) EGF (100 μg $kg^{-1} h^{-1}$ s.c.) followed 30 min later by ASA, TC or stress,
(3) EGF (100 μg kg^{-1} p.o.) followed 30 min later by ASA, TC or stress.

In tests with ethanol and acidified ASA and TC, the biopsies of oxyntic mucosa were taken immediately after the animals were killed to determine the mucosal generation of PGE_2 using RIA-PGE_2 kits (New England Nuclear, Munich, Germany) as described elsewhere (Konturek *et al.*, 1986) and mucosal DNA synthesis *in vitro* as presented before (Konturek *et al.*, 1981a).

Means were compared by Student's *t*-test for unpaired values or many sample, one-way analysis of variance and Duncan's multiple range test. The differences between means were considered significant at $P < 0.05$.

Effects of EGF, DFMO or aminoquanide on acute gastric lesions

The effects of EGF infused s.c. in various doses on the mean ulcer area induced by absolute ethanol in rats with intact and resected salivary glands are shown in Figure 19.1. EGF resulted in a dose-dependent reduction in the mean area of gastric lesions in rats with intact and resected glands, the ID_{50} (dose of EGF reducing the area by 50%) of EGF being, respectively, 41 and 79 μg kg^{-1}. EGF was significantly less effective in the prevention of gastric damage by ethanol in sialoadenectomized rats at both 50 and 100 μg kg^{-1} h^{-1}. Pretreatment with 16,16-dimethyl-PGE_2 also prevented dose-dependently the ethanol-induced gastric damage and the ID_{50} for PGE_2 was similar in rats with intact and resected glands.

The effects of EGF on gastric damage induced by absolute ethanol, acidified ASA, acidified TC or stress are shown in Figure 19.2. EGF infused s.c. 30 min before and during induction of gastric damage effectively reduced the mean area of gastric lesions induced by all four ulcerogens. When administered as a

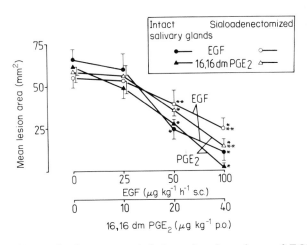

Figure 19.1   Effects of subcutaneous infusion of various doses of EGF (25–100 μg kg^{-1} h^{-1}) and oral administration of 16,16-dimethyl PGE_2 in various doses (10–40 μg kg^{-1}) on the area of gastric lesions induced by absolute ethanol in rats. Each column represents mean ± s.e.m. of 8–20 rats. An asterisk indicates a significant decrease below the control value obtained with ethanol alone

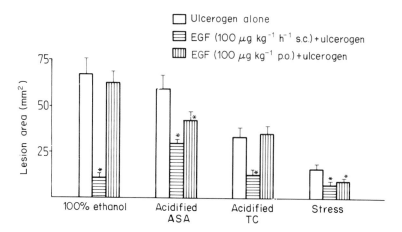

Figure 19.2 Effects of subcutaneous infusion or intragastric administration of EGF ($100 \mu g$ kg^{-1}) on mean ulcer area of gastric lesions induced by absolute ethanol, acidified ASA, acidified TC or water immersion and restraint stress. An asterisk indicates a significant decrease below the control lesion area obtained with ulcerogen alone. Mean ± s.e.m. of 8–12 rats

single bolus dose given intragastrically 30 min before the ulcerogen, it was without any influence on ethanol- or TC-induced gastric lesions, but reduced significantly those produced by ASA and stress.

Following pretreatment with DFMO, the area and the number of gastric lesions induced by absolute ethanol tended to increase, but this was not significant (Figure 19.3). DFMO reversed, in part, the EGF-induced decrease in area and number of ethanol-induced lesions.

Effects of EGF on mucosal PGE$_2$ and DNA synthesis

The values of the gastric mucosal generation of PGE$_2$ in rats with intact stomach and those exposed to absolute ethanol, acidified ASA, acidified TC and stress in tests with vehicle (saline solution) and EGF (as in Figure 19.2) are shown in Figure 19.4. Mucosal PGE$_2$ was significantly elevated in tests with ethanol and acidified TC, unchanged in tests with stress, and reduced by about 90% in tests with acidified ASA. Pretreatment with EGF ($100 \mu g$ $kg^{-1} h^{-1}$ s.c.) failed to affect mucosal prostaglandin generation in rats with intact stomach or in those exposed to various ulcerogens.

As shown in Figure 19.5, DNA synthesis in the gastric mucosa was significantly reduced after exposure to either absolute ethanol or acidified ASA. Pretreatment with EGF significantly decreased the fall in DNA synthesis after exposure to ethanol and almost completely restored DNA synthesis in ASA-treated animals.

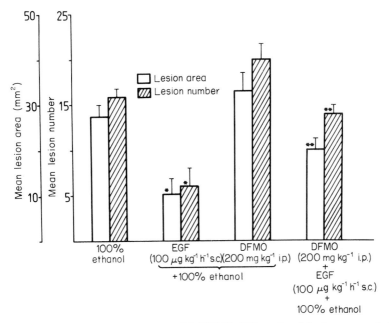

Figure 19.3 Effect of the pretreatment with DFMO (200 mg kg^{-1} i.p.) on mean lesion area induced by absolute ethanol in rats without and with subcutaneous administration of EGF (100 μg kg^{-1}h^{-1}). Mean ± s.e.m. of 8–14 rats. An asterisk indicates a significant decrease below the control value. A double asterisk indicates a significant increase above the value obtained with EGF

Chronic gastric and duodenal ulcers

Chronic gastric and duodenal ulcers were produced in 24 h fasted rats using our modification (Konturek *et al.*, 1987) of the acetic acid method. Briefly, the animals were anaesthetized with ether. The stomach was exposed to 100% acetic acid applied on the serosal surface in an area of 13.8 mm^2 while the proximal duodenum was exposed to 75% acetic acid for 10 s. This resulted in the formation of gastric and duodenal ulcerations which did not perforate or penetrate into the surrounding organs and usually healed within 2–3 weeks. In these experiments, the animals were killed 7 days after the induction of ulcers. The area of gastric and duodenal ulcers (verified histologically) was measured by planimetry.

The following groups of 8–10 rats with chronic gastric and duodenal ulcers were tested:

(1) chronic (gastric and duodenal) ulcers in rats with intact salivary glands treated with vehicle (saline solution) in drinking water (p.o.) or injected s.c.,

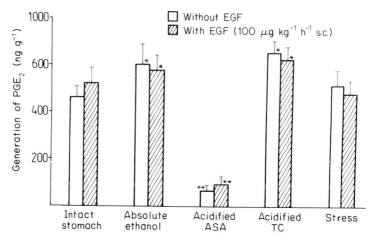

Figure 19.4 Mucosal generation of PGE in the intact gastric mucosa and that exposed to absolute ethanol, acidified ASA, TC or stress in rats without and with pretreatment with EGF ($100 \mu g$ kg^{-1} h^{-1} s.c.). Mean ± s.e.m. of 8–12 rats as in Figure 19.2. An asterisk indicates a significant increase above the value obtained in intact mucosa. A double asterisk indicates a significant decrease below the value obtained in the intact mucosa

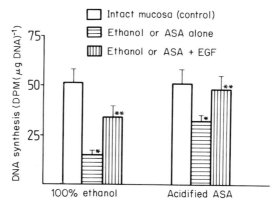

Figure 19.5 DNA synthesis measured as incorporation of [^{3}H]thymidine into DNA in the oxyntic mucosa exposed to absolute ethanol or acidified ASA with and without pretreatment with EGF. An asterisk indicates a significant decrease below the value obtained in the intact mucosa. A double asterisk indicates a significant increase above the value obtained with ethanol or ASA alone

(2) chronic ulcers in rats with submandibular glands removed about 7 days earlier and treated with vehicle,

(3) chronic ulcers in intact or sialoadenectomized rats treated with EGF ($30 \mu g$ kg^{-1} day^{-1}) injected s.c. for 7 days,

(4) chronic ulcers in intact or sialoadenectomized rats treated with EGF ($30 \mu g$ kg^{-1} day^{-1}) given p.o. (added to drinking water) for 7 days,

(5) chronic ulcers in intact rats treated with EGF i.p. (30 μg kg^{-1} day^{-1}) in combination with DFMO (200 mg kg^{-1} day^{-1} i.p.),

(6) chronic ulcers in intact rats treated with DFMO alone (200 mg kg^{-1} day^{-1} i.p.).

The ulcer area in all the test groups was measured immediately after killing the rats. The stomach and the 3 cm segment of the upper duodenum were then dissected out and weighed. About 50 mg of the mucosa was scraped from the resected fundic portion of the stomach and the duodenum (excluding the ulcer area) for measurements of DNA and RNA contents as described before (Dembinski *et al.*, 1982).

Effects of EGF on healing of chronic gastric and duodenal ulcers

The initial area of gastric and duodenal ulcers induced by acetic acid was 13.8 mm^2. In control rats treated with vehicle (saline solution) injected s.c. three times daily or added to the drinking water, the mean area of gastric ulcers was reduced after 7 days to 6.2 ± 1.4 mm^2 and that of duodenal ulcers to 5.3 ± 0.8 mm^2.

In rats treated with EGF administered s.c. for 7 days, there was a significant reduction in the area of both gastric and duodenal ulcers (Figure 19.6). Sialoadenectomy delayed the healing, whereas the administration of EGF reversed this effect (Figure 19.6).

DFMO administered i.p. (300 mg kg^{-1} day^{-1}) throughout the period of experimentation (7 days after ulcer induction) did not influence the mean area of gastric or duodenal ulcerations in rats receiving vehicle (Figure 19.7). When combined with EGF injected i.p., DFMO almost completely reversed the ulcer-healing affects of EGF. In DFMO/EGF-treated rats, the area of gastric lesions was significantly larger than that observed in rats treated only with EGF.

The mucosal weights and DNA and RNA content in rats with intact and resected salivary glands and gastric and duodenal ulcers treated with EGF are shown in Figure 19.8. EGF significantly increased the weights of gastric mucosa and increased the content of nucleic acid in the respective mucosae. Sialoadenectomy reduced the organ weights and nucleic acid content, but the addition of EGF restored to normal values both the weights and RNA and DNA content of gastric but not duodenal mucosa.

MECHANISMS OF PROTECTIVE AND ANTI-ULCER ACTIONS OF EGF

This study confirms that EGF exhibits gastric protective and ulcer-healing actions and suggests that the mucosal growth promoting effect of this peptide may play an important role in these actions.

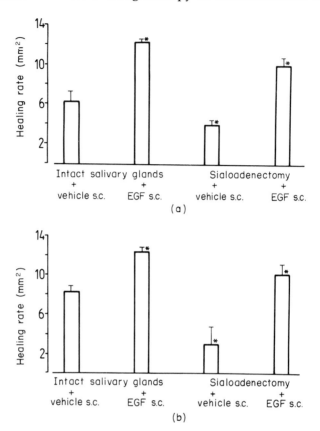

Figure 19.6 The rate of healing of (a) gastric and (b) duodenal ulcers (determined 7 days after ulcer induction) in rats with intact or resected salivary glands with or without s.c. administration of EGF ($30 \mu g$ kg^{-1} day^{-1}). An asterisk indicates a significant difference compared to the value obtained with vehicle in rats with intact glands. Mean $\pm$ s.e.m. of 10–14 rats

Previous studies have shown that EGF protects the gastric mucosa against damage by aspirin (Konturek *et al.*, 1981b), ethanol (Konturek *et al.*, 1983b) and cysteamine (Olsen *et al.*, 1984). In this study, we have confirmed these findings and observed that the mucosal injury by acidified taurocholate and by water immersion and restraint stress are also sensitive to the protective action of EGF. When given subcutaneously, EGF was protective against all four irritants used, whereas oral administration of EGF was protective only against the lesions induced by acidified ASA and stress. The difference in the action of EGF administered parenterally and orally could be attributed to the longer exposure required for orally applied EGF to develop gastric protection. Indeed, in tests with absolute ethanol and taurocholate (when EGF was ineffective), this

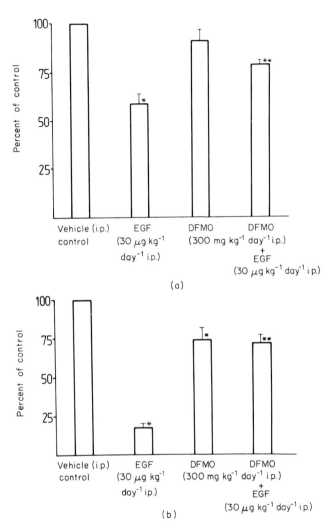

Figure 19.7 Mean area (expressed as percentage of control taken as 100%) of (a) chronic gastric ulcers and (b) chronic duodenal ulcers induced by acetic acid in rats treated for 7 days with DFMO alone, DFMO + EGF and EGF alone. Means ± s.e.m. of 8–10 rats. An asterisk indicates a significant decrease below the value obtained with vehicle, and a double asterisk indicates a significant increase above the value obtained with EGF alone

exposure to orally applied EGF lasted for only 1.5 h while in tests with ASA and stress (when EGF partly protected mucosa) the exposure was 3.5 and 7.5 h respectively.

Although PGE$_2$ mimicked the gastric protective effects of EGF, the fact that this peptide did not influence mucosal generation of PGE$_2$ in the intact or

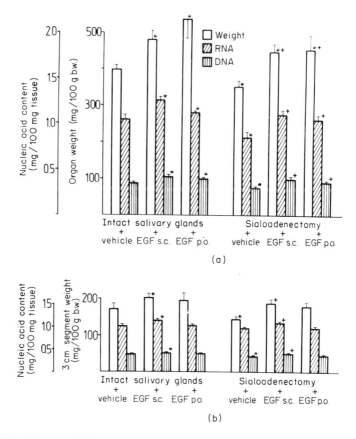

Figure 19.8 Organ weights and RNA and DNA contents in (a) oxyntic mucosa and (b) duodenal mucosa in rats with intact and resected salivary glands treated for 7 days with vehicle (saline solution) or EGF (30 μg kg^{-1} day^{-1}) given s.c. or p.o. An asterisk indicates a significant increase above the values obtained with vehicle in rats with intact salivary glands. A cross indicates a significant increase above the value obtained in sialoadenectomized rats treated with vehicle

injured (by various ulcerogens) stomach militates against the involvement of prostaglandins in the EGF-induced gastric protection as proposed before (Konturek *et al.*, 1981b).

The finding that the EGF-protected mucosa exhibited much higher DNA synthetic activity than that exposed to ulcerogen alone could be interpreted as the result of the protective effect of EGF rather than its cause. Another approach to examine the possible role of mucosal growth in EGF-induced mucosal protection was the use of agents affecting the cellular content of polyamines which appear to play an important role in the early phase of cell proliferative processes (Tabor and Tabor, 1984) and which themselves have been shown to exhibit mucosal protection (Mizui, Shimono and Doteuchi, 1987). Pretreatment with DFMO, an irreversible ornithine decarboxylase (ODC) inhibitor, which is known to cause sustained depletion of polyamines (Luk, Marton and Baylin, 1980), did not influence the damaging effect of absolute ethanol itself, but reversed, in part, the protective action of EGF against this damage. Since EGF is known to stimulate ODC activity in the gastric mucosa (Feldman, Aures and Grossman, 1978) it is likely that the increase in polyamine formation may account for the protective properties of EGF. This notion is supported by the finding that aminoguanidine, which blocks diamino-oxidase, an enzyme responsible for the degradation of polyamines, was highly protective against the mucosal damage induced by absolute ethanol (unpublished data).

The physiological role of EGF in gastric protection may also be related to its mucosal growth-promoting action. This is supported by our finding that sialoadenectomy (to remove the major source of EGF) was accompanied by a significant decrease in the mucosal weight and the content of RNA and DNA (Konturek et al., 1988). The protective effects of exogenous EGF and exogenous PGE_2 (a standard protective agent) were still observed in sialoadenectomized rats but their protective potency was greatly reduced. Thus, the presence of EGF and normal mucosal growth and integrity seems to be a prerequisite of adequate responsiveness of the mucosa to protective agents.

EGF administered exogenously or released endogenously is also an effective stimulant of the healing of chronic gastric and duodenal ulcers in rats. In our model, the ulcers healed spontaneously within 2–3 weeks, and therefore comparison of the action of EGF on the healing rate was determined after 7 days of treatment. EGF significantly enhanced ulcer healing in rats with intact and resected salivary glands. Sialoadenectomy by itself delayed ulcer healing but did not affect the healing effect of exogenous EGF. Since the enhancement of ulcer healing by exogenous EGF was accompanied by the increase in mucosal growth parameters (organ weight and tissue content of RNA and DNA), whereas the delay of this healing caused by sialoadenectomy occurred with the decrease in mucosal growth parameters, it is likely that the growth-promoting effect of EGF contributes to the healing of gastroduodenal ulcers.

This conclusion is in keeping with previous reports showing that EGF enhanced ulcer healing whereas sialoadenectomy delayed the healing process (Olsen et al., 1986a,b). Further support for this conclusion comes from our studies with DFMO, which almost completely reversed the ulcer-healing action of EGF. Although the mechanism of ulcer-healing processes is not fully explained, the stimulation of lateral growth of epithelial cells and fibroblasts in the ulcer area concurrent with the removal of necrotic tissue is considered to play an important role, and the enhancement of this process by EGF could well explain its ulcer-healing properties. The accumulation of endogenous EGF locally in the area of gastric and duodenal ulceration (Konturek et al., 1988) suggests that this mitogenic peptide may be available in higher concentrations at the ulcer site to stimulate the re-epithelialization and tissue repair processes.

REFERENCES

Byyny, R. L., Orth, D. N. and Cohen, S. (1972). Radioimmunoassay of epidermal growth factor, *Endocrinology*, **90**, 1261–6.

Dembinski, A., Gregory, H., Konturek, S. J. and Polanski, M. (1982). Trophic action of epidermal growth factor on the pancreas and gastroduodenal mucosa in rats, *J. Physiol. (Lond.)*, **325**, 35–42.

Feldman, E. J., Aures, D. and Grossman, M. I. (1978). Epidermal growth factor stimulates ornithidine decarboxylase activity in the digestive tract of mouse, *Proc. Soc. Exp. Biol. Med.*, **159**, 400–2.

Gregory, H. (1975). Isolation and structure of urogastrone and its relationship to epidermal growth factor, *Nature*, **257**, 325–7.

Gresik, E. W., Van der Noen, H. and Barka, T. (1979). Epidermal growth-like material in rat submandibular gland, *Am. J. Anat.*, **156**, 83–9.

Heitz, P. V., Kasper, M., Van Noordenn, S., Polak, J. M., Gregory, H. and Pearse, A. G. E. (1978). Immunohistochemical localisation of urogastrone to human duodenal and submandibular glands, *Gut*, **19**, 408–13.

Konturek, S. J., Brzozowski, T., Piastucki, I. *et al.* (1981a). Role of mucosal prostaglandins and DNA synthesis in gastric cytoprotection by luminal epidermal growth factor, *Gut*, **22**, 927–32.

Konturek, S. J., Radecki, T., Brzozowski, T. *et al.* (1981b). Gastric cytoprotection by epidermal growth factor: role of endogenous prostaglandins and DNA synthesis, *Gastroenterology*, **81**, 438–43.

Konturek, S. J., Brzozowski, T., Piastucki, I., Radecki, T. and Dembinska-Kiec, A. (1983a). Role of prostaglandin and thromboxane biosynthesis in gastric necrosis produced by taurocholate and ethanol, *Dig. Dis. Sci.*, **28**, 154–60.

Konturek, S. J., Brzozowski, T., Radecki, T., Piastucki, I. and Dembinski, A. (1983b). Cytoprotective effects of gastrointestinal hormones. In A. Myoshi (ed.) *Gut Peptides and Ulcer*, Biomedical Research Foundation, Tokyo, pp. 411–17.

Konturek, S. J., Cieszkowski, M., Jaworek, J., Brzozowski, T. and Gregory, H. (1984). Effects of epidermal growth factor on gastrointestinal secretions, *Am. J. Physiol.*, **246**, G580–6.

Konturek, S. J., Radecki, T., Brzozowski, T. *et al.* (1986). Antiulcer and gastroprotective effects of solon, a synthetic flavonoid derivative of sophoradin: role of endogenous prostaglandins, *Eur. J. Pharmacol.*, **125**, 185–92.

Konturek, S. J., Stachura, J., Radecki, T., Drozdowicz, D. and Brzozowski, T. (1987). Cytoprotective and ulcer healing properties of prostaglandin E_2, colloidal bismuth and sucralfate in rats, *Digestion*, **38**, 103–13.

Konturek, S. J., Dembinski, A., Warzecha, Z., Brzozowski, T. and Gregory, H. (1988). Role of epidermal growth factor in healing of chronic gastroduodenal ulcers in rats, *Gastroenterology*, **94**, 1300–7.

Luk, G. D., Marton, L. J. and Baylin, S. B. (1980). Ornithine decarboxylase is important in intestinal mucosal maturation and recovery from injury in rats, *Science*, **210**, 195–8.

Mizui, T., Shimono, N. and Doteuchi, M. (1987). A possible mechanism of protection by polyamines against gastric damage induced by acidified ethanol in rats: polyamine protection may depend on its antiperoxidative properties, *Jap. J. Pharmacol.*, **44**, 43–50.

Olsen, P. S., Poulsen, S. S., Kirkegaard, P. and Nexo, E. (1984). Role of submandibular saliva and epidermal growth factor in gastric cytoprotection, *Gastroenterology*, **87**, 103–8.

Olsen, P. S., Poulsen, S. S., Therkelsen, K. and Nexo, E. (1986a). Effect of sialoadenectomy and synthetic human urogastrone on healing of chronic gastric ulcers in rats, *Gut*, **27**, 1443–9.

Olsen, P. S., Poulsen, S. S., Therkelsen, K. and Nexo, E. (1986b). Oral administration of synthetic humans urogastrone promotes healing of chronic duodenal ulcers in rats, *Gastroenterology*, **90**, 911–17.

Skinner, K. A., Soper, B. D. and Tepperman, B. L. (1984). Effect of sialoadenectomy and salivary gland extracts on gastrointestinal mucosa growth and gastrin levels in the rat, *J. Physiol. (Lond.)*, **351**, 1–12.

Tabor, C. W. and Tabor, H. (1984). Polyamines, *Ann. Rev. Biochem.*, **53**, 749–90.

Takagi, K., Kasuya, Y. and Watanabe, K. (1964). Studies on the drugs for peptic ulcer: a reliable method for producing stress ulcers in rats, *Chem. Pharm. Bull.*, **12**, 465–70.

Advances in Drug Therapy of Gastrointestinal Ulceration
Edited by A. Garner and B. J. R. Whittle
Published by John Wiley & Sons Ltd

Chapter Twenty

Strategies for the Development of Novel Anti-ulcer Drugs

A. Garner

Bioscience Department, ICI Pharmaceuticals, Alderley Park, Macclesfield, Cheshire SK10 4TG, UK

INTRODUCTION

Peptic ulcer is a chronic, relapsing disease with current drug therapy based upon either inhibiting acid secretion and peptic activity or stimulating mucosal protection. This approach reflects the popular belief that ulcers occur when there is an imbalance between luminal aggressors and mucosal defence. Inhibitors of acid secretion, exemplified by the histamine H_2-antagonists, cimetidine and ranitidine, have proved to be effective, convenient and safe therapy for both gastric and duodenal ulceration. The increase in rate of ulcer healing over placebo obtained with antisecretory agents probably reflects the fact that normal wound healing is retarded in the acid–protease environment which prevails in the upper gastrointestinal tract. Ulcer healing with inhibitors of parietal secretion or antacids does not influence the tendency of ulcers to recur, although relapse can be markedly attenuated by continuous maintenance therapy at reduced dose levels (Pounder, 1981).

A proportion of duodenal ulcer patients exhibit over-production of gastric acid (Baron, 1978). However, the majority have an acid output within the normal range and some gastric ulcer patients in fact appear to be hyposecretors. These findings are frequently cited as evidence that peptic ulceration is primarily due to breakdown of mucosal protective mechanisms. There are a number of effective anti-ulcer drugs (e.g. sucralfate and colloidal bismuth) which do not inhibit acid secretion and which are presumed to act by stimulating mucosal defences. Although prostaglandins have also been considered in this category, evidence from clinical trials suggests that the ulcer-healing activity of E-type prostaglandins is solely a consequence of their antisecretory activity (Lauritsen and Rask-Madsen, 1986). Recent studies demonstrate that ulcer healing with colloidal bismuth subcitrate (CBS) is associated with a reduced rate of recurrence (Miller and Faragher, 1986). This effect is currently ascribed to the bactericidal actions of CBS against *Campylobacter pylori*, organisms which colonize the mucosal surface, particularly the gastric antrum (Hornick, 1987).

This chapter initially considers the future of anti-ulcer drug development based on current concepts of inhibiting luminal aggressors or stimulating mucosal defences. Whilst a number of opportunities for new agents can be identified in these two categories, it would appear that clinical needs of acute healing are largely fulfilled by currently available drugs. The possibility of developing novel agents based on application of the principles of wound healing together with the opportunity for developing new diagnostic tests are highlighted as worthwhile targets for the future. Finally, it is possible to make fairly accurate short-term predictions about the shape of the anti-ulcer drug market up to the turn of this century by drawing parallels with the similar but more mature antihypertensive therapeutic area. The outcome of this analysis together with a few speculations on the treatment of peptic ulcer disease in the 21st century are also discussed.

INHIBITORS OF ACID AND PEPSIN

Definition of the histamine H_2-receptor by Black *et al.* (1972) arose from discovery of a specific antagonist and culminated 5 years later in the introduction of cimetidine for therapy of peptic ulcer disease. This scientific achievement closely mirrors characterization of β-adrenergic receptor antagonists by Black and Stephenson (1962) a decade earlier which eventually led to the introduction of propranolol for therapy of hypertension. Cimetidine was found to be an effective inhibitor of acid secretion stimulated by histamine, gastrin, cholinergic agonists or food in various laboratory models and man (Parsons, 1980). In patients, the drug proved to be an extremely effective ulcer-healing agent and rapidly rose to become the number one selling pharmaceutical product in the world. A plethora of other antisecretory drugs have been evaluated in clinical trials over the past decade. Ranitidine, famotidine and nizatidine have been successfully marketed, and ranitidine has displaced cimetidine as the world's top selling drug. Although varying in absolute potency, all these compounds behave as competitive antagonists of the histamine H_2-receptor and display a relatively short duration of action when administered at doses on the linear portion of the dose–response curve.

In an attempt to increase duration of action, a series of compounds have been developed which display a sustained (slowly reversible) interaction with the H_2-receptor leading to a prolonged antisecretory action *in vivo* which is most clearly demonstrated following intravenous administration (Figure 20.1).

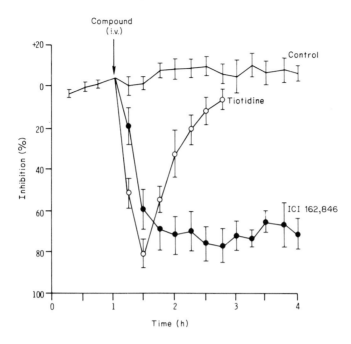

Figure 20.1 Comparison of the antisecretory profiles of tiotidine (ICI 125 211), a competitive histamine H_2-antagonist with a relatively short duration of action, and ICI 162 846, which displays a sustained interaction with the H_2-receptor leading to a prolonged inhibitory response. Compounds were injected i.v. at doses of 0.1 μmol kg^{-1} (tiotidine) and 0.02 μmol kg^{-1} (ICI 162 846) after stimulation of gastric acid secretion with a continuous infusion of histamine in Heidenhain pouch dogs. Mean $\pm$ s.e.m. ($n = 5$)

Unfortunately, these long-acting H_2-antagonists together with the potent competitive antagonist tiotidine have induced gastric tumours during long-term toxicity testing in animals (Betton and Salmon, 1984; Streett, Cimprich and Robertson, 1984; Poynter, Pick and Harcourt, 1985). Enterochromaffin cell carcinoid tumours seem to be one common feature after long-term dosing of potent antisecretory agents and have also occurred in rats receiving the H^+,K^+-ATPase inhibitor omeprazole (Carlsson *et al.*, 1986).

Hypergastrinaemia consequent upon continuous achlorhydria has been proposed as the mechanism responsible for tumour induction by omeprazole. Undoubtedly, gastrin can be demonstrated to act as a tumour growth factor capable of stimulating DNA synthesis in various gastrointestinal tumour cell lines *in vitro* (Watson, Durrant and Morris, 1988). Gastrin has also been reported to stimulate growth of xeno-transplants and chemically induced gastrointestinal tumours *in vivo* (Beauchamp *et al.*, 1985). Whether hypergastrinaemia *per se*, luminal hypochlorhydria, or some other mechanism is responsible for primary induction of gastric tumours with antisecretory agents, is, however, far from clear on the basis of these studies. In this context it seems pertinent to note that tiotidine, which induces adenocarcinoma in rats (Streett, Cimprich and Robertson, 1984) is a structural hybrid comprising the cimetidine side-chain and famotidine ring system (Figure 20.2). Until the primary mechanism of tumour induction has been identified it would seem advisable to use potent inhibitors of acid secretion with caution, particularly since tumours in animals appear only after prolonged dosing.

The therapeutic potential of antimuscarinics or gastrin inhibitors in peptic ulcer disease has received little attention hitherto. Gastrin receptor antagonists in particular could assume importance if the hypergastrinaemia associated with H_2-antagonists and ATPase inhibitors eventually proves a clinical problem. The cholecystokinin antagonist proglumide, which also inhibits gastrin-stimulated acid secretion, is a clinically effective anti-ulcer drug (Weiss and Miederer, 1979). There are various approaches to antagonizing the action of gastrin, including inhibitors of synthesis, antibodies directed against the ligand or receptor, conventional receptor antagonists, and agents such as somatostatin and E-type prostaglandins which inhibit gastrin release. Prostaglandin analogues which retain antigastrin activity but which do not induce diarrhoea and abortion

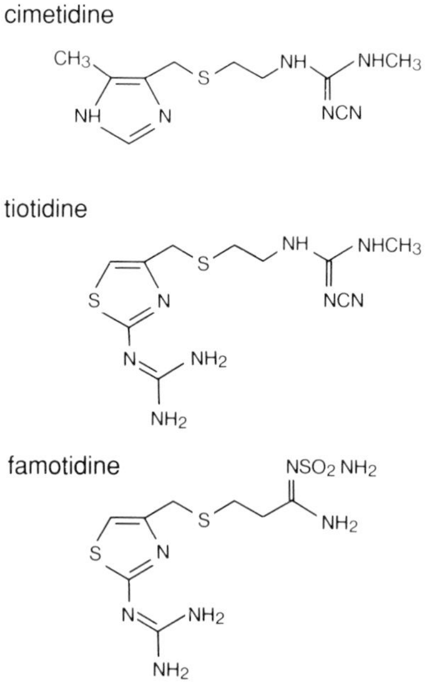

Figure 20.2 Structures of three histamine H_2-antagonists. In 2-year carcinogenic studies, tiotidine induced tumours in the stomach of rats while none were found in animals receiving cimetidine or famotidine. Note that tiotidine is simply a structural hybrid of the other two molecules and contains the cimetidine side-chain and famotidine ring system

or inhibit pancreatic bicarbonate secretion (and thus bulk neutralization in the duodenum) may provide useful anti-ulcer drugs in the future. Inhibitors of pepsinogen biosynthesis and secretion or agents which inactivate luminal pepsin represent alternative targets for new drugs aimed at diminishing the influence of aggressive factors. Whether agents with any of these activities are commercially attractive in the short term is debatable given the overwhelming market dominance of H_2-receptor antagonists. Indeed, the current spectrum of antisecretory drugs, ranging from ranitidine, which induces nocturnal hypochlorhydria and heals 90% of ulcers in 6 weeks (McIsaac et al., 1987), to omeprazole which induces 24 h achlorhydria and heals ulcers in as little as 2 weeks (Prichard, Rubinstein and Colin-Jones, 1984), would appear to satisfy totally medical needs for a range of drugs which act by inhibition of acid secretion. Within the pharmaceutical industry, the expense and disappointment of having to withdraw long-acting, second-generation H_2-antagonists from development as a result of gastric tumour formation should nevertheless focus attention on gastric cancer, a disease where the need for *any* form of drug therapy is unquestionable.

STIMULANTS OF MUCOSAL PROTECTION

Carbenoxolone, a glycyrrhetic acid derivative, has demonstrated unequivocally that ulcer healing rate can be increased by mechanisms other than reduction of gastric acidity, although the presence of a number of side-effects severely limits the use of this drug. Sucralfate, a complex of aluminium and sucrose octasulphate, is widely available and commands some 15% of the worldwide anti-ulcer market. This drug has been variously claimed to heal ulcers by providing a physical barrier over the ulcer crater, binding pepsin and bile acids within the lumen, stimulating prostaglandin biosynthesis, and enhancing mucosal blood flow (Baron and Sullivan, 1970; Peskar, Holland and Peskar, 1976). However, in common with the majority of other mucosal protective drugs, the clinically relevant mechanism of action of sucralfate is unknown and thus no rationale exists on which to base a research programme to discover improved compounds of this type.

Bismuth compounds have a long tradition as anti-ulcer agents and are also devoid of antisecretory activity. Interest in bismuth-containing preparations has recently been re-awakened by the finding of lower relapse rates in patients treated with CBS (Lee, Samloff and Hardman, 1985). Typical 12 month relapse rates of over 80% in patients treated with a healing course of an H_2-antagonist compared with about 60% in those receiving bismuth preparations have been reported from a number of controlled clinical trials. Furthermore, combination of CBS with an antibacterial such as amoxicilin has been claimed to give a further reduction in relapse rate 12 months after treatment to a level which approaches that on continuous maintenance therapy with an H_2-antagonist. The efficacy of these treatments is thought to result from activity against *Campylobacter pylori*, an organism which colonizes the surface of antral mucosa and is associated with active gastritis and inflammation (Marshall *et al.*, 1985). Whether this organism is also an aetiological factor in duodenal ulcer disease remains to be established. Nevertheless, there would appear to be a clinical and commercial opportunity for developing non-systemic antibacterial or bactericidal agents designed to concentrate at the mucosal surface of the stomach and proximal duodenum.

An alternative to inhibiting acid secretion from the parietal cell is to increase the ability of gastric and duodenal mucosae to dispose of luminal acid. This approach has the potential advantage of retaining an acidic pH within the lumen of the upper gastrointestinal tract, thereby overcoming some of the problems associated with conventional antisecretory therapy such as hyper-gastrinaemia, bacterial overgrowth and their sequelae. Three mechanisms of acid disposal have been identified in gastroduodenal mucosa which occur at pre-epithelial, intracellular and interstitial sites (Figure 20.3). Pre-epithelial surface neutralization within the mucus–bicarbonate barrier is readily amenable to pharmacological manipulation (Garner, 1988a). Gastric and duodenal surface epithelial cells transport small amounts of bicarbonate into the overlying mucus gel layer which acts as an unstirred zone and prevents immediate mixing of the mucosal alkaline secretion with luminal acid (Allen and Garner, 1980; Flemström and Garner, 1982). Surface neutralization, demonstrated by advancing microelectrodes from the lumen towards the mucosa, enables pH in the vicinity

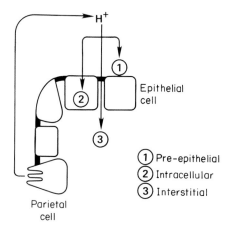

Figure 20.3 Sites of acid disposal in the gastric mucosa. The parietal cell secretes hydrochloric acid into the lumen of the stomach with an H^+ concentration approaching $155\ \mathrm{mmol\,l^{-1}}$. Protection against luminal acid is achieved at three levels: pre-epithelial neutralization occurs in the mucus–bicarbonate barrier, intracellular disposal of hydrogen ions relies on mechanisms present to ensure cytoplasmic homeostasis, and interstitial acid–base balance is maintained by the buffering capacity of the blood

of the apical membrane to remain close to neutrality when the lumen is bathed with $10 \, mmol \, l^{-1}$ HCl (Ross, Bahari and Turnberg, 1981; Flemström and Kivilaakso, 1983; Quigley and Turnberg, 1987). Evidence supporting a protective role for the mucus–bicarbonate barrier is provided by the contrasting actions of ulcerogens, such as non-steroidal anti-inflammatory agents, and prostaglandins, which prevent ulcers in experimental animals (Table 20.1).

The potential attraction of enhancing mucosal protective mechanisms has been undermined of late as a result of the disappointing clinical performance of the prostaglandin analogues. In laboratory experiments, low doses of prostaglandins stimulate mucus and bicarbonate secretions and also mobilize many other elements deemed important in acute mucosal protection (Miller, 1983). Despite this spectrum of activity, prostaglandins display ulcer healing activity in man only at high, antisecretory doses where they also cause an unacceptable incidence of side-effects, notably diarrhoea. As well as an inferior side-effect profile compared with histamine H_2-antagonists, current prostaglandins have a very short duration of action which necessitates multiple daily dosing. A further disadvantage in attempting to stimulate mucosal protective mechanisms is the universal problem associated with use of agonist drugs, namely down-regulation leading to tachyphylaxis. Thus, it is perhaps no surprise that all five of the world's top medicines are antagonists (Table 20.2). The question of which protective mechanism to stimulate and the fact that the relative importance of different mechanisms varies between stomach and duodenum provide added problems for this approach. The ubiquity of many epithelial protective mechanisms at both the cellular and the vascular levels is also likely to lead to problems in obtaining specificity by means other than locally acting formulations. The ability of currently available protective drugs to adhere and therefore accumulate at the mucosal surface probably contributes to their apparent specificity, while the resultant counter-irritant response of the mucosa may contribute to their ulcer-healing activity.

Table 20.1 Pharmacology of the mucus–bicarbonate barrier

Ulcerogenic drugs (e.g. non-steroidal anti-inflammatory drugs)
    Inhibit bicarbonate transport
    Inhibit mucus biosynthesis
    Reduce surface pH (7.4 to 5.3)

Anti-ulcer drugs (e.g. prostaglandin E-type analogues)
    Stimulate alkalki secretion
    Stimulate mucus release
    Increase surface pH (7.4 to 7.9)

Table 20.2 The world's top-value drugs

		1987 sales (£ million)
1	Ranitidine	1000
2	Cimetidine	690
3	Nifedipine	680
4	Captopril	543
5	Atenolol	530

ENHANCING WOUND HEALING

In contrast to the original concept of a 'gastric mucosal barrier' (Davenport, 1972), continuity of the superficial epithelium of the stomach is probably disrupted many times per day. However, mechanisms exist for rapid re-epithelialization of the mucosal surface as a consequence of undamaged cells migrating from within the gastric pits across the exposed basal lamina (Silen and Ito, 1985). This process is complete within a matter of hours in both the stomach and the duodenum (Lacy and Ito, 1984) and thus operates on an entirely different timescale compared with ulcer healing. It is possible, however, that a fault in the mechanism of rapid epithelialization could make gastroduodenal mucosa susceptible to damage and subsequently to development of chronic ulcers. Investigation of the process of superficial repair in individuals prone to ulceration could thus be a profitable line of future research.

In contrast to rapid reconstitution of the epithelium, recovery from peptic ulceration is essentially a problem of wound healing. Repair of a chronic ulcer is initiated by a fully developed inflammatory response and necessitates tissue rebuilding. The remodelling process requires cellular recruitment, proliferation, matrix formation, and establishment of a new microvasculature. Many of the processes involved in tissue repair, including mitogenesis and angiogenesis, are under the control of various peptide growth factors such as epithelial growth factor (EGF), platelet derived growth factor (PDGF) and endothelial derived growth factor (EDGF). Urogastrone (human EGF) is a 53 amino acid peptide which stimulates wound repair at sites throughout the body including the upper gastrointestinal tract where it is present in secretions from salivary glands and duodenal Brunner glands (Gregory, 1975; Olsen *et al.*, 1986).

Current antisecretory agents presumably act by creating an environment which facilitates normal wound healing by inhibiting acid–peptic activity. In terms of ulcer therapy, urogastrone possesses two ideal properties since not only does it enhance epithelial proliferation and repair, it is also a potent inhibitor of acid secretion (Figure 20.4). It seems likely that the same membrane receptor is responsible for these two actions of urogastrone as evidenced by the activity of a series of C-terminal truncated peptides of varying potency which display

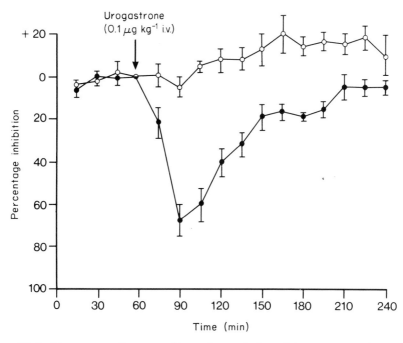

Figure 20.4 Urogastrone (human epidermal growth factor) is a potent antisecretory agent as well as a mitogen and stimulant of wound healing. In this experiment human EFG was injected at 0.1 μg kg^{-1} i.v. into Heidenhain pouch dogs in which acid secretion was stimulated by continuous infusion of histamine. The control response (open symbols) is also shown. Mean $\pm$ s.e.m. ($n = 6$)

identical activity in mitogenic and antisecretory systems (Gregory *et al.*, 1988). The poor oral absorption of peptides has been overcome in other disease areas, e.g. use of LHRH agonists in prostate cancer by administration of a biodegradable depot which allows controlled release of peptide over a period of weeks (Hutchinson and Furr, 1985). A subcutaneous depot formulation is attractive in peptic ulcer therapy where patient compliance can be a problem after disappearance of pain symptoms which normally occurs within 1 week of commencing drug treatment. Application of the principles of wound healing would appear to offer a definable strategy on which to base a search for the next generation of anti-ulcer drugs (Garner, 1988b).

DIAGNOSTIC AGENTS

The diagnosis of peptic ulceration was revolutionized following introduction of the endoscope. However, endoscopy is not a trivial procedure and opportunity exists for a convenient, reliable and rapid diagnostic test. Such a product has implications for studies of epidemiology as well as enabling effective use of maintenance therapy given the dual problems of silent relapse and symptoms in the absence of an endoscopically identifiable lesion. Diagnostics are also commercially attractive in terms of the speed and cost of development when compared with conventional therapeutic agents. Furthermore, a test capable of discriminating between gastric and duodenal ulceration would facilitate development of site-specific therapy compatible with the different aetiology of the ulcers that occur in these two regions. Simple test kits enabling identification of *Campylobacter pylori* have already been introduced based on the high urease activity of this organism. Serum markers associated with peptic ulceration such as elevated levels of acute phase reactants and acid proteases, and procedures to detect the presence of auto-antibodies, are all amenable to development of rapid screening tests. Developments in the field of molecular biology may also enable identification of that proportion of the population with a genetic predisposition for developing the disease.

FUTURE MARKET DEVELOPMENT

A period of 10–20 years frequently elapses between discovery and marketing of a new drug. In the short term, therefore, newly introduced anti-ulcer drugs will come from among compounds which are currently in development. Novel therapeutic agents which may be discovered during the early part of the next century will necessitate exploitation of current basic and clinical research on peptic ulcer disease. Whether any of these approaches will lead to discovery of agents which are clinically superior to existing therapy and which will therefore enjoy the commercial success of cimetidine and ranitidine is highly debatable. Indeed, it could be argued that advances in fields which are not traditionally related to peptic ulcer research, such as developmental biology, differentiation and growth, immunology, and molecular biology are likely to prove more fruitful as a future basis for discovering novel anti-ulcer drugs. The eventual target is a drug which heals ulcer disease following a single course of treatment, without serious side-effects, and without the disease recurring on discontinuation of therapy. In reality, a therapeutic regimen which prolongs the period of ulcer remission past 1 year would represent a clear therapeutic advance on current therapy. The long-term results of trials aimed at eradicating *Campylobacter pylori* will therefore be of great interest to clinical gastroenterologists and basic researchers alike.

Analysis of compounds which are currently under development as potential ulcer therapy reveals the change in emphasis from antisecretory to mucosal protective agents (Table 20.3). Antacids, the previous mainstay of peptic ulcer treatment, have been largely replaced by histamine H_2-antagonists. The antacid market is likely to come under further pressure in the future if and when

Table 20.3 Anti-ulcer compounds currently under development

Status	Antacids	H$_2$-antagonists	Prostaglandins	Others*
Marketed	>30	6	3	11
Registration	—	—	3	11
Suspended	—	>7	2	1
Clinical trial	—	9	9	18
Animal testing	2	11	4	43
Total	>32	>33	21	84

(Data compiled from various sources, notably Pharma Projects (May 1988) and personal communications)
*Mainly non-antisecretory (mucosal protective) agents, but also antimuscarinics, H$^+$,K$^+$-ATPase inhibitors and peptides such as EGF and somatostatin derivatives

cimetidine becomes available as a non-prescription treatment for non-ulcer dyspepsia. Numerous prostaglandin analogues are under development but early clinical results are disappointing and it is unlikely that these agents will challenge the H$_2$-antagonists. Compounds with alternative antisecretory mechanisms, including H$^+$,K$^+$-ATPase inhibitors, antimuscarinics and various peptides such as EGF analogues and somatostatin derivatives, are also undergoing clinical evaluation at present. Of these, the H$^+$,K$^+$-ATPase inhibitor omeprazole could eventually command a significant market share as a result of increased rate of healing provided that concerns over potential long-term toxicity can be dispelled. The largest category of compounds under development comprises agents which have shown activity in acute laboratory models of gastrointestinal injury as a result of their ability to prevent or reduce apparent (macroscopic) damage caused by exogenous chemical ulcerogens. Despite the current enthusiasm for this approach it seems naive to believe that inhibitors of acute chemical injury will heal human peptic ulcers. Indeed, it is difficult to predict whether any of these compounds will have an impact on ulcer treatment or even survive the rigours of clinical and commercial development.

Making comparisons with the similar but more mature antihypertensive market allows various conclusions to be drawn about the future of anti-ulcer therapy. The most realistic scenario would predict that antisecretory agents will continue to dominate peptic ulcer therapy at least for the foreseeable future. Thus the β-blocker propranolol quickly became first-choice therapy for high blood pressure. This drug was eventually replaced by the cardioselective β_1-antagonist atenolol and later by the ACE inhibitor captopril. Similarly, cimetidine, followed by ranitidine and finally omeprazole, has joined antacids in the therapy of ulcer disease. Despite similarities in overall value of the two therapeutic areas (£3–4 billion in 1988) it is neither desirable nor likely that the number of anti-ulcer treatments will attain that of currently registered antihypertensive drugs. Nevertheless, more antisecretory agents will undoubtedly appear. New introductions and consequent fragmentation of the market will lead to further diversification by way of formulation changes, combination therapies, new indications and possibly even hybrid molecules combining two different mechanisms of action, such as acid inhibition and stimulation of mucosal protection, within the same chemical structure.

CONCLUSIONS

A clear strategy for discovering novel anti-ulcer drugs is difficult to define since the primary cause of peptic ulceration is unknown. Current ulcer therapy with antisecretory or mucosal protective drugs has little or no influence on relapse unless administered continuously and the obvious challenge for the future will be to develop an agent that cures the disease. The possibility exists that ulcers are caused by exposure to an environmental ulcerogen or by a bacterial infection, implying that a cure may eventually be found. For the foreseeable future, however, it is likely that therapy will be based upon symptomatic treatment, with inhibitors of acid secretion such as histamine H_2-antagonists continuing to dominate. In view of the concerns over long-term use of potent antisecretory drugs, opportunity exists for developing new mucosal protective agents. However, it is difficult to conceive of a rational approach for identifying improved compounds until the mechanism of action of current protective drugs is established. Agents which act by enhancing the ability of gastric and duodenal mucosa to dispose of luminal acid could provide an alternative to antisecretory therapy. This mechanism has the potential advantage that an acidic intraluminal pH would be maintained in the upper gastrointestinal tract, thereby overcoming some of the problems associated with antisecretory therapy, such as bacterial overgrowth, together with the potential risk of inducing gastric tumours during continuous long-term administration. Recovery from an acute attack necessitates tissue repair and it may be possible to discover a new class of anti-ulcer drugs based on application of the principles of wound healing. Improvement in the quality of mucosal repair may itself have a favourable influence on recurrence rate. Commercial opportunity also exists for development of diagnostic tests which provide a more convenient approach than endoscopy for identifying the presence of a peptic ulcer. Apart from ulcer relapse, however, gastrointestinal cancer and inflammatory bowel disease provide more worthwhile targets on which to focus research effort since the clinical need for effective ulcer therapy is largely satisfied by existing drugs.

REFERENCES

Allen, A. and Garner, A. (1980). Mucus and bicarbonate secretion in the stomach and their possible role in mucosal protection, *Gut*, **21**, 249–62.

Baron, J. H. (1978). *Clinical Tests of Gastric Secretion*, Macmillan, London, pp. 86–119.

Baron, J. H. and Sullivan, F. M. (1970). *Carbenoxolone Sodium*, Butterworths, London.

Beauchamp, R. D., Townsend, C. M., Singh, P., Glass, E. J. and Thompson, J. C. (1985). Proglumide, a gastrin receptor antagonist, inhibits growth of colon cancer and enhances survival in mice, *Ann. Surg.*, **202**, 303–9.

Betton, G. R. and Salmon, G. K. (1984). Pathology of the fore-stomach in rats treated for 1 year with a new histamine H_2 receptor antagonist, SK&F 93479 trihydrochloride, *Scand. J. Gastroenterol.*, **19** (Suppl. 101), 103–8.

Black, J. W. and Stephensen, J. S. (1962). Pharmacology of a new adrenergic beta receptor blocking compound (nethalide), *Lancet*, **ii**, 311–14.

Black, J. W., Duncan, W. A. M., Durant, G. J., Ganellin, C. R. and Parsons, M. E. (1972). Definition and antagonism of histamine H_2 receptors, *Nature*, **236**, 385–90.

Carlsson, E., Larsson, H., Mattsson, H., Ryberg, B. and Sundell, G. (1986). Pharmacology and toxicology of omeprazole with special reference to the effects on the gastric mucosa, *Scand. J. Gastroenterol.*, **21** (Suppl. 118), 31–8.

Davenport, H. W. (1972). The gastric mucosal barrier, *Digestion*, **5**, 162–5.

Flemström, G. and Garner, A. (1982). Gastroduodenal HCO_3^- transport: characteristics and proposed role in acidity regulation and mucosal protection, *Am. J. Physiol.*, **242**, G183–93.

Flemström, G. and Kivilaakso, E. (1983). Demonstration of a pH gradient at the luminal surface of rat duodenium *in vivo* and its dependence on mucosal alkaline secretion, *Gastroenterology*, **84**, 787–94.

Garner, A. (1988a). Stimulants of duodenal alkaline secretion. In S. Szabo and G. Mozsik (eds) *New Pharmacology of Ulcer Disease*, Elsevier, Amsterdam, pp. 37–47.

Garner, A. (1988b). Enhancing mucosal defence and repair mechanisms. In W. D. W. Rees (ed.) *Advance in Peptic Ulcer Pathogenesis*, MTP Press, Lancaster, pp. 225–37.

Gregory, H. (1975). Isolation and structure of urogastrone and its relationship to epidermal growth factor, *Nature*, **257**, 325–7.

Gregory, H., Thomas, C. E., Young, J. A., Willshire, I. R. and Garner, A. (1988). The contribution of the C-terminal undecapeptide sequence of urogastrone–epidermal growth factor to its biological action, *Regulatory Peptides*, **22**, 217–26.

Hornick, R. B. (1987). Peptic ulcer disease: a bacterial infection?, *New Engl. J. Med.*, **316**, 1598–600.

Hutchinson, F. G. and Furr, B. J. A. (1985). Biodegradable polymers for the sustained release of peptides, *Biochem. Soc. Trans.*, **13**, 520–3.

Lacy, E. R. and Ito, S. (1984). Ethanol-induced insult to the superficial rat gastric epithelium: a study of damage and rapid repair. In A. Allen, G. Flemström, A. Garner, W. Silen and L. A. Turnberg (eds) *Mechanisms of Mucosal Protection in the Upper Gastrointestinal Tract*, Raven Press, New York, pp. 49–56.

Lauritsen, K. and Rask-Madsen, J. (1986). Prostaglandins and clinical experience in peptic ulcer disease, *Scand. J. Gastroenterol.*, **21** (Suppl. 125), 174–80.

Lee, F. I., Samloff, J. M. and Hardman, M. (1985). Comparison of tri-potassium di-citrato bismuthate tablets with ranitidine in healing and relapse of duodenal ulcers, *Lancet*, **i**, 1299–301.

Marshall, B. J., McGechie, D. B., Regens, P. A. and Glancy, R. J. (1985). Pyloric *Campylobacter* infection and gastroduodenal disease, *Med. J. Aust.*, **142**, 439–44.

McIsaac, R. L., McCanless, I., Summers, K. and Wood, J. R. (1987). Ranitidine and cimitidine in the healing of duodenal ulcer: meta-analysis of comparative clinical trials, *Aliment. Pharmacol. Ther.*, **1**, 369–81.

Miller, T. A. (1983). Protective effects of prostaglandins against gastric mucosal damage: current knowledge and proposed mechanisms, *Am. J. Physiol.*, **245**, G606–23.

Miller, J. P. and Faragher, E. B. (1986). Relapse of duodenal ulcer: does it matter which drug is used in initial treatment?, *Br. Med. J.*, **293**, 1117–18.

Olsen, S. P., Poulsen, S. S., Therkelsen, K. and Nexo, E. (1986). Effect of sialoadenectomy and synthetic human urogastrone on healing of chronic gastric ulcers in rats, *Gut*, **27**, 1443–9.

Parsons, M. E. (1980). Some speculations on the physiological control of gastric secretion. In A. Torsoli, P. E. Lucchelli and R. W. Brimblecombe (eds) *H₂-Receptor Antagonists*, Excerpta Medica, Amsterdam, pp. 243–50.

Peskar, B. M., Holland, A. and Peskar, B. A. (1976). Effects of carbenoxolone on prostaglandin synthesis and degradation, *J. Pharm. Pharmacol.*, **28**, 146–8.

Pounder, R. E. (1981). Model of medical treatment for duodenal ulcer, *Lancet*, **i**, 29–30.

Poynter, D., Pick, C. R. and Harcourt, R. A. (1985). Association of long lasting, unsurmountable histamine H_2 blockade and gastric carcinoid tumours in the rat, *Gut*, **26**, 1284–95.

Pritchard, P. J., Rubinstein, D. and Colin-Jones, D. B. (1984). Omeprazole: double-blind comparison of 10 mg versus 30 mg for healing duodenal ulcers, *Gastroenterology*, **86**, 1213.

Quigley, E. M. M. and Turnberg, L. A. (1987). pH of the microclimate lining human gastric and duodenal mucosa *in vivo*, *Gastroenterology*, **92**, 1876–84.

Ross, I. N., Bahari, H. M. M. and Turnberg, L. A. (1981). The pH gradient across mucus adherent to rat fundic mucosa *in vivo* and the effect of potential damaging agents, *Gastroenterology*, **81**, 713–18.

Silen, W. and Ito, S. (1985). Mechanism for rapid re-epithelialisation of the gastric mucosal surface, *Ann. Rev. Physiol.*, **49**, 21–35.

Streett, C. S., Cimprich, R. E. and Robertson, J. L. (1984). Pathologic findings in the stomachs of rats treated with the H_2 receptor antagonist, tiotidine, *Scand. J. Gastroenterol.*, **19** (Suppl. 101), 109–17.

Watson, S. A., Durrant, L. G. and Morris, D. L. (1988). Gastric dependence of human colorectal and gastric tumours, *Gut*, **29**, A738.

Weiss, J. and Miederer, S. E. (1979). *Proglumide and Other Gastrin Receptor Antagonists*, Excerpta Medica, Amsterdam.

Index